Praise for *Saving Your Sex Life*

"Dr. Mulhall has written the authoritative guide to erectile dysfunction for the layperson. This book provides understanding and guidance for the man, couple and doctor. Especially valuable for patients are the in-depth discussions of every form of treatment, their use, benefits and cautions. An easy-to-read book about a complex subject."

—Barbara and Ralph Alterowitz
Authors of *The Lovin' Ain't Over* and *Intimacy with Impotence*

SAVING YOUR SEX LIFE

A GUIDE FOR MEN WITH PROSTATE CANCER

JOHN P. MULHALL, M.D.,

*Director, Sexual and Reproductive Medicine Program,
Division of Urology, Memorial Sloan-Kettering Cancer Center*

HILTON PUBLISHING COMPANY • CHICAGO, ILLINOIS

© 2008 by Hilton Publishing Company, Munster, IN

Hilton Publishing Company
Chicago, IL

Direct all correspondence to:
Hilton Publishing Company
1630 45th Street, Suite 103
Munster, IN 46321
219–922–4868
www.hiltonpub.com

ISBN 13: 978-0-9800649-6-4

Notice: The information in this book is true and complete to the best of the author's and publisher's knowledge. This book is intended only as an informative reference and should not replace, countermand, or conflict with the advice given to readers by their physicians. The authors and publisher disclaim all liability in connection with the specific personal use of any and all information provided in this book. References to real people, events, establishments, organizations, or locales are intended only to provide a sense of authenticity and are used fictitiously.

All rights reserved. No part of this book may be reproduced or transmitted in any form or by any means, electronic or mechanical, including photocopy, recording, or any information storage or retrieval systems, including digital systems, without written permission from the publisher, except by a reviewer who may quote brief passages from the book in a review.

Images by Tony J. Riley

Library of Congress Cataloging-in-Publication Data

Mulhall, John P.
   Saving your sex life : a guide for men with prostate cancer / John P. Mulhall.
      p. cm.
   ISBN 978-0-9800649-6-4
    1. Prostate—Cancer—Popular works. 2. Prostate—Diseases—Popular works. 3. Men—Health and hygiene—Popular works. 4. Sex—Popular works. I. Title.
   RC280.P7M85 2008
   616.99'463—dc22
                                                                2008017467

For Cameron—my son—who has been a source of joy and inspiration for every day of his almost 7 years

For John—my grandfather—whose leadership, compassion and fairness touched all he met—a role model each day I strive to emulate

CONTENTS

Acknowledgments xiii

Prologue: How to Use This Book xvii

CHAPTER 1
THE BASICS OF SEXUAL FUNCTION 1

I. Penile Anatomy 1
II. How Erections Work 7
III. Reproductive Organs 9
IV. How Ejaculation Works 11
V. How Libido Works 13
VI. Sexual Difficulties Are Common 14

CHAPTER 2
PROSTATE ENLARGEMENT AND SEXUAL DYSFUNCTION 17

I. Prostate Anatomy 17
II. Prostate Growth—BPH 18
III. Treatment of BPH/LUTS 21
IV. Surgical Treatments of BPH/LUTS 24
V. How Does BPH/LUTS Affect Erectile Function? 27

vii

CHAPTER 3
DECIDING ON A TREATMENT 31

I. Deciding on a Treatment 31
II. Impact of Prostate Cancer Diagnosis on Sexual Function 32
III. Complications of Treatment: Overview 35
IV. Factors to Consider When Deciding on Treatment 38
V. Information You Should Give Your Doctor 42
VI. Questions You Should Ask Your Doctor 45

CHAPTER 4
THE EFFECT OF RADICAL PROSTATECTOMY ON SEXUAL FUNCTION 53

I. What Does the Surgery Involve? 53
II. Nerve Sparing 58
III. What to Expect before and after Your Operation 62
IV. Complications 64
V. Predictors of Erectile Function Recovery 65
VI. Erectile Function Results after Racial Prostatectomy 67

CHAPTER 5
PROSTATE RADIATION AND SEXUAL FUNCTION 73

I. How Does Radiation Work? 73
II. How is Radiation Delivered? 75
III. Side Effects of Radiation 79
IV. Erectile Function Outcomes after Radiation 80

CHAPTER 6
THE EFFECT OF HORMONE THERAPY ON SEXUAL FUNCTION 85

I. What is Androgen Deprivation Therapy 85
II. Side Effects of Hormone Therapy 89
III. The Effect of Hormone Therapy on Sexual Function 91

CHAPTER 7
PENILE REHABILITATION AND PRESERVATION 95

I. Introduction 95
II. What is Penile Rehabilitation? 97
III. Structure of the Penile Rehabilitation Program 100
IV. Other Strategies for Rehabilitation 104

CHAPTER 8
MISCELLANEOUS SEXUAL PROBLEMS IN THE PROSTATE CANCER PATIENT 105

I. Urine Leakage during Sex 105
II. Changes in Orgasm 110
III. Penile Length Changes 114
IV. Penile Curvature 116
V. Fertility Options 121

CHAPTER 9
PILLS 123

I. Viagra and the Like! 123
II. Differences and Similarities in the PDE5 Inhibitors 126
III. Safety of PDE5 Inhibitors 129
IV. Pills for Premature Ejaculation 130
V. Summary 134

CHAPTER 10
INTRAURETHRAL SUPPOSITORIES 135

I. How They Work 135
II. Advantages 137
III. Disadvantages 138

CHAPTER 11
PENILE INJECTIONS 141

I. Historical Perspective 141
II. How They Work 143
III. Injection Technique 143
IV. Medications 147
V. Side Effects 149
VI. Tricks of the Trade 152

CHAPTER 12
VACUUM DEVICES 159

I. How Do They Work 159
II. Advantages 162
III. Disadvantages 163

CONTENTS

CHAPTER 13
PENILE IMPLANTS 167

I. Historical Perspective 167
II. Who Are Candidates for Penile Implant Surgery? 171
III. Device Types 174
IV. Device Selection 175
V. Surgical Technique 177
VI. Complications 183
VII. Summary 189

CHAPTER 14
FUTURE THERAPIES FOR SEXUAL PROBLEMS 193

I. Drugs for Nerve Protection 193
II. Drugs for Erectile Dysfunction 197
III. Gene and Growth Factor Therapy 199
IV. Stem Cell Therapy 200
V. Multimodal Therapy 201

CHAPTER 15
TESTOSTERONE AND THE PROSTATE 205

I. Testosterone 205
II. Hypogonadism 208
III. Symptoms of Low Testosterone 209
IV. Evaluation of a Man with Low Testosterone 211
V. Risks and Benefits of Testosterone Supplementation 212
VI. Testosterone and Prostate Cancer 215
VII. How Testosterone is Supplemented 218
VIII. Monitoring of the Patient Receiving Testosterone Supplementation . 223

CHAPTER 16
GETTING BACK A SEX LIFE 227

I. What Is a Normal Sex Life? 227
II. The Effect of Aging on Sexual Function 229
III. Seeing a Doctor for Sexual Problems...232
IV. Re-establishing a Good Sex Life 236

Suggested Reading 241

Resources 289

Glossary 291

Index 299

About the Author 307

ACKNOWLEDGMENTS

No work of this nature can be accomplished alone. While this book has been written by me, many of its chapters have been reviewed by internationally recognized experts. For the past six years, I have had the distinct honor and privilege of practicing sexual and reproductive medicine at Memorial Sloan-Kettering Cancer Center in New York, a center that I believe offers the best cancer care anywhere in the world. I would like to thank the leadership at Memorial Sloan-Kettering Cancer Center for allowing me to develop a sexual and reproductive medicine program within the Division of Urology, where much of my focus has been the management of patients with sexual problems after prostate cancer treatment. In particular, I would like to acknowledge Dr. Peter Scardino, whose book *Dr. Peter Scardino's Prostate Book* I have used as a reference for this book. I would also like to thank Dr. Scardino for his unerring support and vision in the development of a sexual and reproductive medicine program at MSKCC. I believe that this program over the course of the last six years has made a difference in many people's lives.

I would like to thank Dr. James Eastham and Dr. Jonathan Coleman of the Division of Urology, for reviewing the chapter on radical prostatectomy. These two highly recognized surgeons have made sure that the information on surgery is both accurate and up-to-date. I would like to thank Dr. Michael Zelefsky and Dr. Marisa Kollmeier from the Department of Radiation Oncology for their review of the chapter on radiation therapy. While I see many patients who have had radiation therapy, I am not a radiation oncologist and they have ensured accuracy of the information presented.

I would like to thank Dr. Michael Morris, an expert in the management of advanced prostate cancer, for reading the chapter on hormone therapy. I owe a debt of gratitude to Chris Nelson PhD, a clinical psychologist, for his review of the chapter on sexual intimacy. I have had the distinct pleasure of working with Dr. Nelson in my daily clinical practice for the past 5 years. Joe Narus, nurse practitioner on the sexual & reproductive medicine team and the coordinator of the penile rehabilitation program, graciously and expertly reviewed the chapter on penile injection therapy.

I would like to thank Mrs. Vicky Frohnhoefer for her expert transcription of this manuscript, Rockelle Henderson from Hilton Publishing, and Clarence Haynes, whose insightful editing has helped me deliver critical and often complex medical information in a reader-friendly way. The illustrations drawn by Tony Riley BFA, a medical artist at Memorial Sloan-Kettering speak for themselves. Many thanks to him for the beautiful images.

Mention must be made of some of my mentors. My introduction to Urology occurred during my earliest years as a surgery resident in Ireland under Professor John Fitzpatrick at the Mater Hospital in Dublin. Indeed, it was Professor Fitzpatrick who encouraged me to seriously explore Urology as a career. I am forever grateful to him for his guidance. My career in the United States started under Dr. Myron Walczak, then Chief of Urology at the University of Connecticut Medical Center. While he has since passed away, I am eternally grateful to him for his foresight and guidance. My original interest in sexual medicine was inspired by Dr. Jim Graydon at Hartford Hospital, while my sexual medicine training was conducted under Dr. Irwin Goldstein and Dr. Robert Krane (RIP) and my infertility training under Dr. Robert Oates, all three of whom were at Boston University Medical Center. I would like to thank Dr. Robert Flanigan from Loyola University Medical Center for his mentorship during my early years as an academic urologist. It was he and his patients who sparked my interest in sexual health following the treatment of prostate cancer.

I would like to recognize the physicians and surgeons, famous and not-so-famous, who have contributed to the field of prostate cancer treatment over the course of the last 50 years. We must not forget those physicians whose shoulders we stand on, who have made great efforts and sacrifices before our time. I am also indebted to my sexual medicine colleagues alongside whom I have worked over the course of last decade. Your curiosity in and critique of my research has only made me a stronger surgeon-scientist.

ACKNOWLEDGMENTS

I would like to pay particular tribute to two such scientists who have been a source of great inspiration to me, namely Dr. Irwin Goldstein and Dr. Tom Lue. These founding fathers of modern sexual medicine within urology have been a constant driving force for me in my efforts to conduct the best research and to deliver the best clinical care to patients.

I am indebted also to my clinical and support staff at Memorial Sloan-Kettering Cancer Center, especially all of the nurses/nurse practitioners with whom I have had the privilege to work. They have worked tirelessly to educate and support my patients. I would also like to thank the residents and fellows that have trained under me, for working with me to construct and refine the penile rehabilitation program.

Finally, I would like to pay tribute and offer my sincerest gratitude to the patients whom I cared for over the course of my 12 years in the practice of sexual and reproductive medicine. I have strived to offer nothing short of the best, most state-of-the-art medical care, and this has been driven by their honesty, by their needs, by their curiosity and inquisition. I believe that at Memorial Sloan-Kettering Cancer Center, the Sexual & Reproductive Medicine Program has made large contributions to the field of medicine over the course of last several years and this is in no small part due to these patients.

PROLOGUE
HOW TO USE THIS BOOK

Prostate cancer is the most common form of cancer in American men other than skin cancer. It is estimated that about 185,000 new cases of prostate cancer will be diagnosed in 2008 in the USA alone. Almost 30,000 men will die of the disease this year alone in this country. It is the second leading cause of cancer death in men after lung cancer. While a man has a 15% chance of being diagnosed with prostate cancer in his lifetime, only 3% die of the disease. In the modern era, the vast majority of men live for very long periods of time.

Over the course of the last 20 years, numerous discoveries and refinements in management have occurred in this disease. There have been refinements in prostate biopsy technique, in imaging of prostate cancer, in surgical technique (for example, the introduction of laparoscopic and robotic prostatectomy), in the delivery of radiation therapy and in the treatment of advanced disease. Furthermore, the use of PSA as a screening tool has resulted in a far greater number of men being diagnosed with prostate cancer at its earliest stages. This has also translated into younger men being diagnosed with prostate cancer. Thus, a man's long-term sexual function has become an even bigger issue now, given these factors.

Being diagnosed with cancer for any person, and prostate cancer for any man, is a major stressor in one's life. It is easy in the early stages after diagnosis to become overwhelmed with decisions. These decisions often center on what treatment to choose, surgery or radiation therapy or watchful waiting? Each of the three has its respective pros and cons.

So, why have I written this book? The simple fact of the matter is that most physicians and patients do not talk about sexual health in a routine medical interview. Both are uncomfortable with the topic and avoid it. Secondly, physicians treating patients sometimes shy away from discussing in detail the side effects and complications of a treatment and so patients are left with unrealistic expectations. Thirdly, there is a dire need for the dissemination of credible information on the sexual effects of prostate cancer treatments, whether it be surgery, radiation or hormone therapy. While there are excellent books written by physicians and patients on prostate cancer in general and its treatment, this is the first book written entirely about sexual function in the prostate cancer patient. We know prostate cancer is common and treatment with surgery or radiation occurs in the majority of patients. Thus, sexual problems in this population are common, some short-lived, some permanent. Finally, this is an area of medicine to which I have devoted most of my 12 years in academia, both in treating patients and in research. In my practice at Memorial Sloan-Kettering Cancer Center, I see more than 600 radical prostatectomy patients, around 150 radiation patients and about 100 hormone therapy patients per year.

This book is not designed to be a resource in your decision-making about your treatment nor will it give a comprehensive account of what's involved in radical prostatectomy or radiation therapy treatment. Rather, this book is aimed at giving you state-of-the-art, up-to-date, comprehensive information on the impact of prostate cancer treatments on your sexual function and what options are available to you for the treatment of such sexual problems.

The book opens with a chapter on the basics of sexual function: how do erections, libido, and ejaculation work? The next chapter discusses benign prostate enlargement and lower urinary tract symptoms. This chapter discusses the treatments available for benign prostate enlargement (BPH) and their effect on your sexual function. The ensuing chapters deal with the impact of radical prostatectomy, radiation therapy and hormone therapy on your sexual function. There is an important chapter on penile rehabilitation and preservation of erectile function. This concept is unheard of by most patients and, indeed, is alien to many doctors and even to some urologists. There is accumulating evidence that using medications in the early stages after treatment, whether it be surgery or radiation, and while on hormone therapy, may positively impact the health of erectile tissue and thus maximize the chances of a man retaining long-term sexual function. A chapter on miscellaneous problems discusses the non-erection sexual problems that occur after these treatments, including orgasm and penile length problems, and the development of Peyronie's disease. The ensuing five chapters are devoted to discussing treatments available to you for erection problems. These include pills (Viagra and the like), suppositories, vacuum devices, penile injections, and penile implants. The book ends with a chapter on future therapies for sexual dysfunction, a chapter on the very controversial subject of testosterone supplementation and a final chapter on restoring your sex life.

The advice offered in this book is based on my own research, my interpretation of other people's research, and my clinical experience over the 12 years that I have been practicing sexual and reproductive medicine. I have tried to be comprehensive, but where I believe a better resource exists I have mentioned it. Furthermore, at the end of the book, there is a *Suggested Reading* list. There is also a section on *Resources*, including books, websites, and organizations that have expertise or interest in sexual health in the prostate cancer patient.

The goal of the sexual medicine physician is to ensure that the couple (should one exist) or the patient has the ability to resume satisfactory sexual relations. My goals are as follows: (i) to provide you with well-researched, well-thought-out educational material so that you can make a rational decision regarding your treatment, (ii) to give you the tools necessary to ensure that you get the best care possible, and (iii) to encourage you to be proactive about your sexual health, all in an effort to maximize your sexual function recovery. At this moment, it is easy to feel overwhelmed. You are worried about surviving your cancer, you are worried about being incontinent after surgery, and you are worried about the sexual function consequences of radiation therapy, surgery, and hormone therapy. The good news is that almost 90% of men who walk into my office with sexual dysfunction related to prostate cancer are treatable. That is, 90% of men can resume satisfactory sexual intercourse with a partner using available treatments. You should finish reading this book with a sense of optimism with regard to your future sexual function. You can be helped! Good luck!

JOHN P. MULHALL, M.D.

CHAPTER 1

THE BASICS OF SEXUAL FUNCTION

> I. Penile Anatomy
> II. How Erections Work
> III. Reproductive Organs
> IV. How Ejaculation Works
> V. How Libido Works
> VI. Sexual Difficulties Are Common

I. Penile Anatomy

Leonardo da Vinci described the penis as follows: ". . . it disputes with the human intellect, and sometimes has intellect itself, and although the will of a man may wish to stimulate it, it remains obstinate and goes its own way, sometimes moving on its own without the permission or thought of the man. Whether he is asleep or awake, it does what it desires, the penis having a mind of its own." This organ has been a source of fascination for thousands of years. It facilitates not just urination and sexual activity, but is the seat of masculinity and virility in many cultures. This organ is perfectly designed for its functions and is composed of multiple types of tissues and structures, which, like a good orchestra in concert, function perfectly together in the healthy male.

About two-thirds of the penis is external (that is, outside of the body) and one-third is internal (Figure 1). The erection chambers are paired cigar-shaped structures that travel from the head of the penis into the body and run along the bony structures known as the ischiopubic rami. These bony structures are what we sit on when we sit on a bicycle seat, for example. The paired erection chambers are technically known as the corpora cavernosa (singular: corpus cavernosum). They are composed of two major types of tissue. The outer lining, which is approximately 2mm in thickness, is known as the tunica albuginea, more commonly called, simply, the tunica. Housed within the tunica is the erectile tissue, which itself is composed of numerous types of tissues (Figure 2). This tissue includes muscle, blood vessels, nerves, elastic tissue, collagen, and a tissue very important to erectile function known as the endothelium. I will talk more about this tissue toward the end of this chapter and you will see it pop up again and again in this book.

The erectile tissue is fashioned into a lattice-work of spaces. The simplest way to think of it is that erectile tissue is like Swiss cheese; you have solid tissue interspersed with spaces. In the flaccid (soft) state, these spaces are tiny. However, when men are aroused, these spaces expand, become large, and actually fill with blood to allow an erection to occur (Figure 3). Each of these spaces (known as sinusoids or lacunar spaces) is lined on its inside by endothelium. The endothelium is a major regulator of blood flow into the penis. It produces numerous chemicals, the most important one of which is nitric oxide, which I will discuss in greater detail shortly. Outside of the endothelium is the muscle. This muscle is similar in nature to the bladder and bowel muscle in that it is not under your direct control. In the flaccid state, it is kept contracted to make sure the spaces are tiny, but under arousal, it relaxes greatly and allows these spaces to expand significantly. Coursing outside of the smooth muscle between the spaces are blood vessels and nerves, which, of course, are essential to erection.

The third chamber inside the penis is known as the corpus spongiosum. This sits beneath the paired erectile bodies and houses the urethra (the urine channel). It travels from the opening of the bladder (bladder neck) as the urethra passes through the prostate, all the way out to the head of the penis. In fact, the head of the penis (known as the glans) is in direct continuity with the corpus spongiosum and has no direct connection with the erectile bodies. Strictly speaking, the corpus spongiosum is not a true erectile body as it has very little spongy tissue in contrast to the corpora cavernosa. The corpora cavernosa are tightly joined along their external two-thirds and share an

THE BASICS OF SEXUAL FUNCTION

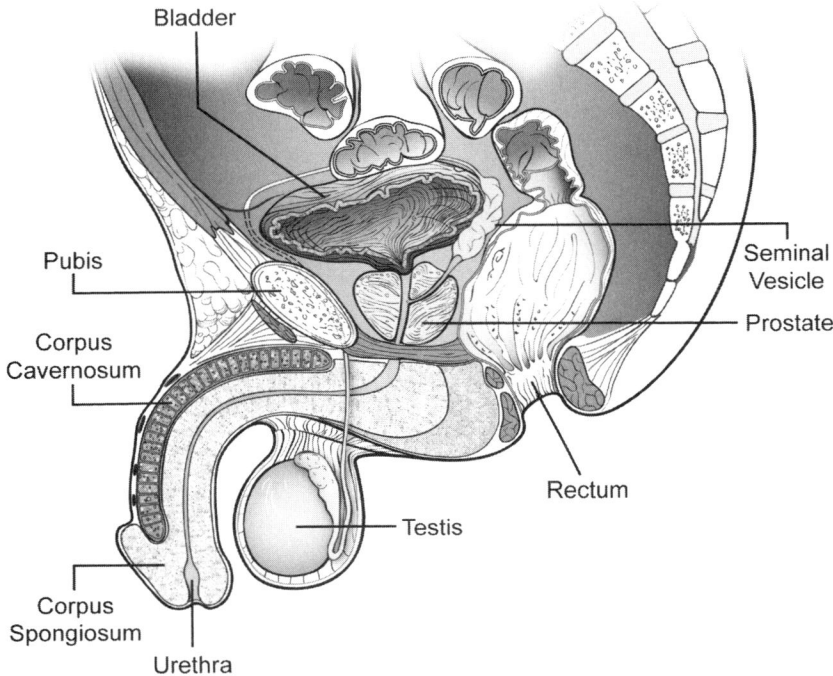

Figure 1 • Side view of the male pelvis illustrating relationship between the bladder, prostate, and penis (corpora cavernosa).

intervening wall known as the septum. This septum has numerous channels passing from right to left side so that there is equalization of blood flow and pressure between the two erectile bodies. For example, with a penile injection (where a patient injects his penis to get an erection; see Chapter 11), an injection on the left side of the penis causes an erection in both right and left erectile bodies.

Outside the erectile bodies, there are numerous layers of tissue, but most importantly, on the top surface of the penis (that is, the surface of the penis that a man looks down on), there is a vein (dorsal vein), a right and a left artery (dorsal artery), and a right- and left-sided set of nerves (dorsal nerves). The deep dorsal vein is a major route of blood flow leaving the penis. The dorsal arteries supply the penile shaft, skin, and subcutaneous tissue, as well as the head of the penis, with fresh blood. They also have some branches that travel into the erectile chambers as the dorsal artery passes from the base to the head of the penis. In some men, these arteries (known as perforators, as

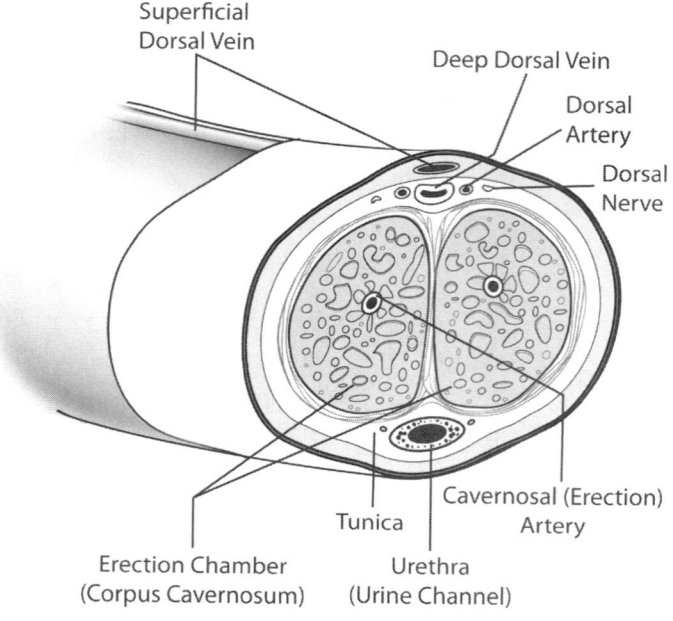

Figure 2 • Cross section of the penis demonstrating the corpora cavernosa and corpus spongiosum. The outer lining of the tunica albuginea is a multi-layered structure. The erectile tissue has a honey-comb appearance.

they perforate the tunica) are significant contributors to erectile function. The nerves running on the surface of the penis beneath the skin, known as the dorsal nerves, are sensory in nature. That is, they supply sensation and only sensation to the penis. Thus, they are not intrinsically involved in erectile function.

Blood Supply

The major source of blood flow for erection is the deep or cavernosal artery. Given how erections work (to be discussed later), increased blood flow during erection is critical to gaining maximum rigidity and maximum sustaining capability. The cavernosal artery starts its journey in the pelvis, where it is known as the internal pudendal artery. This artery takes a circuitous course and travels underneath the ischiopubic ramus (remember, that bony structure

THE BASICS OF SEXUAL FUNCTION

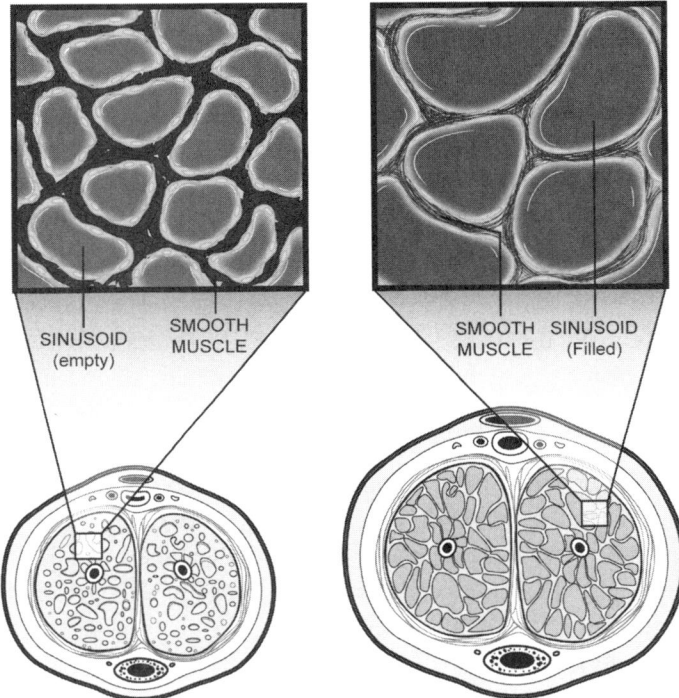

Figure 3 • High power view of erectile tissue. The lacunar spaces are lined by endothelium beneath which is smooth muscle. In the space between the lacunar spaces run the nerves.

that we sit on while on a bicycle seat). It travels in a special canal along with the dorsal (sensory) nerves. The right artery travels on the right side, the left artery travels on the left, and they pass about one-third of the way into the erection chamber and give off numerous branches to supply blood to the lacunar spaces inside the erection tissue. This artery at rest is approximately 0.5 mm in diameter and during erection dilates (expands) to approximately 1 to 1.2 mm in diameter. When you appreciate that the coronary arteries are 1.5 to 3 mm in diameter, you can appreciate why we now believe that there is a link between penile blood flow problems and hidden or future coronary artery disease. There is accumulating evidence to suggest that men who have erectile problems are more likely currently or in the future to develop blockage of their heart arteries, which, of course, is a risk factor for heart attack.

To make matters more complicated, there are a series of arteries that travel very closely to the prostate, known as accessory pudendal arteries. It is important to understand that the prostate sits on a layer of muscle known as the urogenital diaphragm known officially as the levator ani muscles but more commonly referred to as the pelvic floor. The two erection arteries, the cavernosal arteries, sit beneath this and cannot be injured at the time of prostatectomy. However, with radiation, these arteries fall into the field of radiation exposure. The accessory pudendal arteries, on the other hand, sit above the pelvic floor muscles and travel very close to the prostate. They are also potentially threatened and injured at the time of prostatectomy and during radiation therapy. How common these arteries are is variable. It is generally believed that somewhere in the range of one in four men have an accessory pudendal artery, and in a majority of these men, these arteries are contributors to erection. Indeed, in some, these blood vessels are the major source of arterial blood flowing into the penis for the purpose of erection. Thus, you can see that, if they are injured at the time of radical prostatectomy or exposed to radiation, this may, in fact, impair erection function recovery after both of these treatments.

The anatomy of the venous drainage from the penis is complicated and highly variable. There are numerous veins that leave the penis traveling on the top and bottom surfaces. These veins carry blood from exits the lacunar (erection) spaces through the emissary veins. These veins are tiny veins that travel from the erection tissue through the tunica albuginea into the subcutaneous veins that drain blood back into the general circulation.

Nerve Supply

I previously mentioned the dorsal nerves of the penis, which are purely sensory. However, erection nerves are entirely different. While the sensory nerves travel with the erection artery underneath the ischiopubic ramus, the erection nerves travel very much like the accessory pudendal arteries I mentioned earlier alongside the prostate. Many men equate penis sensation or even orgasm with erection nerve function. In fact, the erection nerves can be completely damaged and sensation will be unaffected.

The complex neuro-anatomy was only first described in great detail for surgeons in the early 1980s, and this is how Dr. Patrick Walsh at Johns Hopkins Medical Institutions first developed the nerve sparing (also known as the anatomical) prostatectomy. Prior to 1982, all prostatectomies were conducted with little attention paid to the erection nerves. These erection nerves, known as the cavernosal nerves (also known as the cavernous nerves), start their journey from the spinal cord. They start at the lowest portion of the spinal cord known as the sacral area, and then travel out of the spinal cord and the vertebral column to join a plexus of nerves. Think of an old telephone switchboard with numerous wires traveling in multiple directions, and this best describes a pelvic nerve plexus. From this pelvic nerve plexus sitting along the front of the rectum, they travel forward alongside the prostate, pass under the pubic bone into the penis to supply the erection tissue that I previously described. While the nerve anatomy is somewhat variable, it is well accepted that the major fibers travel in intimate contact with the prostate.

The simplest way to think of it is if you imagine an orange that represents the prostate, covered on its top half with Saran Wrap. Inside the Saran Wrap layer are the cavernous erection nerves. Thus, during dissection and removal of the prostate, one can easily see how these nerves can be injured. Even in the hands of a highly experienced and skilled surgeon who does excellent nerve sparing, when these nerves are handled, their response is to go to sleep. This dormancy period can last 12 to 24 months. This is why men after radical prostatectomy often have a highly delayed recovery of erectile function. These nerves supply the smooth muscle in the penis, and they supply this tissue with nitric oxide, which is the main factor that causes the smooth muscle to relax, allowing the lacunar spaces to expand and fill with blood. During radiation therapy for prostate cancer, the nerves are in the field of radiation as they are in close contact with the prostate; radiation is usually delivered not just to the prostate but also to a margin of about 1cm around the prostate.

II. How Erections Work

The simplest way to think of an erection is to think of a simple hydraulic process like the inflation of a bicycle tire. To inflate a bicycle tire, you need a hose to transfer air into the tire, and when the hose is removed, there is a valve that is closed tightly to maintain that air pressure. I have already described the two erection arteries that carry blood into the penis (the hoses), and as the blood fills up the lacunar spaces and they expand, the previously mentioned emissary veins get trapped and compressed (the valve). The valve mechanism is critical to the generation of good rigidity and maintenance of an erection. Indeed, the most common cause of men losing an erection in the middle of intercourse is because this muscle, under adrenaline control, contracts precipitously allowing the veins to carry blood out of the penis rapidly.

So for erection to function, there are a number of key elements that need to be in working order. Firstly, the arteries need to be healthy. Next, the nerves need to be functioning. And finally, the erectile tissue needs to be in good condition. Arterial blockage will reduce the blood flowing into the penis, and this will lead to erection dysfunction. Cavernous nerves that are injured will not supply nitric oxide to allow an erection to occur, and erection tissue which is injured due to diabetes, cigarette smoking, radiation therapy or the chronic absence of erections will also lead to erectile dysfunction.

The nerves are not the only source of nitric oxide, as the endothelium also supplies nitric oxide and is a key regulator of maintenance of erection. In addition to erectile smooth muscle needing to be healthy, so too must the endothelium. It is now known that conditions such as high blood pressure, high cholesterol, diabetes, and cigarette smoking, all cause endothelial dysfunction and this is why these men have a higher incidence of erectile dysfunction than the general population. There are more than 20 neurotransmitters (chemicals that come from the nerves) that are involved in erectile function, but the most important ones are nitric oxide, which is a pro-erection chemical, and adrenaline, which is the world's most potent anti-erection chemical. Adrenaline, which is known as the "fight or flight" hormone, is released by the adrenal glands during periods of stress, such as being in a fight or running away from something. Increased adrenaline levels are noted in men during high stress, chronic fatigue, and when they are anxious, irritated, annoyed, upset, or worried. This is why stress is a cause of erectile dysfunction.

When a man is aroused, areas within the brain and within the spinal cord increase nerve signals, which causes increased blood flow through the cavernosal arteries. These signals also cause relaxation of the erectile tissue with an increase in the size of the lacunar spaces. As the blood flows into these spaces, the erectile tissue expands in a three-dimensional fashion, compressing the emissary veins, and a rigid erection occurs. Upon removal of the sexual stimulus (generally after orgasm), the nitric oxide level drops precipitously and adrenaline assumes its usual role of keeping the penis flaccid. Then the erectile tissue contracts, blood makes its way back into the general circulation, and erection dissipates.

III. Reproductive Organs

Besides the penis, there are a number of other reproductive organs that should be considered, including the seminal vesicle and the prostate itself. The prostate is a small, walnut-shaped sized organ in the healthy male that sits beneath the bladder and surrounds the urethra. It is separated from the erectile bodies by a muscle layer (the urogenital diaphragm), which is about 1 cm in thickness. The prostate is composed of two major types of tissue: glands, which secrete fluid that is part of semen, and the tissue between the glands known as a stroma. Within the stroma is muscular tissue, and the tone of this tissue in some men dictates urinary function. The prostate produces an acidic fluid, which makes up about 20 to 25% of the seminal fluid (that is, the fluid that is ejaculated). Sitting behind the prostate are two sets of paired structures, the seminal vesicle on the outside and the vas deferens on the inside (Figure 4). The vas deferens travels from the testicle up through the scrotum and the inguinal hernia canal into the pelvis and enters the prostate. This, of course, is the delivery mechanism for sperm. Much to people's surprise, sperm constitute only 5 to 10% of the volume of the semen that is ejaculated. By the way, normal men produce about 50 million sperm in each cc of semen!

The seminal vesicles are paired structures, which on x-ray look a little like rabbit ears. These structures are glands that produce the vast majority (approximately 70 to 85%) of the seminal fluid. The fluid produced by the seminal vesicle is alkaline in nature and, thus, semen is generally alkaline, as the seminal vesicle fluid amount is larger than the acidic prostate fluid. The seminal vesicles and the vas deferens on each side actually join to form the ejaculatory duct. A right- and left-side ejaculatory duct is present. The ejaculatory duct travels through the prostate and opens into the urethra. The urethra travels through the prostate much in the same way as if you core a whole apple so that there is a channel running through the apple.

At the time of radical prostatectomy, not only is the prostate removed, but the seminal vesicles are also removed. Also during the procedure, the vas deferens is cut and ligated (closed off with suture or metal clips) behind the prostate. This is why patients who have had a radical prostatectomy do not ejaculate despite the fact that most of them achieve a normal orgasm. Furthermore, patients who have had a radical prostatectomy are sterile, although they do produce sperm which is made by the testicles and travels into the vas deferens within their scrotum. This sperm can be extracted at a

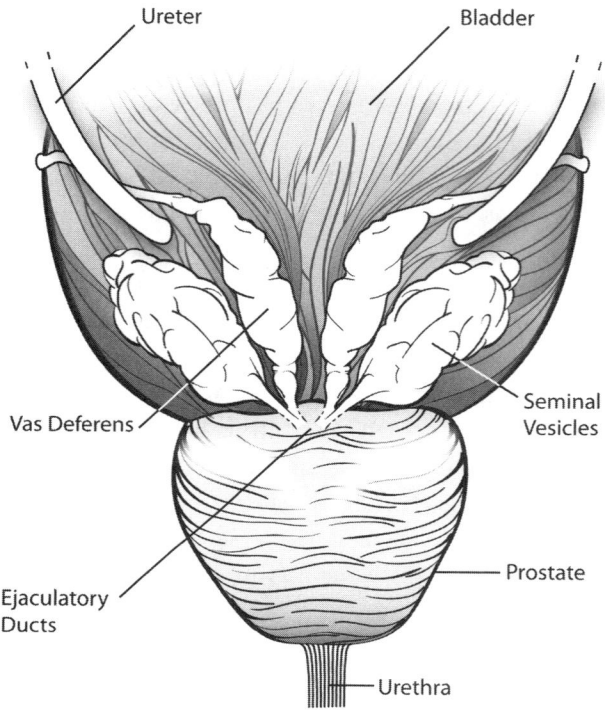

Figure 4 • Rear view of the prostate. Sitting behind the prostate are the seminal vesicles (one on each side) and inside these the vas deferens (one on each side). The seminal vesicle and vas deferens join to form the ejaculatory duct, which passes through the prostate.

later date, and this can be utilized with a woman's eggs using in-vitro fertilization (IVF). For patients who want to continue to have children, it is recommended that, prior to radical prostatectomy or prostate radiation, semen be banked for purposes of future attempts of in-vitro fertilization. Saying that, if a man has not banked sperm and decides that he wants to increase the size of his family after radical prostatectomy, a simple procedure can be performed to extract tissue from his testicle which has a very high likelihood of providing enough sperm for the purposes of IVF. Following prostate radiation, the ejaculation ducts and prostate ducts often undergo scarring with time (nothing with radiation occurs immediately), and over the course of one to five years after the completion of radiation, there is a very high likelihood that the man will notice a significant reduction in the amount of fluid ejaculated and may eventually end up with a very similar situation to patients after prostate surgery where there is no ejaculation whatsoever. Again, most patients—post-radiation therapy for prostate cancer—are capable of achieving an orgasm even if they are not ejaculating.

IV. How Ejaculation Works

Much in the same way that the multiple tissues of the penis act in concert to achieve erection, the aforementioned reproductive organs—prostate, seminal vesicles and vas deferens—function together to ensure normal ejaculation. During sexual activity, after a threshold amount of stimulation (this varies dramatically from person to person), ejaculation occurs. The ejaculatory process starts by increased nerve signals coming from the brain to the spinal cord. The ejaculation control center is at the junction of the thoracic and lumbar spinal cord. Nerves travel from the spinal cord and travel to the prostate, seminal vesicle and vas deferens. Interestingly, these nerves use adrenaline (the anti-erection chemical) as their major neurotransmitter for the purposes of ejaculation. The neurotransmitter in the brain that is most intimately involved in ejaculation is serotonin. During arousal, prior to ejaculation, the seminal vesicle and the vas deferens contract and deposit semen into the urethra as it runs through the prostate. At the same time, there is simultaneous closure of the bladder neck, which is the opening between the bladder and the urethra sitting above the prostate, and the urethral sphincter, which sits below the prostate. This causes a high-pressure zone inside the urethra within the prostate. This is followed by the sudden opening of the urethral sphincter combined with rhythmic contractions of the muscles around the urethra, which forces semen out through the urethra, resulting in ejaculation. In patients who have had radical prostatectomy surgery, of course, there is no ejaculatory apparatus to produce or deliver semen, and so they fail to ejaculate. Likewise as previously mentioned, radiation therapy can cause damage to the ejaculation ducts, such that these patients either have a significant reduction in the amount of ejaculate or have a complete absence of ejaculate. In patients after surgery or radiation, the muscles surrounding the urethra still contract at the time of orgasm, so the genital throbbing sensation that men experience at orgasm should remain.

In men who have a benign prostate disease (BPH), the enlarged prostate may, in fact, interfere with this ejaculatory process, and if they are using certain prostate medications for their prostate enlargement (medications known as alpha blockers, such as Flomax, Uroxatral, Hytrin, or Cardura) or if they've had surgery for the prostate, the bladder neck will not close properly and they will experience retrograde ejaculation. This is a condition where the semen, rather than traveling out through the urethra and ejaculate, passes back into the bladder and is then passed out in the first urination after orgasm. Patients who have this problem because of medications can stop the medication, and it is fully reversible.

However, patients who have had surgery for benign prostate enlargement (such as TURP, green light laser, microwave therapy) cannot generally be cured of this, as it is a structural problem. It is surprisingly common for patients not to be informed that after radical prostatectomy and after radiation therapy that there will be significant interference with their ejaculation. For the majority of older men, this is not a major concern, as they are not interested in fertility, and most older men do not assign any major significance to the production of semen. However, in younger men, the production of semen and the process of ejaculation may for some be significant contributors to sexual satisfaction, and the loss of this may impact upon the quality of their sexual lives. This is not a physical process, but more a psychological one. It is very common to produce a tiny amount of clear sticky fluid at urethral meatus (opening of the urethra). This should be of no concern, as this fluid (known as pre-cum) is fluid that is produced by glands inside the urethra which are not interfered with by surgery or radiation. Most importantly, this fluid contains no sperm.

Orgasm is, in the words of Captain James Kirk, the final frontier. Little is known about the physiology of orgasm in comparison to the physiology of erection or ejaculation. Orgasm is a brain event and it has been shown at the time of orgasm that men and women have brain activity that is as close to a seizure as possible without there being an actual seizure. The ability to achieve orgasm, as well as its intensity, is mediated by many different factors, predominantly psychological, but some physical. Most patients after radical prostatectomy and radiation therapy achieve an orgasm, although many will say that it is different, particularly after surgery. Indeed, interestingly, about 10% of them will say that their orgasm intensity is better after surgery than before. What is surprising to most people is that, even in the complete absence of any erection whatsoever, they are capable of achieving an orgasm, and this is routine. I will discuss problems with orgasm later on in Chapter 8.

V. How Libido Works

Libido is yet another brain event. (The brain is the biggest sex organ after all!) The most important factor for libido in men is the presence of testosterone. This is also somewhat true for women and may be a reason as to why women lose their sex drive after menopause. The next chapter deals with testosterone in far greater detail, but in the absence of testosterone, there is a significant reduction in sex drive. There are other factors, of course, which impact upon this. There are some men, for example, who have perfectly normal testosterone levels who constitutionally have a low sex drive. Whether this is related to prior sexual experiences or cultural factors is not well defined. How much testosterone is actually needed for sex drive is not well understood, but if a man over the course of his third, fourth and fifth decades of life has a significant reduction in his testosterone level, this will manifest in a variety of ways, one of which is low sex drive.

Saying this, the majority of men reporting low sex drive do not, in fact, have low testosterone, but have psychological reasons for this. A testosterone level is easy to check. It is an early morning blood test for which a man does not need to fast. It is generally recommended that the blood work be performed as early as possible in the morning, but certainly before 10 o'clock. The reason for this is that there is a circadian rhythm of testosterone production, with the levels being highest in the morning and lowest in the late afternoon.

Any external stressor or psychological disorder (such as depression and anxiety) and certain medications, in particular those that interfere with testosterone and those that have an impact upon the brain (for example, those used for depression and psychotic disorders), can negatively impact a man's sex drive. In the general population, one of the most common reasons for loss of sex drive is, in fact, erectile dysfunction. It is very common for men who have erection problems over the course of time to lose their sex drive. This is explained very simply through avoidance behavior. Men do not like to pursue activities at which they fail, and when a man fails to get an erection that satisfies him and his partner, he will avoid sexual scenarios. For many men that includes intimacy activities, such as kissing, cuddling and hugging, because there is a concern for men that these activities will lead to sexual relations, which is an anxiety-inducing event for men with erectile dysfunction. Thus, when a man presents with low sex drive, the routine response from the physician should be to have an early morning testosterone level checked. If this is normal, then it is safe to presume that the man's libido problems are psychologically based, and the decision should be made whether that patient should be seeing a psychologist or if there is an obvious reason that can be corrected by the physician. If the testosterone level is low, then a comprehensive discussion should be held with the patient regarding the pros and cons, risks and benefits of testosterone supplementation. In the patient with a diagnosis of prostate cancer, this is an extremely complicated discussion. See Chapter 15 for a detailed discussion of this.

VI. Sexual Difficulties are Common

It is estimated that 50% of men over the age of 40 have erectile dysfunction. This is defined as the persistent inability to get and/or keep an erection sufficient for satisfactory sexual relations. The older a man gets, and the more medical problems he has (in particular, conditions such as high blood pressure, diabetes, high cholesterol, coronary artery disease and cigarette smoking exposure), the more likely he is to develop erectile dysfunction. Erectile dysfunction rates are estimated to be approximately 20% at 40 years of age and 70% at 75 years of age, with about 5% of 40–year-olds being completely unable to have sexual intercourse and 25% of 75–year-olds likewise. In contrast to what most people think, most men who have erectile dysfunction do not have a complete inability to have sexual intercourse. Indeed in the ED drug (Viagra, Levitra and Cialis) trials, something in the range of 25 to 30% of attempts before a man went on the trial drug resulted in the ability to have intercourse. However, the presence of erectile dysfunction is associated with a dramatic reduction in the man's quality of life, which doesn't just affect his function in the bedroom, but also affects his self-esteem and self-confidence and may carry over into his activities of daily living.

By far, the medical condition that is worst to have for erectile function is diabetes. Diabetes affects not just the blood vessels, but the erection nerves also, causing failure of the nerves to function properly and the health of the erectile tissue, which undergoes scarring. All of these issues cause problems with erection.

Other causes of erectile dysfunction include hormone problems, such as low testosterone and thyroid disease, neurological problems such as Parkinson's disease, stroke, and lumbar disc disease, medications (in particular blood pressure medications and depression medications) and, of course, surgery. The surgeries that are most likely to cause erection problems are

THE BASICS OF SEXUAL FUNCTION

radical prostatectomy, radical cystoprostatectomy (for bladder cancer) and radical rectal surgery (for rectal cancer). Having described the anatomy previously, it is easy to understand how these surgeries may have a negative impact upon erections given the interference with the blood flow and nerves supplying the penis. The incidence of erectile problems after radical prostatectomy and pelvic radiation is very variable depending upon which literature you read. For example, after prostatectomy for prostate cancer, the erectile dysfunction rates in the literature range from 20 to 90%. Saying that, it is routine for the vast majority of patients in the early stages after radical prostatectomy to have some significant reduction in erectile function, at least temporarily. Recovery of erectile function after surgery may take 12 to 24 months and probably only 15% of men will have recovery of the same erection hardness after surgery that they had before surgery, at least without the use of medication. Likewise, the literature tells us that the incidence of erectile dysfunction after radiation therapy is highly variable, with rates ranging from 30 to 70%.

As I do not have a vested interest in which treatment you choose (as I do not perform prostatectomies or coordinate prostate radiation), throughout this book, I will call it as I see it! I believe that the medical literature is not likely, in its current format, to represent the true extent of erectile dysfunction after radiation therapy for prostate cancer. In contrast to surgery, it is the minority of patients in the first year after radiation who run into erectile function problems, but erectile dysfunction rates peak probably somewhere between three and five years after the completion of radiation. Understanding that there are no studies that compare radiation to surgery at the same center (absence of a randomized study), my review of the current literature suggests that the incidence of erectile dysfunction three years after both radical prostatectomy and prostate radiation are approximately the same. Thus, when I see patients who are deciding which intervention to pursue, surgery or radiation, I always tell them the same thing, "You should never base your decision on which intervention to choose on your future sexual function as it appears that the chances of you developing erection problems three years after both is approximately the same."

CHAPTER 2

PROSTATE ENLARGEMENT AND SEXUAL DYSFUNCTION

> I. Prostate Anatomy
> II. Prostate Growth—Benign Prostatic Hyperplasia
> III. Treatment of BPH/LUTS
> IV. Surgical Treatment of BPH/LUTS
> V. How Does BPH/LUTS Affect Erectile Function

I. Prostate Anatomy

The prostate gland is classically described as a walnut-sized structure that lies behind the pubic bone in the pelvis (see Figure 1, Chapter 1). This analogy is somewhat misleading as the prostate varies dramatically in size, practically being nonexistent in a young child to being very small in the young adult and increasing in size as we age. This increasing size, which we will talk about further later, is predominantly related to hormonal surges that occur. It is a structure known as a gland, which is filled with cells and tissues that produce fluids. Running through the tissue of the prostate are ducts (pretty much in the same way that your home's air conditioning system has ducts) and the purpose of these ducts is to deliver the prostatic fluid into the urethra.

The prostate lies below the bladder and it surrounds the urethra, which passes from the bladder out through the penis. If you think of an apple that you have just cored, the apple itself is the prostate and the cored portion is the urethra. The prostate gland secretes fluid from many ducts into the urethra. Directly in front of the prostate is the pubic bone, and directly behind it is the rectum. It is important to understand that the pelvis, and particularly the male pelvis, is a relatively tight area with multiple organs and structures in very close communication. The prostate lies directly against the front surface of the rectum, and this is why when a physician places his or her finger in the rectum, the prostate can be easily felt and examined.

The primary function of the prostate is to produce a portion of semen. You will remember from Chapter 1 that semen is a combination of fluids coming from the seminal vesicles, the prostate and the vas deferens. The latter is the structure that transports sperm from the testicle. The seminal vesicles produce the vast majority of the semen, but a significant portion of it is produced by the prostate. The purpose of this prostate fluid is to balance the pH of the semen. The seminal vesicle fluid is predominantly alkaline and the prostatic fluid is predominantly acidic, so there is a balance once these two are mixed together. This balance is critical to the nourishment and protection of sperm as they are being stored and delivered into the vagina during sexual intercourse. The prostate, or more accurately the cells (epithelial cells) in the gland, produce an enzyme called prostate specific antigen (PSA). PSA is a chemical which gets delivered into the blood and is used as a screening test for prostate cancer. PSA has a vital function in semen in that it dissolves the semen clot once it is deposited in the vagina and allows sperm to swim out from the liquid toward the cervix.

II. Prostate Growth—Benign Prostatic Hyperplasia (BPH)

In a boy, the prostate weighs about 5 gm and in a young man it grows to approximately 20 gm. Beyond the fourth decade in life, it is inevitable that the prostate will grow, and prostates have been removed which are in excess of 200 grams. Increase in size is due to increase in the size and number of the glands within the prostate itself. As the prostate grows, it impinges upon the urethra, which results in an obstruction of urine flow from the bladder. This leads to symptoms known as lower urinary tract symptoms (LUTS).

Table 1 • **Symptoms of Lower Urinary Tract Symptoms (LUTS) Associated With BPH**

- Decreased urine stream
- Having to strain to empty bladder
- Frequent urination (frequency)
- Getting up at night to urinate (nocturia)
- Urine stream stopping and starting (intermittency)
- Difficulty starting urine stream (hesitancy)
- Feeling bladder is not empty at end of urination (incomplete emptying)

BPH (benign prostatic hyperplasia) is the pathological entity that causes the symptoms known as LUTS. Now, it is important to understand that BPH is a benign process and by no means does it infer prostate cancer. In fact, many prostate cancers occur in small glands with very small amounts of BPH. Hyperplasia is a word that means overgrowth of cells. It is important to understand that BPH is not a precursor to the development of prostate cancer.

The classic lower urinary tract symptoms include (Table 1): 1) incomplete emptying of the bladder—patients will often complain that they go to the bathroom, and five to ten minutes later, they need to return because they feel their bladders are not completely emptied; 2) frequency of urination—patients often complain about having to go to the bathroom very frequently, some men every thirty minutes during the day; 3) intermittency—this refers to a urine stream that is interrupted as you are urinating, in a staccato style; 4) urgency of urination, which implies that the patient has to get to the bathroom very quickly once he gets the first sensation that his bladder is full; 5) weak stream—men will notice that the force of their streams have decreased from when they were young men and they will have to strain to empty their bladders fully; 6) nocturia—this means having to get up in the middle of the night to pass urine. Some men have to do this more than every hour during sleep. You can imagine how sleep deprived these men can be. Appended to this chapter is the questionnaire which your physician is most likely to give you if you have symptoms consistent with LUTS. This questionnaire is known as the International Prostate Symptoms Score (IPSS). Below the questionnaire are scores which indicate level of symptoms. You can score yourself at the end of this chapter and see exactly where you stand. This is a useful test to do periodically to see what the progress of your BPH might be.

Prostate growth is related to hormone production. I previously talked about testosterone and its important role in male sexual development. Within the prostate, the testosterone is degraded to a hormone called dihydrotestosterone (DHT). It is DHT which causes most of the prostate growth. In fact, in men who have no testosterone and cannot produce DHT, the prostate is generally underdeveloped and fails to increase in size. Testosterone is degraded to DHT by an enzyme called 5–alpha reductase, and this enzyme is important because it is one of the targets of medical therapy for BPH and LUTS. There are likely to be other contributors to benign prostate growth, but the bottom line is that how the prostate grows is not well understood. Furthermore, why some men have very aggressive growth of the prostate and others do not remains a mystery.

One of the most serious problems associated with BPH is called urinary retention. This means that a man can no longer pass urine, that his prostate has become so swollen that it has essentially blocked off his urine channel completely. This can be extremely painful. The normal male bladder holds approximately 400 ml or about 13 oz of urine. We see men in the emergency room with urinary retention who, when they have catheters placed, have more than a litre of urine (33 oz) in their bladders and this, as you can imagine, is excruciatingly painful. When a man is in urinary retention, he needs to have his urine drained, and this is most frequently accomplished with the placement of a catheter through the penis, via the prostate, into the bladder. The most common catheter used is known as the Foley catheter, but there are a variety of catheters that urologists have at their disposal to bypass the blockage. Sometimes a man can have such enlargement of the prostate that placing a catheter through the penis is impossible and he needs one placed through the abdominal wall, known as a suprapubic catheter. Most men who have histories of urinary retention are going to require some significant intervention, usually surgery, for their prostates. One of the more common causes of older men passing into urinary retention is the use of over-the-counter cold medicines, which cause over-contraction of the prostate and bladder neck. So be cautious using these medications if your prostate is enlarged.

Another problem that BPH causes is changes in the bladder muscle. We know that when the bladder is contracting against increased pressure at the level of the prostate, over the course of time, it will undergo hypertrophy (bulking up) and scarring (collagen deposition). This scarring is probably a major factor in the development of symptoms such as nocturia, frequency of urination and urgency. Most importantly, when the BPH is treated, whether medically or surgically, if a man has had long-standing prostate enlargement, then it is likely that these symptoms mentioned above, known as irritative symptoms, will remain even if the prostate no longer exists as a result of the irreversible structural changes in the bladder.

Yet another problem that men with very large prostates may experience is the development of bladder stones. The chronic obstruction causes failure to empty the bladder, minerals will deposit in the urine that is left behind in the bladder, and these will eventually form stones. These may require a surgical procedure to be removed or fragmented. Finally, in extreme cases, pressure build-up can get so great that kidney damage can occur. It is common for urologists to see men who have urinary retention who also have reduced kidney function, although this is generally reversible. However, if left unattended for a long enough period of time, the kidney function can be irreversibly damaged.

If you have symptoms consistent with LUTS, then a conversation with your physician is important. Much of what is done regarding BPH and LUTS is related to the patient's "bother index." How bothered is he? If a man has a very large prostate gland, has normal urinary function, does not have much nocturia and has normal kidney function, then no treatment may be the best course of action. However, for men with even mild enlargement of the prostate gland who have tremendous symptoms (for example, getting out of bed five times every night and going to the bathroom once every hour during the day) even with normal kidney function, even without bladder stones, or a history of urinary retention, a medical or surgical option may be appropriate. Surgical therapy is generally reserved for patients who have failed medical therapy.

III. Treatment of BPH/LUTS

Most patients who have BPH and LUTS are encouraged to limit their caffeine intakes as well as their alcohol intakes. Alcohol is a diuretic, and caffeine is a well recognized bladder-irritant. The first line treatment for BPH/LUTS is medication. There are two classes of drugs that are used for the treatment of BPH; the first is known as alpha-blockers (also known as alpha-adrenergic antagonists), and the second is known as 5–alpha reductase inhibitors. Alpha-blockers (Table 2) are drugs that have been around for many decades, but in their most current form are very effective treatments for BPH and LUTS. Drugs in this class include doxazosin (Cardura), terazosin (Hytrin), tamsulosin (Flomax) and alfuzosin (Uroxatral). These medications have a dual action in that they can reduce LUTS as well as treat a man's blood pressure. The newer prostate drugs, such as Flomax and Uroxatal, have very little effect on blood pressure and are more specific to the prostate. The belief is that these medications work through reducing muscle tone in the prostate, bladder neck, and urethra. Interestingly, there are many men who have relatively small prostate glands who have tremendous symptoms, and it is proposed that this is not a mechanical obstruction in the sense that the prostate is not large enough to compress the urethra; however, the muscle tone inside the prostate is very high. These are patients who are generally highly sensitive to alpha-blocker therapy.

Another difference between the older (Hytrin, Cardura) and newer alpha-blockers (Flomax, Uroxatral) is that the older ones needed titration, that is, a tweaking of the dose in a sequential fashion to find the correct dose. This is not true for Flomax or Uroxatal. Approximately 60% of men with LUTS will have significant improvement in their symptoms with the use of alpha-blockers. These drugs typically act rapidly (in contrast to 5–alpha reductase inhibitors), but are associated with some side effects. These side effects include lethargy, nasal congestion and, with the older agents, blood pressure drop when the patient moves from a lying or sitting to a standing position (known as postural hypotension).

Another side effect that is worth noting is that they can cause retrograde ejaculation. As I mentioned in Chapter 1, semen is deposited through the ejaculatory ducts and prostate ducts into the urethra as it runs through the prostate. At the same time, the bladder neck closes and the external sphincter below the prostate closes also. This causes the development of a high-pressure zone within the prostate. The external sphincter then opens and the semen is propelled out of the urethra through the penis by rhythmic contractions of the muscles surrounding the urethra. However, in men who have a bladder neck that does not close properly, such as those men who are on alpha blockers, there is a propensity for the semen to travel in a retrograde fashion back into the bladder rather than out through the urethra. This is not a dangerous situation, but it does result in the presence of a dry orgasm, which is alarming for some men.

5–alpha reductase inhibitors (Table 2) are a fairly new drug class available to physicians. They were first introduced to the US in 1996. There are two

Table 2 • **Medications for LUTS**

Alpha-Blocking Agents
Doxazosin (Cardura)
Terazosin (Hytrin)
Tamsulosin (Flomax)
Alfuzosin (Uroxatral)
5–Alpha Reductase Inhibitors
Finasteride (Proscar)
Dutasteride (Avodart)

drugs that are currently available in the United States: finasteride (Proscar) and dutasteride (Avodart). These work in an entirely different fashion to alpha-blockers. They actually shrink the prostate by blocking the production of 5–alpha reductase. Remember that 5–alpha reductase is that enzyme that degrades testosterone to DHT, the latter being the primary hormone that causes prostate growth. These agents can take between three to six months to effect any significant reduction in prostate size and usually, at best, men have a 30 to 50% reduction in their prostate size. It is also important to understand that 5–alpha reductase inhibitors will reduce the PSA level by approximately 50%, and therefore, it is critical that a man have his PSA level checked before starting one of these drugs. 5–alpha reductase inhibitors are also used for male pattern baldness. In fact, the first commercially available male baldness drug, Propecia, is low-dose finasteride.

Most urologists tend to reserve the use of 5–alpha reductase inhibitors as a first-line treatment for men with very large prostates. For men with small to medium prostates, alpha-blockers are typically first-line. However, there is recent evidence that the combination of both may, in fact, be even more effective than the single agent alone.

There is great interest in the concept that 5–alpha reductase inhibitors might prevent prostate cancer. There is a single trial which was conducted, known as the Prostate Cancer Prevention Trial (PCPT). This was published a few years ago and demonstrated that the regular use of finasteride reduced the incidence of prostate cancer, but when prostate cancer was present, the Gleason grade (the assessment of the aggressiveness of the tumor) was

Table 3 • **Surgical Options for BPH**

Open
Suprapubic (simple) prostatectomy
Transurethral
Transurethral resection of the prostate (TURP)
Transurethral incision of the prostate (TUIP)
Minimally Invasive
Laser prostatectomy
Laser vaporization (TUVAP)
Transurethral microwave therapy (TUMT)
Transurethral needle aspiration (TUNA)

increased. There remains confusion regarding this data and at this point in time most authorities suggest that 5–alpha reductase inhibitors should not be used as a prostate cancer prevention strategy.

The side effects of 5–alpha reductase inhibitors are not very common. Approximately 5% of men will complain of loss of libido, and approximately 1% of men will have some problems with erectile function. It is not uncommon for men to note some change in the volume of ejaculate. While beyond the scope of this book, there is a lot of interest in the use of herbal supplements (phytotherapy) for the treatment of benign prostate enlargement, and there are some, in particular saw palmetto, which have been shown in controlled trials to result in some improvement in urinary symptoms in men with BPH/LUTS.

IV. Surgical Treatment of BPH/LUTS

When medications are no longer effective in reducing the symptoms associated with BPH, most men are faced with the decision regarding surgery. Surgery is broken down into three categories (Table 3): 1) open surgery (where an incision is made in the abdomen), 2) transurethral surgery (where a telescopic device is passed through the urethra) and 3) minimally invasive procedures (usually performed in a doctor's office or as an out-patient).

Historically, prostatectomy was performed through an abdominal incision, either through the capsule of the prostate (known as a simple retropubic prostatectomy) or through the bladder (known as transvesical prostatectomy). In modern urology, these procedures are reserved for patients who have very large prostate glands that are believed not to be amenable to transurethral procedures. Another situation in which the surgeon may opt for an open prostatectomy is if a patient also has bladder stones at the same time. Then the open procedure will enable the urologist to take care of the prostate enlargement as well as the bladder stones at the same time.

When the prostatectomy is effective, irrespective of how it is performed, virtually every man will have retrograde ejaculation. In fact, surgeons previously used this as an assessment of the effectiveness of their surgeries. Open surgery is associated with more bleeding than transurethral surgery usually, and as with any open operation, it is associated also with a low incidence of wound infections, blood clots (deep venous thrombosis) in the legs or lungs (pulmonary embolus) and pulmonary embolism. The incidence of erectile dysfunction occurring after prostatectomy for BPH is low.

The gold standard of treatment from the 1970s to the 1990s for BPH is known as TURP (transurethral resection of the prostate). Most patients who have had this procedure will tell you they have had Roto-Rooter procedures. With the patient under anesthesia and in stirrups, an instrument (known as a resectoscope) is passed with a video camera into the urethra and through the prostate, and then a cautery loop is used to scoop out the prostate from inside out. TURP surgery is done far less commonly today than it was 20 years ago. When I was in residency in the early 90s, one of the most common procedures performed on a daily basis in the operating room by urologists was the TURP. The decrease in use of this procedure has been due to improvement in medications for BPH as well as the introduction of minimally invasive technologies. It is a highly effective treatment for large prostate glands. In the hands of a well-trained surgeon, it is also a very safe procedure. A patient are required to spend a day or two in hospital afterward, will have a catheter in and will generally have blood in the urine for a couple of days, sometimes requiring continuous bladder water irrigation to make sure that no clots are formed. The procedure results in a dramatic improvement in urinary symptoms in men who have large prostate glands. It is not a good option for men who have small prostate glands but significant lower urinary tract symptoms.

Bleeding is not an uncommon problem with the TURP, but transfusion rates are generally less than 5%. Urinary infections occur in approximately the same percentage of people. There is an uncommon syndrome known as the TUR syndrome, whereby the fluid that is used to irrigate the bladder and prostate during the procedure gets absorbed into the blood stream and can result in significant problems with the chemicals (electrolytes) in the blood. The longer the procedure takes to finish and the deeper the prostate resection is, the more likely this is to happen. As you will read a number of times in this book, experience is a key factor in avoiding this complication.

A more modern form of TURP is known as transurethral vaporization of the prostate (TUVAP). Rather than a cautery loop, a specially designed roller ball electrode is used, which generates very high temperatures to vaporize the prostate tissue. This is associated with less bleeding and can be used with safety in men who are on blood thinners, for example, for cardiac disease.

Minimally invasive prostatectomy includes laser prostatectomy, transurethral incision of the prostate (TUIP), transurethral microwave therapy (TUMT) and transurethral needle ablation (TUNA). The incidence of performing TURP has dropped dramatically as the role for lasers in prostate surgery has increased over the course of the last decade. There are several laser types that are used, the most common being the KTP laser and the green light laser. These procedures tend to be associated with shorter hospital stay, generally no more than overnight, and a more rapid removal of the catheter than that with the TURP. The incidence of bleeding is far lower, and for patients on blood thinners, this is an excellent option. In contrast to the TURP, where the tissue is actually scooped out and removed, the tissue is destroyed by the laser, and it may take one to two months for all of the dead tissue to fall off and make its way out of the urethra. Therefore, it will be common for you, if you have this procedure, to see small pieces of tissue coming out in your urine for some time after the procedure. During this phase, it is not uncommon for the bladder to be somewhat irritated, and patients frequently have persistent voiding symptoms (frequency and urgency) after this procedure.

TUIP is generally reserved for young men with a very small prostate gland who have significant symptoms. It uses a cautery loop, but rather than scooping out the entire prostate, a channel is dug at the 6 o'clock position in the prostate. In a carefully selected patient, it results in significant improvement in urinary symptoms and has a far lower incidence of retrograde ejaculation than any of the other procedures.

There are several microwave devices available on the market for TUMT. As an outpatient, a catheter is placed into the penis and microwave energy is transmitted through the catheter into the prostate. A cooling system prevents the urethra from being damaged during this procedure. In very much the same way as with laser prostatectomy, the prostate tissue is irreparably damaged and then sloughs off over the course of the ensuing few months.

TUNA is a procedure where the prostate is heated directly by microwave needles. This is different from TUMT, where there is a catheter placed through the middle of the prostate. In TUNA, needles are placed directly into the prostate through the urethra, using a telescope. Beyond the scope of this book are the relative values, advantages and disadvantages of these various procedures. It is essential that if you are exploring one of these, that you see a surgeon who does this regularly, who has a lot of experience with a particular procedure and who feels comfortable that you are a good candidate for whichever procedure you opt for. Having a frank discussion with the surgeon about the sexual function consequences of each procedure is worthwhile.

V. How Does BPH/LUTS Affect Erectile Function?

BPH is a very common condition, with more than six million men over 50 years of age suffering from it and symptoms associated with it. The estimate is that these figures are going to double over the next 20 years, largely related to the aging of our population and the increased risk of BPH as we age. As previously mentioned, age is the number one factor associated with the incidence of BPH. Patients between 60 and 69 years of age have a two-fold increased risk of acute urinary retention, and that jumps to a four-fold risk of urinary retention for men over 70 years of age. When the International Prostate Symptoms Score is 8 or greater, there is a two-fold risk of acute urinary retention. Score yourself at the end of this chapter. Men with prostate sizes over 40 grams are three times as likely to have moderate to severe symptoms, twice as likely to be bothered by these symptoms and twice as likely to experience interference with normal daily activities.

In a very large study known as the MTOPS (Medical Treatment of Prostate Symptoms) study, finasteride was associated with a 34% reduction in risk for progression of BPH, doxazosin, an alpha-blocker, was associated with a 39% reduction in risk of BPH progression, and the combination of doxazosin and finasteride was associated with 67% reduction in risk for BPH progression. Previously it was thought that men with BPH/LUTS had erectile dysfunction because BPH typically occurred in older men, and older men

Table 4 • **Incidence Of ED in men with and without LUTS (Modified after Braun, et. al.)**

	30–39y	40–49y	50–59y	60–69y	70–80y	Total
Percentage of men with LUTS who have ED	38	43	72	79	75	72
Percentage of men without LUTS who have ED	20	31	41	62	64	38

In each age group, the proportion of men with LUTS who have ED is far higher than those without LUTS

are likely to have conditions such as high blood pressure, high cholesterol and coronary artery disease, or to have undergone radical prostate surgery, and therefore, it was believed that age was the real link. However, it has now been shown in several medical studies that LUTS is an age-independent risk factor for the development of erectile dysfunction.

A large study from Cologne, Germany, showed that for each decade of life over 30 years of age, men who had LUTS had a two-fold higher incidence of erectile dysfunction than men who did not have LUTS (Table 4). Another very large study called the MSAM-7 study demonstrated that there was both an age and severity of LUTS relationship. That is, that the older men were and the more severe their lower urinary tract symptoms, the more likely they were to have erectile problems.

It is not fully understood exactly why lower urinary tract symptoms are associated with the development of erectile dysfunction. There is no doubt that men who have severe LUTS have a significant interference with their quality of life. Imagine a man who has to get out of bed five times every night. His sleep deprivation will be such that he will have a significant reduction in his quality of his sleep. It is well known that anything that reduces life satisfaction may, in fact, impact negatively upon erectile function. Much animal and human research is ongoing at the moment which demonstrates that BPH-associated LUTS is a cause for sympathetic nervous system hyperactivity. The autonomic (involuntary) nerves are combined sympathetic and parasympathetic. Sympathetic nerve fibers transmit signals which result in a variety of bodily functions including stress-related symptoms. This increased sympathetic nerve discharge may be a factor in why men have urgency and frequency of urination during the day time. If a state of sympathetic overactivity is present, this is well known to be associated with erection problems as sympathetic nerve fibers are anti-erection. While other theories exist, it is not yet fully understood how LUTS results in erectile dysfunction.

So for the 45–year-old man who has no medical conditions other than BPH and the LUTS associated with it, he is at increased risk for the development of erectile dysfunction. In men with LUTS, the increased risk of erection problems developing is somewhere in the range of 2– to 11–fold, depending on the severity of the lower urinary tract symptoms. Interestingly, it is now understood that the enzyme PDE5 (see later for the story about PDE5 inhibitors) is present within the prostate. PDE5 inhibitors are a class of drugs that includes Viagra, Levitra and Cialis, and it has now been shown that all three drugs not only result in improved erections in many men, but also improved urinary function in men with BPH/LUTS. While these drugs are not yet approved for the treatment of LUTS, it is likely that sometime in the future, one of these drugs will be or that the newer PDE5 inhibitors coming down the road will be used as a medical treatment for BPH.

It is my practice in men who present with the complaint of erectile dysfunction who also have an elevated International Prostate Symptom Scores to inform them that they may not only see improvement in their erectile function but also in their urinary symptoms when using a Viagra-like medication. There are now some physicians in the country who are exploring the use of Viagra, Levitra and Cialis in patients with LUTS without erectile problems, for the purpose of urinary symptom improvement.

APPENDIX

The International Prostate Symptoms Score (IPSS)

	Never	Less than 1 time in 5	Less than half the time	About half the time	More than half the time	Almost always
1. Over the past month or so, how often have you had a sensation of not emptying your bladder completely after you finished urinating?	☐	☐	☐	☐	☐	☐
2. Over the past month or so, how often have you had to urinate again less than two hours after you finished urinating?	☐	☐	☐	☐	☐	☐
3. Over the past month or so, how often have you found you stopped and started again several times when you urinated?	☐	☐	☐	☐	☐	☐
4. Over the past month or so, how often have you found it difficult to postpone urination?	☐	☐	☐	☐	☐	☐
5. Over the past month or so, how often have you had a weak urinary stream?	☐	☐	☐	☐	☐	☐
6. Over the past month or so, how often have you had to push or strain to begin urination?	☐	☐	☐	☐	☐	☐
7. Over the last month, how many times did you usually get up to urinate from the time you went to bed at night until the time you got up in the morning?	never	1	2	3	4	≥5

<7 mild symptoms
8–19 moderate
>19 severe

CHAPTER 3

DECIDING ON A TREATMENT

> I. Deciding on a Treatment
> II. Impact of Prostate Cancer Diagnosis on Sexual Function
> III. Complications of Treatment: Overview
> IV. Factors to Consider when Deciding on Treatment
> V. Information You Should Give Your Doctor
> VI. Questions You Should Ask Your Doctor

I. Deciding on a Treatment

After the initial shock of being given a diagnosis of cancer, you will need to start grappling with decisions regarding treatment. The treatments outlined in this book include watchful waiting (where no specific therapy is undertaken), radical prostatectomy surgery and radiation therapy, either in the form of implantable seeds (brachytherapy) or external beam radiation in a number of forms.

It is prudent to take your time when making decisions about prostate cancer treatment. While patients are understandably stressed and distressed by their diagnoses, the good news is that prostate cancer is a relatively slow-growing cancer in the vast majority of cases. Once you have been biopsied, your surgeon will be able to tell you how many of the cores on the biopsy were positive and what the volume of cancer is within each core and in the entire set of specimens.

The pathologist will also grade the cancer. The grading system most frequently used is the Gleason grading system, which identifies the major and the minor patterns and is scored from 1 to 5, where 5 is the most aggressive cancer and 1 is the least aggressive cancer. The majority of men are in the Gleason 6 (3+3) range, a large number are 7 (3+4 or 4+3), very uncommonly we see Gleason 8, 9 and 10, and likewise, rarely do we see Gleason 5 or 4. Gleason cancers that are 5 or 6 are moderately differentiated. Gleason 7 cancers are deemed to be of intermediate aggressiveness, and Gleason 8, 9 and 10 are highly aggressive cancers. In general, the higher the Gleason grade, the greater the concern the physician will have about the prostate cancer growth.

It is important to understand that the vast majority of men who have prostate cancer are curable and may go on to live many years after treatment. These men may also live with the complications of their treatments. The literature comparing radiation, surgery and watchful waiting is largely murky. There is evidence from a large Swedish study that shows that there is a survival advantage to men undergoing radical prostatectomy. There is also evidence that seed implantation is less effective for patients with intermediate-or high-grade cancers, Gleason grades 7 through 10.

Only you and your partner, should you have one, can make the final decision. It is likely that a good physician will give you options and you will have to make decisions regarding these based on a risk-benefit analysis. Risk benefit analysis means that you will review the extent and the aggressiveness of the cancer and compare it to the side effects of the respective treatments.

II. Impact of Prostate Cancer Diagnosis on Sexual Function

I have outlined the mechanisms by which erections occur in the first chapter of this book, but to recap, blood flows into the penis under the stimulation of a chemical known as nitric oxide. Nitric oxide comes predominantly from the erection nerves and results in relaxation of the erectile tissue, which is combined smooth muscle and endothelium. Blood flows into the penis, the penis enlarges, the valve mechanism closes and erection occurs. Therefore, erection nerves, erection tissue and a properly functioning valve mechanism are critical to the generation of a good erection. The penis is kept flaccid during non-aroused states, and after orgasm it returns to flaccidity by the action of adrenaline. The erection nerves supply adrenaline, which is the most potent anti-erection chemical that exists. It is not unusual for a prostate cancer patient soon after diagnosis to experience fear, anger, stress, frustration, thus leading his life in a state of high adrenaline. In the bedroom, adrenaline is the enemy of good erections, and in this high-stressed state, it is very common for men to notice significant reduction in their erection hardness during sexual relations.

As previously stated, the confidence that a man has in his erectile ability is critical to his erectile function. Clinical experience has shown me that as men, we often believe that we are only as good as our last erection, and if our last erection is not good, the majority of men will walk into the bedroom on the next occasion remembering the failed attempt and being worried about the next attempt. This lack of confidence leads to high levels of adrenaline in the penis. This restricts blood flow into the penis, opens up the valve mechanism, and a man has difficulty getting an erection or just gets a short-lived erection (often this erection comes and goes during the sexual event). As many men take several months to make a final decision regarding treatment, they may experience several months of poor erections.

What is interesting about erectile dysfunction is that the longer it goes on, the greater the degree of distress, the greater the adrenaline level and the lower the confidence a man has in his erection. The typical male response to such a scenario is avoidance behavior, which often appears the same to a partner as a reduced libido. Men hate to fail, especially in the bedroom, and when a man lacks confidence in his ability to get and keep an erection, he will avoid any possible sexual encounter. Not only will he avoid sex, but he will also avoid any physical intimacy, such as kissing and cuddling and sometimes even hand-holding. The reason for this is simple. It is essentially ingrained in our male biology that such activities as adults often lead to a sexual scenario. Given the low level of confidence in such men, they are concerned that such activity will lead to sex, and they will be frustrated and embarrassed, and their partners will be upset. Thus, it is common in my practice to see couples after surgery where the partner complains about the absence of any physical attention by the other partners.

Adrenaline can also cause premature ejaculation. Secondary premature ejaculation is a condition where men acquire rapid ejaculation at some point later in life when they previously experienced normal ejaculation. One of

CASE HISTORY 1
Impact of Diagnosis of Prostate Cancer on Sexual Function

Brian is a 55-year-old man who is married to Joan, his 40-year-old wife. Brian is generally healthy, although he has mild high blood pressure for which he uses a medication. He has been having his PSA level checked annually for the past five years, and this has always been normal. His prostate exams have also been normal, but this year his family doctor found a nodule on the right side of his prostate. He was referred to his local urologist, who did prostate biopsies and found a small area of cancer within one of the cores. He had been trying to make up his mind whether he should proceed with watchful waiting, radical prostatectomy, or radiation therapy. He comes to see me saying that, over the course of the last month since the diagnosis of prostate cancer, his erections are worse. Prior to his diagnosis of prostate cancer, he says his erection hardness was a 10/10 and currently it is 6–7/10, just about good enough for penetration. He has also noticed that he has had a significant reduction in his sex drive. Hormone blood tests and a duplex Doppler ultrasound of his penis are both normal, suggesting that his erectile problems are psychologically based. He was prescribed Viagra and responded beautifully to this. Brian eventually chooses to undergo radical prostatectomy surgery.

This case history illustrates the negative impact of any stressor, including a new diagnosis of prostate cancer, on a man's erectile function. Adrenaline, which is generated under stress, during anxiety or in association with frustration, has a potent negative impact on erectile function.
The penile ultrasound demonstrate normal blood flow confirms the diagnosis of psychologically based erection problems. This case also illustrates the negative impact of erection problems on a man's libido; roughly two-thirds of men having erection problems will have loss of libido also. His normal testosterone blood test confirms that there is no hormonal cause for his low sex drive.

the most common reasons for this in my practice is the presence of erectile dysfunction. Practically two-thirds of the patients in my practice who have lost erection sustaining capability have developed decreased ejaculation time. Once the erectile dysfunction is adequately treated, the majority of men will improve, if not completely correct, their ejaculatory function.

Some men may experience the exact opposite problem, retarded orgasm, where they have difficulty reaching orgasm or find it impossible. Any distraction during sex, for example, worrying about the ability to get or keep an erection, may actually reduce or decrease the ability to obtain an orgasm. I see men who routinely spend more than 30–60 minutes thrusting away in an effort to achieve an orgasm and fail. Some of these men achieve an orgasm only with masturbation, which suggests that the cause is likely psychological in nature. For the post-menopausal woman, who has vaginal lubrication problems even when using an external lubricant, 30 minutes of penetration will often result in vaginal pain during or after sex.

A diagnosis of any kind of cancer is not good for the sexual function of men or women, and you should not be alarmed if you experience some erectile problems after your diagnosis of prostate cancer. A supportive partner will go a long way toward helping this. The last thing a man with erectile dysfunction needs is increased pressure or resentment from his partner, as this will just increase the adrenaline level during sexual encounters. My recommendation to you is that should you be experiencing weakening of your erections after your prostate cancer diagnosis even prior to your treatment, you speak to your physician. Your doctor may consider starting a medication to boost your erection hardness as soon as possible. This may be combined with a suggestion that you speak with a psychologist. Initiating treatment early will "stop the rot" and may limit the severity of the decrease in erectile dysfunction. Interestingly, about 15% of my patients who have pure psychogenic erectile dysfunction (normal blood flow, normal hormone levels) do not respond to Viagra-like drugs. This is a testament to how important adrenaline is in turning off erections. When it is present at high enough levels, it will result in inhibition of the effect of these medications.

III. Complications of Treatment: Overview (Table 1)

While watchful waiting is not associated with any specific complications, it does require that a man be comfortable not treating his prostate cancer and keeping a close eye on his PSA with perhaps repeated prostate biopsies

Table 1 • **Overview of Long-Term Complications of Prostate Cancer Treatments**

	Radical Prostatectomy	Radiation Therapy	Hormone Therapy
Erectile dysfunction	+++	+++	++++
Painful ejaculation	++	++	-
Blood in semen	-	++	-
Urine leakage at orgasm	++	+	-
Loss of libido	+	+	++++
Penile shortening	++	+	+++
Urinary incontinence	++	++	-
Urinary frequency	+	++	-
Blood in urine	+	++	-
Osteoporosis	-	-	+++
Hot flashes	-	-	++++
Loss of muscle	-	-	++++
Weight gain	-	-	+++

++++ expected
+++ common
++ occasional
+ rare
- never

conducted periodically. Men often opt for a treatment because of the anxiety of knowing that a cancer is present within the body and is not being treated. Both surgery and radiation share erectile problems and urinary problems, but otherwise, they each have their own individual potential complications. Understanding these complications is critical to making a decision as to which treatment you will choose.

For example, surgery is an operation, and therefore, men are exposed to anesthesia and its potential risks. The older and more unhealthy a man is, the greater the risks are from anesthesia, whether it is a general or spinal anesthetic. Likewise, surgical procedures of this nature are associated with the development of clots in the veins of the legs (deep venous thrombosis, or DVT) and potentially dislodging one of these clots into the lung (pulmonary

DECIDING ON A TREATMENT

embolus). These concerns are serious and sometimes life threatening. They are, however, very uncommon today with the use of compression boots that are worn on the operating table during the operation and for sometime after the procedure. An incision is made in the abdomen whether the surgery is done in an open fashion, laparoscopically (using a telescope passed into a small incision in the abdomen) or robotically (using a telescope as above but with the surgeon sitting away from the patient and using a robot to perform the operation), and whenever an incision is made, there is a risk that a wound infection may occur. Wound infection, again, is currently very uncommon.

At the time of radical prostatectomy, the lymph glands (nodes) are generally removed, and sometimes this can lead to the collection of lymph fluid in the pelvis area, known as a lymphocele. It is not well known what percentage of patients actually have a lymphocele present. To answer this question, every patient undergoing radical prostatectomy would need to have a CT scan or an MRI in the first weeks after surgery, and this is not done. However, lymphoceles, for the most part, do not cause any symptoms, but some do cause problems (some lymphoceles may get infected and others may cause leg swelling) and need to be drained for complete resolution. This involves the placement of a narrow tube through the abdominal wall into the fluid collection; sometimes, this tube will need to stay for a few days to ensure complete drainage.

Because the prostate is removed, the bladder at its neck needs to be joined to the urethra (the urine channel). Where these structures are joined is called an anastomosis. This is achieved by using sutures. Sometimes one of these sutures breaks, and a leak of urine occurs behind the bladder. This is known as an urinoma. Again, this is very uncommon in the hands of an experienced and technically proficient surgeon, but all the same it is a recognized complication. More common in the old era and rare now is injury to the rectum. Remember, the prostate sits on top of the rectum as you lie on your back and upon its removal, particularly if there is a lot of scarring around the back side of the prostate, an injury to the rectum can occur. In the vast majority of cases, this can be repaired at the same time in the operating room without any problems.

These complications are generally experienced in the early stages after surgery and, after several weeks, most of these are fully resolved, with the exception of erectile dysfunction and, sometimes, urinary incontinence. However, some people are innately adverse to the concept of surgery because of the fear of needles, incisions or bleeding.

Radiation therapy, whether external beam or seed implantation, is also associated with erection and urinary problems. There are others that are specific to radiation as well. Because of the close proximity of the rectum to the prostate, radiation to the prostate and the surrounding 1 cm will include the front wall of the rectum. This can result in a condition known as proctitis. Proctitis is typically associated with mucous passage in the stool, some bleeding and urgency for passing stool.

One of the differences in complications between surgery and radiation therapy is that proctitis and urinary problems with radiation therapy may occur early on (the latter particularly with seed implantation) and may take several months to resolve as opposed to the several weeks that most men after surgery take to resolve any potential complications. In contrast to surgery, when most men in the earliest stages after surgery have erection problems, most men in the first year after radiation do not have erection problems but may develop these erection problems between years one and five after treatment. In fact, the low point in erectile function after radiation probably is between three and five years after completion of the radiation therapy. The reason for such a delayed effect on erectile function is due to the slow and progressive damage that radiation can cause in the endothelium (lining of the blood vessels). This may lead to a steady reduction in blood flow into the penis over the first five years after treatment.

IV. Factors to Consider when Deciding on Treatment

The first factor that needs to be given consideration to when diagnosed with prostate cancer is the availability of treatment. For example, there are medical centers where expertise in IMRT is extremely limited. The equipment required for this is not available at every single medical center in this country. Likewise, a particular region may have little expertise in seed implantation. Likewise, certain areas of the country may have surgeons who have limited experience or expertise in nerve sparing radical prostatectomy. Even if you opt for watchful waiting, you need to be monitored by somebody with significant expertise in this approach for prostate cancer. And so, you have to decide, if all options are not available to you in your area, whether you wish to pursue one of the available options or you are willing to travel to an area where other options are available.

In trying to identify whether there are experts in your area, utilizing the list of physicians covered under your insurance plan is generally not an excellent way to define this. Even though all urologists are trained in the performance of radical prostatectomy, for instance, not all of them do it in practice. Indeed, the majority of urologists in the USA perform none or very few radical prostatectomies. It is estimated that if a surgeon performs more than 10 prostatectomies a year, he is in the tenth percentile for performance of radical prostatectomy in the United States. Likewise, there are radiation oncologists who have a particular focus on an area other than the prostate, such as head and neck cancer, bowel cancer or breast cancer, and may have had little experience in the management of prostate cancer after they graduated from residency training. Finding out who the top-level experts are is not difficult. Most major medical centers have at least one expert in surgery or radiation. Scanning through "Best Doctors" lists may also help you find an expert. This is not to say that physicians not on these lists are not excellent doctors; however, most doctors who make these lists are superior in the eyes of their peers. I would certainly never remove a surgeon or radiation oncologist from your list because he or she did not appear on one of these lists.

While checking out the medical literature (www.pubmed.org) may help you see who has written papers on prostate cancer treatments, this does not guarantee that the surgeon or radiation oncologist with the most papers is the best in his or her chosen field, nor does it mean that physicians who do not publish papers are not capable of giving you state-of-the-art medical care.

Asking your primary care clinician who he or she recommends you speak to is also sometimes fraught with problems. For example, the clinician that you are speaking to may be good friends with the local urologist or radiation oncologist, or may have a very close working relationship with him or her, so your clinician bias in favor of a particular physician may not be based upon outcomes after the treatment. It is said in medicine that the plural of anecdotes is not evidence, and by this, it is meant that speaking to family members or friends who have positive experiences from a particular surgeon does not necessarily mean that your outcomes will be identical.

Many world-class radical prostatectomists or radiation oncologists are difficult to make an appointment with, some do not take any form of insurance, their businesses are purely cash-based. However, it is not absolutely essential for you to see a world-renowned surgeon to obtain good outcome, provided that the physician who is conducting your treatment has good experience and significant expertise in the procedure that he or she is performing. Sometimes getting the best treatment requires that you move away from home base, and while there is a certain comfort level in using the medical center that you routinely use for your general medical care, this does not always translate into the best outcome for surgical or radiation treatment.

Another factor that is important to evaluate involves cancer statistics. On prostate biopsy there are three major factors that need to be evaluated. The first one is the Gleason grade, as we previously mentioned. The higher the Gleason grade, the more aggressive the cancer is, the more likely it is to spread rapidly, the more likely it is to be outside of the prostate, and the lower the survival is in general terms. Ten years after the diagnosis of prostate cancer, dying from the disease occurs in about 5% of men with a Gleason 5 tumor, 15% with a Gleason 6 tumor, 50% with a Gleason 7 tumor, and with a Gleason 8 cancer, it approaches 80% of men. It is also important to understand that in approximately one-third of cases, the Gleason score will be upgraded when the pathologist looks at the radical prostatectomy specimen if you have had surgery. That is, there are many men who have a Gleason 6 tumor on prostate biopsy examination, but when the surgery is performed, and the prostate is surveyed in its entirety, in fact, have a Gleason 7 cancer. This is very simply due to the fact that there is tremendous sampling error when the needle is placed into the prostate for biopsy, particularly if the prostate is large.

Historically, 10 to 20 years ago, six cores were obtained; now, at least 12 to 14 cores are routinely obtained during a prostate biopsy. Nevertheless, there are areas of the prostate that may harbor cancers that are not touched by the needle during biopsy. The extent of the cancer is important. This is often difficult to define on prostate biopsy and much more easily defined if the patient has had a radical prostatectomy and the pathologist examines the entire prostate. However, the volume of the prostate biopsy cores that are involved with cancer should be easily measured by the pathologist. It is important that you define how many cores are positive, and within each core, what is the volume of the cancer. Both of these factors can be factored into a prediction model (nomogram) that gives you an idea of whether the prostate cancer is confined to the prostate. As previously mentioned, a large Swedish trial recently found that radical prostatectomy had an advantage over watchful waiting in men with localized tumors of intermediate or high grade. Furthermore, the medical literature suggests that seed implantation may be less effective in patients with high-risk prostate cancers.

Another factor to consider is your life expectancy. This is impacted upon by many factors, probably the most important one of which is your general health. Medical conditions such as other cancers, coronary artery disease, diabetes, high blood pressure, high cholesterol or any other chronic illness may significantly negatively impact your life expectancy. A 40–year-old man has approximately a 37–year life expectancy. A 60–year-old man, on the other hand, has a life expectancy of about 20 years, and an 80–year-old has a life expectancy of about 7 years. These are purely statistics, and these figures may not apply directly to you depending on your genetic makeup, your family history of longevity and your medical and surgical history.

Your choice of treatment for prostate cancer may be further impacted upon by your current sexual function and sexual activity. For men who have poor sexual function before treatment and for men who are not particularly sexually active, sexual dysfunction tends not to be a major concern or factor that they consider when choosing a treatment. Patients see me frequently before they choose whether to have surgery or radiation and want to know which I would recommend. I say to all of them that they should never base their decisions regarding treatment on their future sexual function. While there does not exist any study directly comparing surgery and radiation in a randomized, controlled fashion, my review of the literature suggests at this time that the erectile dysfunction rates at three years after surgery and three years after radiation are approximately the same.

You should be very wary of a radiation oncologist who touts radiation therapy as being associated with lower rates of sexual dysfunction. Saying that, good radiation is probably better than poor surgery, and good surgery is probably always better than poor radiation. So choose a physician that has experience and expertise in whichever treatment you are receiving. Likewise, be cautious of robotic prostatectomy surgeons who tell you that erectile function recovery is better or quicker using the robot compared to the open approach. At this point in time, there is zero evidence to support that statement, although these statements appear on some robotic prostatectomy websites. My research of these websites has shown that about 50% of the sites devoted to robotic prostatectomy state or infer that erectile function recovery is better after robot surgery than open surgery. This is not true based on the best available evidence at the moment.

The older the patient, the less likely sexual function will play a role in deciding which treatment to undertake, as older men often have more baseline erectile problems and are generally with partners who are less interested in sex. However, for older men who have younger partners, sex often has a significant impact on the choice of treatment. If you have erectile dysfunction at the time of diagnosis and should sexual intercourse be an important part of your life, it may be worthwhile having this investigated and treated before you undergo treatment for prostate cancer. If you have been diagnosed with prostate cancer, you have several months at least to make a decision regarding which treatment to pursue, unless the cancer is very high grade. If you have erection problems during this "decision-making" time period, you may want to consider trying erection pills. If you try them and have significant side effects or they do not work, then you may wish to pursue some other treatment such as penile injection therapy or urethral suppositories. Men for whom pills and suppositories and/or shots fail and for whom sexual intercourse is important, may be considered candidates for simultaneous radical prostatectomy and placement of a penile implant reservoirs (see Chapter 13).

Another factor that plays a role in your decision is your lifestyle. For example, there are men who run small businesses, are self-employed and have a small number of employees, for whom taking four to six weeks off after radical prostatectomy would be problematic for their businesses. Under these circumstances, these men may consider robotic prostatectomy, after which they can get back to work sooner, perhaps within the week depending on the line of work they are in, or they may choose to undergo seed implantation, which is a one-day procedure, for the same reason. For the same reason, having external beam radiation therapy over the course of two months may also be significantly burdensome from a job standpoint. For men who are very physically active and who do not want to take a break in this activity, then seed implantation is a reasonable option. However, the majority of patients with prostate cancer are going to put their prostate cancer therapy ahead of everything else, including their careers, and taking a few weeks to recuperate from surgery is usually not a major concern for most men.

V. Information You Should Give Your Doctor

Whether you see one, two, or 10 doctors for a discussion regarding prostate cancer treatment, the information that you give them may significantly impact upon their advice to you regarding your management. Under these circumstances it is important that you are totally honest with the physician, whether surgeon, radiation therapist or medical oncologist, as his or her decision may vary based on your medical history and profile. These discussions are not the time and place to bury information regarding your medical history. Be honest and forthright with the physician and do not be afraid to ask questions and challenge the physician. Many physicians are put off by patients who walk into the office with large numbers of medical papers under their arms who have been on the internet daily for weeks and come in with a barrage of questions. Even though physicians are under major time constraints in the current health care environment, these conversations do not have to be completed in one session. In fact, it is not unreasonable for you to return to the same physician to ask more questions after your first discussion. Physicians who become defensive or argumentative are probably not a good match for you as a patient. However, it is worthwhile for you to be considerate of the physician and listen to what he or she has to say in response to each question before asking your next question. Prioritize your questions and keep less important ones for a second or third visit.

Besides your prior medical, surgical and medication history, getting the message across to your physician how important your urinary and sexual function is in the future is critical to him or her making a recommendation to you (Table 2). Many a physician will have a script (speech) to use for patients who walk into the office and will give you this spiel during your time with him or her. However, I advocate that all patients be proactive in their discussions with physicians regarding prostate cancer therapy and what is right for them as individuals.

There is no reason in the world why you cannot bring notes to make sure that all of your questions are answered if time allows, and likewise, it is perfectly reasonable for you to take notes during the discussion. Occasionally I have patients who come into the office with voice recorders so that they can go over the information given to them by physicians. Some physicians are turned off by this. I personally have no problem with it, and this is something for you to consider. If you do bring a recorder, it is always a courtesy to ask the physician if he or she would mind you using it to record the conversation. This is particularly useful if your partner could not come to the appointment with you.

Having confidence in your physician, irrespective of his or her specialty, is critical to your long-term satisfaction. It is important that you give informed consent for whichever procedure you choose, and so you should get an excellent feel from the physician what each of these procedures entails and what you are to expect. Often a patient bonds with a physician and chooses therapy based on this. However, whether you like your doctor or whether he or she is a nice person should be secondary to his or her experience and expertise in the management of prostate cancer. If any physician discourages you from having a second opinion be very wary. Expert physicians frequently

Table 2 • **Questions You May Be Asked by a Doctor about Your Sexual Health**

- For how long have you had difficulties?
- Were these difficulties sudden or gradual in onset?
- Have the difficulties been getting worse?
- How often do you have sex with a partner?
- How often do you masturbate?
- How hard does your penis get during sex/masturbation?
- Is there a difference in erection hardness between sex and masturbation?
- How difficult is it for you to get an erection?
- How difficult is it to maintain an erection?
- How often do you fail to penetrate because you lose the erection?
- Is erection painful for you?
- Is penetration painful for your partner?
- Does your penis bend/curve?
- Do you ejaculate (semen)?
- Do you ever see blood in your semen?
- Do you have an orgasm (climax)?
- Is it difficult for you to achieve an orgasm (climax)?
- Is orgasm painful?
- Do you leak urine at orgasm?
- Have you noticed any loss of penis length?
- How would you grade your sex drive?
- How would you grade your partner's sex drive?

see patients who have seen several other physicians for the treatment of a problem and should be accustomed to this.

Having your partner with you if you have one is sometimes helpful. Indeed, even having a family member with you, if you are comfortable discussing urinary and sexual issues in front of them, is of some benefit. I tell patients that most patients remember no more than 50% of what is said to them during a medical interview and if the patient has somebody with them, then that will probably increase the amount of the discussion that is remembered. Under the stress of the diagnosis of prostate cancer and discussion regarding incontinence and erectile function, patients often forget what is told to them. If all the ground has not been covered in a single encounter, then a return visit to that physician is definitely worthwhile. Many physicians will be reluctant to conduct such a conversation by phone as a face-to-face encounter is usually far more effective in communicating key issues.

VI. Questions You Should Ask Your Doctor

Patients often ask us what would we do if we were in their shoes. This is not a useful question, particularly in the setting of prostate cancer. Unless the physician has had prostate cancer himself which has been treated, it is not likely that this question will yield any useful information. However, asking the physician what he or she would recommend to his or her brother or father is sometimes valuable. Remember that physicians are human and they will have biases toward or against particular treatments. It is important that you be the judge when talking to the physician.

Experience is a critical factor in outcome, particularly when it comes to sexual and urinary function recovery. So simply asking the physician how many brachytherapies, external beam radiation treatments or radical prostatectomies he or she has performed annually is a good starting point. Another major factor is how long he or she has been doing this. It is well recognized that there is a learning curve in all of these treatments. For example, it is recognized that the positive margin (some cancer cells left behind) rates at the time of radical prostatectomy are higher during a surgeon's first 100 prostatectomies compared to those during surgeries performed afterwards. So if a surgeon is performing 20 prostatectomies a year, which is a significant number, and has only been doing it for a couple of years, then this is not the same level of experience as somebody who does 20 a year but has been doing it for a decade.

It is also worth asking about or finding out about the physician's training, including the center he or she trained at and who he or she trained under. The experience with radical prostatectomy surgery or prostate radiation is highly variable from one residency training program to another. Asking your physician about his or her change in philosophy over time is also potentially useful. For example, for a physician who has been in practice for 10 years, has he or she changed his or her opinion regarding the role of prostatectomy versus brachytherapy if he or she is a urologist, or if your physician a radiation oncologist, has he or she changed their opinion regarding seed implantation versus IMRT? This may give you a sense of his or her ability to keep up with new techniques and medical literature.

The surgeons work as part of a team, so asking them about the facilities at the medical center is also important. The surgeons work in an operating room alongside residents or fellows as well as alongside operating room nurses and anesthesiologists. It may be worthwhile asking the physician for a reference of one, two or three names of anesthesiologists that he or she likes to work with. Unfortunately, historically, there have been surgeons who spend very little time in the operating room other than being present for the most important part of the procedure and much of the surgery is done by a resident or fellow. As an academic physician, I am fully committed to the training of residents and fellows, and it is my intention to train future leaders in sexual medicine and urology. However, there are critical portions of the operation that an experienced surgeon should be closely involved in, for example, the nerve sparing portion of a radical prostatectomy. As for the radiation oncologist, he or she works very closely with a physicist and radiologist, and asking about the experience of these personnel may also be of some benefit.

While experience is important, it is not the only factor important in defining outcomes or complications with these treatments. Indeed, it has now been well documented that even surgeons with high volume may have poor outcomes. The concept is that you either do good nerve sparing at the time of surgery or you don't. And whether you are doing 20 or 200 radical prostatectomies a year may not impact directly upon this. To do nerve sparing, for example, at the time of radical prostatectomy requires a very meticulous nature and great patience. The top surgeons at Memorial Sloan-Kettering take anywhere from two and a half to three and a half hours to perform nerve sparing surgery. Much of this time is spent teasing the nerves away from the prostate, not using any electrocautery, and applying nothing more than gentle traction to the nerve bundles. Thus, expertise is a critical factor, although admittedly, this is particularly difficult to glean from a discussion with the physician. I recommend that you ask your treating physicians what the specific figures on continence, erectile dysfunction and PSA recurrence are in their particular patients. It is easy to quote the literature, but remember that this literature is usually generated from so-called centers of excellence with vast experience. Such figures may not be replicated at smaller centers. Along with that, they should be able to define what they believe to be the potential outcomes for somebody of your age, your medical condition and with the cancer factors that were previously mentioned. Experienced physicians should be able to tailor the discussion and the risk for complications and outcomes to your particular case.

I encourage all of my patients who are undergoing a surgical procedure performed by me to speak to one of my patients who has previously undergone that procedure. I think it is entirely reasonable for you to ask the surgeon or radiation oncologist if you can speak to patients who have undergone such treatment. Speaking to a single patient may be of limited benefit, however, as it is not likely that the physician is going to have you speak with a patient who had a less than excellent outcome. The quality of the physician is not just assessed in his or her ability to evaluate a patient or conduct the procedure. It is also directly linked to how he or she manages any complications that occur during or after the procedure, and his or her accessibility and willingness to spend time in discussion with you. When choosing a surgeon, it is important to evaluate not just the erectile function recovery rates in his or her experience, but also the surgical margin positivity rate. High rates of erectile function recovery can be obtained at the risk of leaving cancer behind along the nerve, and likewise, excellent cancer control with very low levels of positive margins can be accomplished at the risk of causing significant nerve damage and future erectile dysfunction.

There are a number of prediction models used to predict survival with prostate cancer that are beyond the scope of this book. Memorial Sloan-Kettering Cancer Center, in particular Michael Kattan PhD and Dr. Peter Scardino, has been at the forefront of the development of these prediction models known as nomograms. I encourage you to go to our website at www.nomograms.org to survey the nomograms available for a variety of cancers, including prostate, bladder, kidney and breast. We have developed a prediction model for erectile dysfunction after radical prostatectomy and are in the process of developing one for radiation therapy also.

Appended at the end of this chapter are three nomograms. The first is a preoperative nomogram which helps men who come into the office before their surgeries to define what the long-term erectile function will be. The second is a postoperative nomogram used when a patient comes in after surgery knowing what his nerve sparing status has been. And finally, the 12–month nomogram is for men who return 12 months after surgery, and this uses their 12 month-function to predict their long-term erectile function. These nomograms predict erectile function recovery 24 months after surgery and all of them include the patient's age at the time of surgery, the patient's erectile function at the time of surgery, the number of other medical problems (high blood pressure, cholesterol problems, diabetes, coronary artery disease) a patient has, the nerve sparing status of the patient for the postoperative nomogram and the erectile function at 12 months after surgery for the 12–month nomogram.

The erectile function before surgery and the predicted erectile function at two years after surgery is based on the score from the International Index of Erectile Function, which has been appended to this chapter. This is a six-question questionnaire, which asks you about your ability to get and keep erection as well as your confidence in your ability to function sexually. Each question is scored on a 15–point scale, and the higher the overall score (maximum score is 30), the better the erectile function. To be able to have sexual intercourse consistently, a score of around 24 is required. While the official normal score is 26, there are many patients who are able to have intercourse with scores just below this level. You can score yourself and then you can use the nomograms to predict what your long-term erectile function recovery will be. It is important to understand that there is approximately a 10% error rate in nomograms, but they give you at least a crude guide as to what the potential is for erectile function recovery after surgery.

Thus, you can already get a feel for the complexities that go into not just the decision about which treatment you will pursue, but also whom you are going to have perform the procedure. I recommend you sit and make a decision in a thoughtful manner without rushing to get rid of the cancer, which is often the gut reaction immediately after the diagnosis of prostate cancer has been given to you.

DECIDING ON A TREATMENT

APPENDIX 1
International Index of Erectile Function (IIEF)

OVER THE PAST 4 WEEKS DURING SEXUAL ACTIVITY
(including sexual intercourse or self-stimulation)

1. How often were you able to get an erection during sexual activity?
   - 0 = No sexual activity
   - 1 = Almost never/never
   - 2 = A few times (much less than half the time)
   - 3 = Sometimes (about half the time)
   - 4 = Most times (much more than half the time)
   - 5 = Almost always/always

2. When you had erections with sexual stimulation, how often were your erections hard enough for penetration?
   - 0 = No sexual activity
   - 1 = Almost never/never
   - 2 = A few times (much less than half the time)
   - 3 = Sometimes (about half the time)
   - 4 = Most times (much more than half the time)
   - 5 = Almost always/always

3. When you attempted sexual intercourse, how often were you able to penetrate (enter)?
   - 0 = Did not attempt intercourse
   - 1 = Almost never/never
   - 2 = A few times (much less than half the time)
   - 3 = Sometimes (about half the time)
   - 4 = Most times (much more than half the time)
   - 5 = Almost always/always

continued on the next page

continued from the previous page

4. During sexual intercourse, how often were you able to maintain your erection after you had penetrated (entered) you partner?
    - 0 = Did not attempt intercourse
    - 1 = Almost never/never
    - 2 = A few times (much less than half the time)
    - 3 = Sometimes (about half the time)
    - 4 = Most times (much more than half the time)
    - 5 = Almost always/always

5. During sexual intercourse, how difficult was his to maintain your erection to complete intercourse?
    - 0 = Did not attempt intercourse
    - 1 = Extremely difficult
    - 2 = Very difficult
    - 3 = Difficult
    - 4 = Slightly difficult
    - 5 = Not difficult

6. How do you rate your confidence that you could get and keep an erection?
    - 1 = Very low
    - 2 = Low
    - 3 = Moderate
    - 4 = High
    - 5 = Very high

Grading system:

No erectile dysfunction (ED)	26 or greater
Mild ED	17–25
Moderate ED	11–16
Severe ED	10 or less

DECIDING ON A TREATMENT

APPENDIX 2
Nomograms for the prediction of recovery of erectile function after radical prostatectomy

For each nomogram, the left-hand side has the factors that you will need to plug into the prediction model. Your baseline IIEF score you can glean from Appendix 1 in this chapter. My advice is to use your IIEF score based on your erection function during sexual sactivity (partner of self) from a time-point before your prostate cancer diagnosis. Your age should be age in years (rounded up) at the time of surgery. You should then add up how many comorbidities (medical conditions associated with erectile dysfunction) you have. For example diabetes, high blood pressure, cholesterol problems, coronary artery disease, stroke, cigarette smoking. Add this number up and this is the number of comorbidities you have (having diabetes and cigarette smoking, now or in the past gives you a score of 2). For the postoperative and the 12–month nomogram an added factor is your nerve sparing score. For a guide on the Memorial Sloan Kettering Cancer Center nerve sparing score see the text in this chapter. If you have been told you had nerve sparing surgery your score should be between 2 (perfect nerve sparing) and 4 (reasonable nerve sparing). Finally for the 12–month nomogram there is one further extra factor, which is the 12 month IIEF score (that IIEF score at 12 months after surgery).

Each factor will give you a point score by drawing a vertical line from each horizontal line up to the points line at the top of the nomogram. For example, in the preoperative nomogram, an age of 50 years at the time of surgery will give approximately 73 points, an IIEF score of 24 will yield 46 points and 3 comorbidities will yield 0 points. Next, add up all of these points (for the example above, a total of 119 points). Then draw a line down from total points line to the 24 month IIEF score. For the example cited above, this gives an IIEF score of 19 (mild erectile dysfunction). This is your predicted erectile function 2 years after surgery.

Pre-Operative

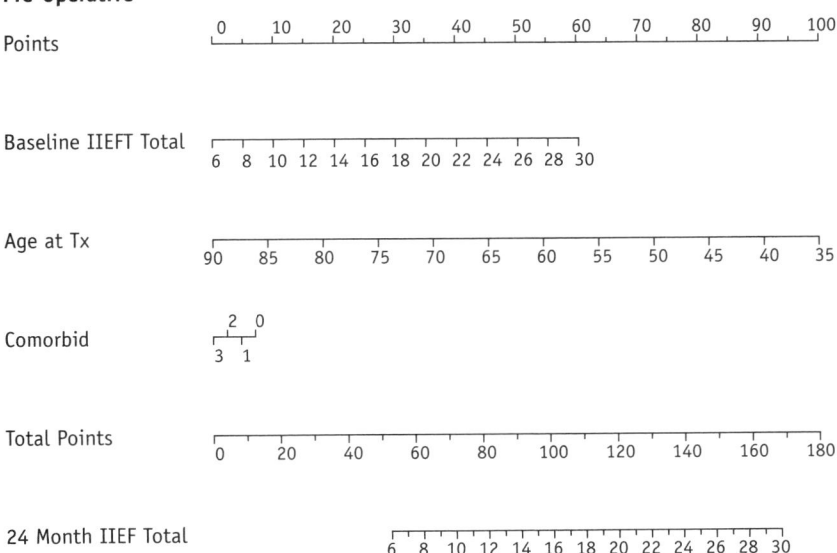

Post-Operative

Points 0 10 20 30 40 50 60 70 80 90 100

Baseline IIEFT Total 6 8 10 14 18 22 26 30

Age at Tx 90 85 80 75 70 65 60 55 50 45 40 35

Comorbid 2 0 / 3 1

Nerve 7 5 3 / 8 6 4 2

Total Points 0 20 40 60 80 100 120 140 160 180 200 220

24–Month IIEF Total 6 8 10 14 18 22 26 30

12-Month Post-Operative

Points 0 10 20 30 40 50 60 70 80 90 100

Baseline IIEFT Total 6 10 16 22 28

Age at Tx 90 85 80 75 70 65 60 55 50 45 40 35

Comorbid 2 0 / 3 1

Nerve 7 5 3 / 8 6 4 2

Month12IIEFTotal 6 8 10 12 14 16 18 20 22 24 26 28 30

Total Points 0 20 40 60 80 100 120 140 160 180 200 220

24–Month IIEF Total 2 4 6 8 10 12 14 16 18 20 22 24 26 28 30 32

CHAPTER 4

THE EFFECT OF RADICAL PROSTATECTOMY ON SEXUAL FUNCTION

> I. What Does the Surgery Involve?
> II. Nerve Sparing
> III. What to Expect Before and after Your Operation
> IV. Complications
> V. Predictors of Erectile Function Recovery
> VI. Erectile Function Results after Radical Prostatectomy

I. What Does the Surgery Involve?

The surgical treatment of prostate cancer involves what is known as a radical prostatectomy. Don't be turned off by the term "radical," as all this means is that not only is the prostate being removed, but so too are other adjacent structures, such as the vas deferens, the seminal vesicles behind the prostate, as well as some of the tissue surrounding the prostate.

Patients frequently ask why is it that we are not able to remove the prostate cancer from the middle of the prostate, and there are very good reasons for this. Prostate cancer tends to be present in multiple sites within the prostate. This is known as multifocality. When a pathologist examines the prostate after radical prostatectomy, there will be on average five separate small tumors present within the gland, and these are distributed in a very unpredictable fashion. Modern technology is not yet accurate enough to determine precisely where these tumors lie. Also, most are too small to feel on prostate examination, and they may not even be discovered on biopsy. For example, just a tiny fraction of the prostate tissue (approximately 1% of the prostate) is sampled using the small needles used during a biopsy. Even modern technology such as color Doppler ultrasound and MRI (magnetic resonance imaging) cannot detect a malignant tumor within the prostate in a way that a mammogram can pinpoint a cancer within the breast or CT (computerized tomography) scan can localize a tumor within the lung accurately.

Modern prostatectomy is a relatively new surgery in historical terms. Dr. Billroth from Germany made the first attempt to remove a prostate in 1867. It was not until 1904, in the United States, when Dr. Hugh Hampton Young did the first prostatectomy at Johns Hopkins. The early procedures were done using a perineal approach, where an incision is made between the scrotum and the anus. In the early part of the 20th century, this method resulted in relatively low blood loss and patients usually recovered quickly. Despite this, the surgeon's view of the most important structures during this approach, particularly the erection nerves, is highly restricted. In these early years, the incontinence and impotence rates were very high.

In 1945, an Irish surgeon named Terence Millin working in the United Kingdom pioneered a new technique involving a vertical abdominal incision, and this was the first report of a radical retropubic prostatectomy. While this procedure resulted in more blood loss, it did provide surgeons with a far better view of the prostate and greater access to the critical structures. However, it was not until the early 1980s that the concept of nerve sparing was introduced by Drs. Donker and Walsh at Johns Hopkins. Prior to this, radical retropubic prostatectomy was associated with severe bleeding; 25% of men remained incontinent and most had no ability to have erections after surgery. The introduction of an anatomical approach to radical prostatectomy (nerve sparing) and further refinements of these techniques have resulted in continued lowering of the rates of incontinence and erectile dysfunction, while still maintaining excellent cure rates.

For a radical prostatectomy, patients are usually admitted the day of the operation. They are told not to eat or drink anything after approximately midnight preceding the day of surgery. This is very important, as anything present in the stomach may result in problems if the patient vomits during the induction of anesthesia, resulting in the condition called aspiration, where the acid contents of the stomach get into the lung and cause severe lung injury. I would recommend to all patients that they see their surgeons, even if briefly, immediately prior to the operation. This time can be used for addressing any last-minute issues or questions that either you or your partner have regarding the procedure. Most importantly, it is usually reassuring for the patient to see the person who is about to remove his prostate.

While patients frequently spend much time poring over which surgeon to use, they spend very little time researching which anesthesiologist will be taking care of them. It is important to have at least your surgeon's reassurance that the anesthesiologist who is going to take care of you is excellent and that the surgeon has worked with him or before. If you meet with an anesthesiologist during your preadmission testing the week before surgery, it is likely that this will not be the same anesthesiologist who will put you to sleep for the procedure. The purpose of pre admission testing is to ensure that there are no concerns about your medications and current medical conditions. Some medical conditions might prompt the doctor or nurse seeing you at this time to order further testing before you undergo surgery. The anesthesiologist has the responsibility for the vital functions of the patient (respiration, blood pressure, etc.) during the operation, not the surgeon. Anesthesia for radical prostatectomy can be administered by a general, spinal or epidural anesthetic, or any combination of any these. When I operate on patients, I tell them that the decision regarding the type of anesthesia is based on a discussion between them and the anesthesiologist. Spinal problems, prior back surgery and other conditions will make an anesthesiologist less willing to perform spinal or epidural anesthesia. Likewise, certain neck and airway problems will decrease his or her willingness to perform general anesthesia.

The operation itself takes anywhere from one and a half to four hours, depending on the surgeon's approach and technique, and your anatomy and the type of cancer that you have. Most surgeons still perform a lymph node dissection, which removes the lymph glands on the side of the pelvis surrounding the prostate. Removing the lymph nodes may provide valuable information for planning treatments if they prove necessary in the future. The fact that your surgeon takes longer to do a procedure than another surgeon does not imply that he or she has inferior technique. In fact, if anything, it may be associated with greater care being taken to preserve the erection nerves at the time of surgery.

There are several ways to do a radical prostatectomy: open, laparoscopic, and robotic. An open procedure uses a vertical incision in the abdomen that is usually about four inches in length, starting just above the pubic bone and heading toward the belly button. Special instruments are used to keep the tissues apart so that the bladder, pelvic lymph nodes, and prostate can be visualized. The surgeon then very carefully dissects the erection nerves from the prostate if she is planning to do a nerve sparing procedure. Think of the erection nerves as being like microscopic fiber-optic cables buried within a layer of Saran Wrap that surrounds the top surface of the prostate. The surgeon needs to peel back this layer, making careful efforts not to injure the fiber optic cables. Once this has been done, the urethra is divided below the prostate, the seminal vesicles are freed up, the vas deferens is cut and ligated behind the prostate, and the prostate is then scooped out of the front surface of the rectum. Most surgeons examine the prostate once they remove it to see if there are any areas where the prostate cancer has extended beyond the capsule of the prostate, in which case further tissue may need to be excised to ensure complete removal of the cancer. Once the lymph glands, the prostate, seminal vesicles and vas deferens have been removed and bleeding has been controlled, the urethra needs to be joined to the bladder neck. Sometimes the bladder neck needs to be reconstructed, and then this is joined to the urethra using dissolvable stitches. This joining is called an anastomosis. Once this is done, the muscles of the abdomen and the skin incision are closed, anesthesia is ceased, and the patient is transported to the recovery room.

It is common for a patient to see me before he makes a final decision regarding the type of surgery and ask me whether he should have an open, laparoscopic, or robotic prostatectomy. There are two important factors in the preservation of erectile function that are based on the surgeon. First is the surgeon's experience. It is likely that it takes a surgeon about 100 prostatectomies to become fully proficient with the procedure. This concept has recently been confirmed, as surgeons who were well known for their open prostatectomy experience, who have switched to robotic prostatectomy, have shown that the incidence of positive margins (that is, cancer being left behind) is far higher in the first 100 cases than those that follow this. So, when speaking to a surgeon regarding prostatectomy surgery, whether it is open, laparoscopic or robotic, getting a sense for the surgeon's experience level is important.

The other surgeon factor and, unfortunately, one that you cannot assess before surgery is your surgeon's technical ability to do nerve sparing surgery.

THE EFFECT OF RADICAL PROSTATECTOMY ON SEXUAL FUNCTION

At Memorial-Sloan Kettering we have shown through our research that the surgeon him or herself is a critical factor in determining whether erection function recovers or not (Table 1). That is, whether the surgeon is doing 50 or 200 prostatectomies a year is not the critical factor, but rather it is their technical expertise and level of meticulousness that is critical to the erectile function recovery. As previously mentioned in the chapter on deciding which treatment and which surgeon to use, having a frank discussion with the physician about his or her personal figures with regard to erectile function is important.

It is common for surgeons to quote medical literature (Table 2), and that is usually generated from evidence that comes from so-called centers of excellence, medical centers that have top-level surgeons who do many prostatectomies and have done so for many years. However, these figures are often not replicated by surgeons in general urologic practice. Ask about the surgeon's personal figures. If he or she is reluctant to give these to you, my suggestion is that you should seek another opinion. Patients are often embarrassed to quiz physicians, and you need to be prepared that certain physicians will be defensive when you ask such probing questions. This to me is an indication that that surgeon is probably not a good match for you as a patient. In summary, asking the surgeon how many prostatectomies he or she have performed and asking about his or her specific erection recovery results are valuable things to accomplish during your interview.

While there are surgeons who continue to perform the perineal radical prostatectomy, most authorities now perform the surgery retropubically. In the late 1990's, surgeons in France and the USA attempted the first laparoscopic prostatectomies, and this has become a readily accepted form of prostatectomy. Laparoscopic surgery involves the placement of instruments through very small incisions (less than half an inch) at several places on the abdomen and the introduction of a camera and surgical instruments through the other holes (ports). Despite the lack of a large window, the laparoscopic surgeon has an excellent view of the internal structures at 10– to 15–fold magnification so that the procedure can be performed with ease by someone with expertise in this procedure. The abdomen is inflated with carbon dioxide gas to make room for insertion of the surgical instruments, and then the procedure is performed in a similar fashion to the open prostatectomy.

Robotic prostatectomy takes laparoscopic surgery one step further in the sense that the instruments that are present within the abdomen are moved by a robot. The surgeon does not stand at the side of the patient by the operating table, but sits at a console somewhat removed from the operating table itself. The surgeon then controls the instruments using a three- or four-arm robot. The most commonly used robot is known as the Da Vinci robot, although others exist. The difference between pure laparoscopic and robotic-assisted laparoscopic surgery is that the robot has a very high level of flexibility and agility, and surgeons who perform robotic prostatectomy claim that this is an advantage over pure laparoscopic prostatectomy. There are also highly experienced laparoscopic surgeons who claim that robotic surgery offers no significant advantage over the classic laparoscopic approach.

As you will hear me say several times in this book, there currently exists no data to suggest that there is any difference in urinary or sexual function outcomes between open, laparoscopic, and robotic prostatectomy. There is no doubt that there are advantages to laparoscopic and robotic prostatectomies for the physician, including 3D imaging, greater flexibility of movement of the surgical instruments, and the ability to sit rather than stand for the surgery. For the patient, there is usually a shorter hospital stay, a more rapid recovery, more rapid return to work, reduced blood loss, less postoperative pain, and generally a quicker return to a normal level of activity. However, the complications of radical prostatectomy (see later in this chapter) are identical for all three approaches. I suggest that two of the factors that should be involved in choosing a surgeon is to make sure that you are comfortable with him or her and that he or she performs the radical prostatectomy using the approach with which he or she is most comfortable.

Several centers have shown that prostate cancer outcomes, that is, the PSA recurrence rate and excision of the cancer in its entirety, are identical for open, laparoscopic and robotic prostatectomy in the hands of an experienced surgeon. In contrast to a decade ago, most urology residents in training are exposed to at least laparoscopic if not robotic prostatectomy nowadays. Therefore, when they start in practice, they have significant experience in at least seeing this technique. There are training programs in the United States where the residents actually do not do hands-on surgery, and therefore, once again, asking the surgeon about his or her personal experience in doing the procedure is critical.

II. Nerve Sparing

As hard as it is to believe, despite the advances in technology that occurred over the 1960s, '70s, and '80s, it wasn't until the early part of the 1980s that nerve sparing prostatectomy was developed. The exact anatomy of the erection nerves was not well appreciated. In fact, many experts thought that the erection nerves actually traveled through the prostate, when in fact, Drs. Donker and Walsh showed that the nerves travel alongside the prostate. This allowed these erection nerves to be gently teased off the prostate, which resulted in a significant increase in the number of men who retained their erections after surgery compared to those patients who had surgery prior to nerve sparing.

The erection nerve is bundled together with blood vessels, and this combination is known as the neurovascular bundle. You will often hear surgeons talk about the neurovascular bundle, and if you read the medical literature you will see the neurovascular bundle mentioned frequently. The erection nerves are autonomic nerves in nature; that is, they are involuntary in their function. This is as opposed to sensory nerves, which supply sensation to your body parts, or motor nerves, which cause your muscles to function. Autonomic nerves connect to organs whose function is not directly under our control, for example, the heart, rectum, bladder and penis. These nerves are difficult to see with the naked eye. However, most surgeons during open prostatectomy now use magnifying glasses to help identify them. And, of course, with the magnification used in laparoscopic and robotic surgery, these nerves are readily identifiable.

The erection nerves are best thought of as a series of fiber optic cables with hundreds of tiny fibers clumped together. In contrast to many other animals, it is not a single nerve on either side but more like a leash of nerve fibers. These nerve fibers are distributed over a relatively large area over the surface of the prostate. If you think of the prostate as being like a clock, with 12 o'clock being the front and 6 o'clock being the back portion, 3 o'clock being the left side of the prostate and 9 o'clock being the right side of the prostate, these nerve fibers typically are present all the way from 4 o'clock around to 8 o'clock in a clockwise fashion, although the density of these nerves is greatest between 3 and 1 o'clock on the right side and 9 and 11 o'clock on the left side.

Erection function recovery is heavily dependent upon the volume of this nerve tissue that is left behind. When you speak to your surgeon on the day following the operation or when your partner speaks to the surgeon the day of surgery, it is important for you to know how much nerve tissue was actually left behind. Historically, nerve sparing has been classified as being bilateral (both nerve bundles saved), unilateral (one nerve saved) or non-nerve sparing (where all nerve fibers are cut, usually because of concerns over excising all of the cancer in men with large tumors). However, this concept of bilateral versus unilateral versus non-nerve sparing is an historical one and does not have a lot of clinical meaningfulness. For example, if 60% of the right neurovascular bundle and 40% of the left neurovascular bundle are saved, is this bilateral, unilateral or non-nerve sparing surgery? So, speaking to the surgeon about quantifying how many nerve fibers have been saved is probably a more accurate way to judge the nerve sparing.

Certain centers use nerve sparing grading systems. For example, at Memorial Sloan-Kettering, there are four grades of nerve sparing which the surgeons utilize. Grade 1 is perfect preservation of the nerves. In Grade 1, the nerves have been minimally handled and have been entirely pushed back from the prostate, and none of the fibers have been injured. Grade 4, on the other hand, is complete removal of the nerves. Once again, this is usually for cancer control, and the nerve fibers are usually visible to the pathologist when he or she examines the prostate microscopically after surgery. It is important to understand that surgeons are not necessarily 100% accurate at defining the nerve sparing status. That is, if they say that the nerves are perfectly preserved, sometimes they are not. If the surgeon says the nerves have been completely removed, in approximately 10% of these patients, there is nerve tissue left behind which may allow the man to become a pill (Viagra, Levitra, Cialis) responder after surgery. Using this system, Grade 2 means minimal damage to the nerves and this usually means less than 25% of the nerve fiber has been trimmed away. Grade 3 is moderate damage, which usually implies that a greater percentage of the nerve has been excised.

The medical literature clearly indicates that men who have bilateral nerve sparing have higher rates of erection function recovery and higher rates of responding to Viagra-like drugs than patients with unilateral nerve sparing. We have shown at Memorial Sloan-Kettering that patients who have a Grade 1 nerve preservation on both sides do better with erection function recovery than patients with Grade 2 preservation on both sides, and this is significantly greater than the erection function recovery capabilities for patients who have Grade 3s or 4s.

It is not always possible to preserve the erection nerves. The main goal of radical prostatectomy, of course, is to cure cancer, and this depends on removing the entire tumor and leaving no cancer behind. If the pathologist finds cancer at the border of the prostate (positive surgical margins), there is clearly an increased risk that the tumor will spread and eventually become incurable. Prostate cancer can extend through the capsule of the prostate (this is known as extracapsular extension), and sometimes this impinges upon the nerves or close to the nerves, and therefore the nerves may need to be excised for the purposes of curing the cancer.

The concept of nerve grafting (also known as cavernous nerve interposition grafting) was introduced by Dr. Peter Scardino and his team while he was at Baylor College of Medicine in 1997. He demonstrated that when patients required both erection nerves to be deliberately removed, the use of a nerve graft between the two cut ends of the neurovascular bundle on either side resulted in improved erectile function outcomes. There are two main sources of nerve grafts. One is the nerve from the side of the foot, known as the Sural nerve, and the other is in the pelvis, known as the Genito-femoral nerve. In a man who has both nerves completely excised and does not have nerve grafting, he has almost certainly a zero percent chance of having recovery of natural erections. Thus, there is good rationale for bilateral cavernous nerve grafting.

While the initial study suggested that 50% of men having bilateral cavernous nerve grafting have recovery of erectile function, the Memorial Sloan-Kettering data would suggest that 30% of men get back to functioning sometimes with or without the use of a Viagra-like drug, but only 10% of men function well with or without the use of the medication. While these figures do not seem very high, they are, in fact, much higher than the zero percent chance that a man will have recovery of natural erections without nerve grafting. Patients frequently ask me before they have their operations whether they should consider nerve grafting. I believe that the procedure is worthwhile because it has such a low complication rate and gives the patient at least a small chance of getting a natural erection back or becoming a pill responder.

There are several centers that are exploring the use of unilateral nerve grafts; that is, when men are having one nerve excised, they undergo grafting on that side. However, at present, there is no clear evidence to show that unilateral nerve grafting is of any significant benefit with regard to erectile function recovery. One of the two downsides of nerve grafting is that it adds more time in the operating room, anywhere from 30 to 60 minutes. The nerve grafting is typically done by a plastic surgeon or a neurosurgeon with expertise in nerve grafting techniques.

The other downside is that it typically adds significant cost to the procedure, and in some circumstances, the cost of the nerve grafting is not covered by insurance. It is important that you confirm this prior to your surgery. If the sural nerve is used, it is not uncommon for a man to have a small area of numbness on the outside of the top surface of the foot. This often improves over the course of the first 24 months after surgery, and approximately 1% of men will develop pain in this area because of the nerve trauma. If the genitofemoral nerve is used, there may be a small area of numbness at the top of the scrotum and inner thigh, but other than these effects, nerve grafting is a very safe procedure.

There are three other therapies that have been explored for the treatment of prostate cancer. Combined they are known as focal or minimally invasive therapy. The first is called cryotherapy, or cryosurgery, which involves the placement of a probe into the prostate through the perineum (that area between the scrotum and the anus). Gas is used to freeze the gland and surrounding tissues by creating an ice ball. This ice ball can be seen by an ultrasound probe placed in the rectum at the time of the procedure, and so the surgeon has control over the extent of tissue damage. Over time, after freezing the prostate tissue dies (thus, hopefully killing the cancer) and the prostate shrinks. This technology has advanced over the course of the last decade and initially was introduced for the treatment of men whose prostate cancer had recurred after radiation therapy, but has now received greater attention for the primary treatment of prostate cancer. The precise outcomes from cryosurgery from a cancer control standpoint are beyond the scope of this book. However, it is safe to say that there exist no studies that accurately assess erectile function recovery in patients undergoing cryosurgery.

Two other therapies that have been explored are high-intensity focus ultrasound (HIFU) and photodynamic (light) therapy. Both of these technologies are in their infancy and their long-term effectiveness in curing prostate cancer is not clear at this point in time, and more importantly, for the purposes of this book, their effect on sexual function is also unclear. However, it has to be said that any therapy that can spare the nerves and the arteries surrounding the prostate from injury may lead to better erectile function recovery. This is always at the potential risk of leaving cancer cells behind in the prostate.

III. What to Expect before and after Your Operation

Most surgeons will advocate waiting about six weeks after your prostate biopsy before having radical prostatectomy surgery. This short delay will in

THE EFFECT OF RADICAL PROSTATECTOMY ON SEXUAL FUNCTION

no way endanger your life or reduce the chances of cure. You will be seen sometime before your operation (usually one to two weeks beforehand) by an anesthesiologist or nurse practitioner for preadmission testing. At this time you will have blood work performed, and this is the point when you must disclose all of your medications, including alcohol intake as well as any recreational drugs. With the explosion in over-the-counter nutritional herbal supplements, it is also important to mention which of these you are taking. It may be beneficial to bring these bottles along with you so that the clinicians can look at the exact ingredients of these supplements as many of them contain several ingredients. Vitamin E, aspirin or any anticoagulant medications will need to be stopped quite some time before surgery, so check with your preadmission testing clinician as to when you should do this. All of these agents decrease blood clotting and increase the likelihood of significant bleeding at the time of surgery or afterwards.

Whether or not you proceed with autologous donation of blood (that is, where you bank your own blood) is an important consideration that you should discuss with your surgeon. Most patients are put on a clear liquid diet the day before surgery, and many are told to take a self-administered enema at home the night before surgery. In contrast to bowel surgery, it is not necessary to do a rigorous bowel preparation because injury to the rectum at the time of prostatectomy is now very rare. This occurs in less than 1% of patients, and most often, when this occurs, the rectal injury can be repaired immediately. If you are over 50 years of age at the time of preadmission testing, you will also have a chest x-ray and an EKG to make sure that you are fit enough for surgery. If you have a cardiac history, the surgeon and anesthesiologist will almost certainly insist on you having what is called cardiac clearance, where your cardiologist examines, evaluates or tests you to make sure that you are fit enough for anesthesia and surgery.

Once the surgery is complete, you will be transferred to the recovery room, and you will spend a few hours there being monitored to make sure that your vital signs (blood pressure, breathing, pulse) all normalize after surgery. With regard to postoperative pain, some men tolerate pain better than others, and usually the patient's partner is well aware which category he falls into. Most men tolerate the pain of the surgery very well, and if this is an issue after surgery, the surgeon may consult one of the pain management physicians (who are usually anesthesiologists) to try to control it. It is in the surgeon's interest to have your pain control excellent so that you are more likely to breathe deeply and move around as soon as possible after surgery.

Most men spend no longer than three days in hospital, and many of our patients at Memorial Sloan-Kettering after open prostatectomy go home on postoperative day two or three. It is routine for patients who have had robotic prostatectomy to go home on the first postoperative day, and patients having laparoscopic surgery to go home on the first or second postoperative day. The catheter in your bladder (known as a Foley catheter) will be removed anywhere from seven to fourteen days after surgery. Most patients are prescribed antibiotics to be taken around the time of catheter removal so that the removal of the catheter doesn't cause the leakage of bacteria into the blood. Pain killers are very constipating. It is important that you use something to allow your stools to stay soft, and I generally recommend the over-the-counter laxative Colace for a period of four weeks after the procedure. Your surgeon will give you instructions with regard to limitations on activity and lifting, and you should pay particular attention to these instructions.

IV. Complications

As with any major surgery, there is an increased risk of blood clotting in the veins of the legs (known as deep vein thrombosis, or DVT) and sometimes if these are large enough and occur in the pelvic veins, the patient is at risk for flipping a clot off into the lung, known as a pulmonary embolus (PE). With modern surgical approaches and modern surgical care, in particular the use of compression boots applied to the patients legs during the procedure to keep the blood within the leg veins from becoming stagnant, the incidence of DVT and PE are very low.

Also, whenever an incision is made anywhere in the body there is a risk of infection of that wound. Wound infection rates are very low in patients undergoing open or laparoscopic/robotic prostatectomy. Nevertheless, good wound care is important and your surgeon and/or his or her nurse or nurse practitioner will go over how to deal with the incision after surgery.

Swelling and discoloration of the skin over the penis and scrotum are common after radical prostatectomy. While this may cause anxiety in the patient, this swelling is usually mild and can generally be relieved by elevating the area with a towel under the scrotum while sitting or lying in bed and by the use of a scrotal (athletic) support when walking. It is not uncommon for men to gain some weight in the days after surgery. This is usually due to the fluid that is given intravenously to keep the patient hydrated during and after the operation. It is common between days two to five after surgery that

THE EFFECT OF RADICAL PROSTATECTOMY ON SEXUAL FUNCTION

Table 1 • **Factors Predicting Erectile Function Recovery after Radical Prostatectomy**

- Patient age at time of surgery (younger better)
- Patient erectile function before surgery (harder better)
- Amount of nerve tissue preserved (more spared better)
- Blood flow into and out of penis after surgery (better blood flow better)
- Erection tissue health
- Surgeon results (specific to him or her)
- Surgeon volume (how often the surgeon does a radical prostatectomy)
- Number and severity of comorbidities (diabetes, high blood pressure, high cholesterol, etc.)

this fluid is excreted, and the patient starts urinating large amounts of urine and loses the weight over this course of time. Thus, you can see that radical prostatectomy is a safe procedure in the hands of an experienced and technically proficient surgeon.

V. Predictors of Erectile Function Recovery (Table 1)

There are five major predictors of recovery of erectile function after radical prostatectomy: 1) patient age at the time of surgery, 2) erectile function before surgery, 3) nerve sparing status, 4) erectile tissue health and 5) erectile blood flow after surgery. It has been well documented in many series that younger men typically have better erectile function recovery than older men. Firstly, this is likely due to the fact that older men tend to have more medical conditions than younger men, and likely their erectile function even before surgery is not as strong. Secondly, older men likely have poor ability to regenerate their erection nerves than younger men. At Memorial Sloan-Kettering, the men who get back to the exact same level of erection hardness after surgery that they had before surgery, are typically under 50 years of age. The better a man's erections are before surgery, the more likely he is to recover his erection function after surgery.

I have already alluded to the concept that the volume of nerve tissue spared at the time of surgery is critical to recovery of erectile function. In Chapter 7, I discuss the concept of penile rehabilitation and preservation.

The purpose of penile rehabilitation is to protect erectile tissue from damage as the health of the erection tissue is critically important to recovery of erections. For example, there are men who have 100% recovery of their erection nerves after the trauma of surgery, but whose erectile tissue has degenerated so they will then no longer be able to get erections on their own or with oral medications. Thus, while the surgeon is heavily focused on nerve sparing at the time of surgery, he or she should also be heavily focused on protection of erection tissue while the nerves are recovering over the course of 12 to 24 months after surgery.

Finally, there is new evidence coming to light that the blood flow status in the penis in the early stages after surgery may, in fact, be critical to recovery of erection function. I have already spoken about injury to accessory pudendal arteries and the development of venous leak (where the valve mechanism within the erection chambers fails to function properly), and both of these can be diagnosed using a duplex upper ultrasound of the penis. This is a procedure where a patient is given an injection of medication into the penis using a tiny needle which generally feels like a mosquito bite. The man develops an erection, and a probe is used to measure the blood flow velocity into and out of the penis. The presence of low blood flow into the penis results in lower likelihood of long-term recovery of erections. Furthermore, the presence of venous leak gives a poor prognosis for the recovery for natural or medication-assisted erections. It is estimated that less than 10% of men who develop venous leak after radical prostatectomy ever recover natural erections after surgery. So, venous leak is clearly a bad thing to have occur, and rehabilitation, which I will discuss in great detail in Chapter 7, is aimed to prevent venous leak occurring. Saying that, 25% of men with venous leak get good erections with Viagra-like drugs, and the majority are able to have sexual intercourse using penile injections. Thus, all is NOT lost!

The predictors of the development of venous leak after surgery include older age (patients over 60 years of age are more likely to develop venous leak early than those who are under 60), minimal or non-nerve sparing surgery, poor erections before surgery, and most importantly, delay in treatment after surgery. The latter is very important and is the reason why we encourage patients to come in to see us six weeks after surgery to start rehabilitation as soon as possible. We know, when men delay more than six months after surgery if they are obtaining no erections, that they have a significantly increased risk of developing venous leak. It is extremely uncommon for men to develop venous leak within the first three months of surgery, but the group of men who are most likely to experience this terrible problem are those men who have had non-nerve sparing surgery.

VI. Erectile Function Results after Radical Prostatectomy (Table 2)

As simple as it would seem to be to report erection function recovery rates after this operation, the literature is highly confusing, not just to patients but also to physicians. The erectile function recovery rate ranges anywhere from 20 to 90% after surgery depending on which literature you read. This begs the question, "Could it be that one center does radical prostatectomy so much better than others?" The answer to this question is not a simple one, but probably rests as much in how data are reported as in the technical expertise of any given surgery. When reviewing the literature, the erectile function recovery rates tend to be higher at so-called centers of excellence by well-established surgeons compared to studies that look at many centers lumped together.

It is important that you understand that this literature is highly variable, particularly in how data is acquired and reported, which populations are studied, and how high levels of variation are in the actual definition of erectile dysfunction after surgery. The key elements to understanding erectile function outcomes after radical prostatectomy include who the men were who were studied, how the data was obtained by the surgeon, when patients were questioned after surgery, erection function before surgery and how the surgeon defined adequate erectile function after surgery.

You will see from Table 2 that the number of patients included in some studies is tremendously variable from less than 100 to more than 25,000. The greater the number of patients, the more likely we are to be able to come up with accurate information because this gets around the natural variability that is seen in erectile function recovery. Another factor to look at is the patient age in the study. Most studies have patients around 60 years of age, but there are some that have patients with an average age younger than this, and some that have an average age older than this. As previously mentioned, this will impact significantly upon erectile function recovery as younger men have better erection function recovery.

There is evidence to show that erection function recovery is dependent to some extent on the number and severity of comorbidities that the patient has at the time of surgery. Despite this, on review of the 24 most recent

Table 2 • Incidence of Erectile Dysfunction after Radical Prostatectomy

Author	Year of Publication	Type of Surgery	Patient Number	Patients Returning to Same Erectile Function as Before Surgery	Capable Of Having Sexual Intercourse (%) BNS	Capable Of Having Sexual Intercourse (%) UNS
Kubler	2007	O	265	NR	60	NR
Kaul	2006	R	154	NR	96	NR
Ficarra	2006	O	75	NR	65	NR
Mulhall	2005	O	132	NR	52	NR
Montorsi	2005	O	42	100%	52	NR
Gallo	2005	O	58	NR	14	NR
Chien	2005	R	56	NR	50	44
Ahlering	2005	R	318	NR	47	46
Rozet	2005	L	231	NR	43	NR
Shimuzu	2005	O	66	NR	17	0
Saranchuk	2005	O	647	NR	62	NR
Korfage	2005	O	123	NR	12	NR
Penson	2005	O	1,288	NR	28	NR
Kundu	2004	O	2,415	NR	76	53
Karakiewicz	2004	O	2,415	NR	25	NR
Steineck	2002	O	187	NR	20	NR
Noldus	2002	O	366	NR	52	16
Katz	2002	L	143	NR	12	36
Rabbani	2000	O	314	NR	76	30
Benoit	2000	O	25,561	NR	78	NR
Walsh	2000	O	70	NR	86	NR
Stanford	2000	O	1,291	NR	44	41

O: open RP; L: laparoscopic RP; R: robotic RP;
NR: not reported; BNS: both nerves spared; UNS: one nerve spared

journal articles reporting on post-prostatectomy erectile function, only five of these actually quoted the percentage of patients who had the presence of medical conditions such as diabetes, high blood pressure, high cholesterol and coronary artery disease, all of which impact on erection function.

Another key issue is how erectile function data are actually acquired. Has the data been acquired by a telephone call to the patient, by an interview with the patient or using a special questionnaire designed for the assessment of erectile function? Furthermore, who acquired the data? Who ran the interview or administered the questionnaire? The involvement of the primary surgeon in the acquisition of this data is fraught with problems, not the least of which is the concept of social desirability. This is the idea that patients may tell their physicians what they think their physicians want to hear. Thus, if a patient has been promised bilateral nerve sparing surgery by an eminent prostatectomist and has been told both nerves were saved during surgery, is there a chance that the patient will be reticent to own up to the fact that his postoperative erections are poor? Some patients will shy away from telling the surgeon such, and this is one way in which questionnaires administered by another person may improve the quality and accuracy of this information. Plus, given that it may take 24 months at least for the full recovery of erectile function, it is important that patients are evaluated long enough after surgery to define the true recovery of erectile function.

Probably the most critical and yet complex issue is how adequate erectile function is actually defined by the surgeon. There are many surgeons who say a man is potent if he responds to a Viagra-like pill or even if he is responsive to penile injection therapy. However, the National Institutes of Health consensus conference definition of erectile dysfunction is "the consistent inability to obtain and/or maintain an erection sufficient for satisfactory sexual performance," and nowhere in this definition appears any reference to the use of medication. When surgeons quote recovery of erections to patients and fail to divulge that what they are really talking about is the ability to have an erection with medication, this is somewhat disingenuous.

You will see from Table 2 that the variability in recovery of erectile function is great. Very few surgeons ever report on men getting back to normal function or returning to their preoperative erectile function. This is critically important, especially for younger men, as the quality of erection is directly linked to the patient's confidence and sexual self-esteem and sexual satisfaction. A much ignored concept is erection quality, that is, erection hardness. Let's say we use a 10–point rigidity scale, where 0 is completely flaccid, 10 is fully rigid and 6/10 is adequate for vaginal penetration; now, let's look at the case of a 54–year-old man who undergoes radical prostatectomy, who had preoperative erection hardness of 9/10 (that is almost fully rigid), and 24 months after surgery, he has a rigidity level of 6/10. Yes, he is capable of having sexual intercourse, but the patient has experienced a 33% reduction in his erection hardness. If a man has not been using a medication, he will start using a medication, and if he is using a medication, he will switch that medication because this level of erection hardness reduction results in sexual dissatisfaction. So, erection quality is a critical factor that most surgeons never discuss. The majority of men over 50 years of age will have some reduction in erection hardness without the use of erection pills after surgery.

The final issue is consistency of erections. There are patients who tell me that the surgeons deem them to be potent despite the fact that only one out of every five erections allows them to have sexual intercourse. This concept of consistency is important, as very low levels of consistency translate into low levels of confidence in one's ability to get and keep an erection. This is a tremendously negative factor when it comes to sexual confidence. It is likely that young men require consistency levels of 90% and above, but even for older men, consistency levels of 75% or greater are required to maintain their sexual confidence. This is rarely reported in the literature that you will read.

As I have mentioned on more than one occasion in this book, there is no evidence to show that open surgery is any better or worse than robotic or laparoscopic surgery prostatectomy when it comes to urinary or sexual function outcomes. Despite this, some surgeons have a tendency to suggest that erection function recovery is better after robotic prostatectomy than the other approaches. There clearly is, at this point in time, no evidence to support this statement. On review of 75 robotic prostatectomy websites and 20 open prostatectomy websites, we were surprised to find that only approximately one-half of these sites actually ever mentioned erectile dysfunction. Even more staggering is that we found that only one-fifth of the robotic prostatectomy sites and one-third of the open sites were actually giving accurate erectile recovery function. Furthermore, only 1% of the robotic and only 10% of the open sites were comprehensive in the information that was given to patients. More than one-half of the robotic prostatectomy sites stated or inferred that erectile function recovery was better after robotic than open prostatectomy, while only 5% of open sites inferred that their rates were better than robotic prostatectomy. This level of misinformation only fuels the confusion and unrealistic expectations that patients have prior to surgery.

Finally, I want to remind you about nomograms, which I mentioned in the previous chapter. These mathematical models factor in all the relevant data in prediction of risk and are far better in gauging outcomes than a single physician's impression or opinion of the literature. Memorial Sloan-Kettering has been pivotal in the development of nomograms for the prediction of PSA recurrence after radical prostatectomy, as well as in many other cancers. I direct you to www.nomograms.org, which is the official website at Memorial Sloan-Kettering for nomograms for a variety of cancers. These nomograms are likely to be more accurate in predicting erection function recovery than a surgeon's opinion or the internet.

CHAPTER 5
PROSTATE RADIATION AND SEXUAL FUNCTION

> I. How Does Radiation Work?
> II. How Is Radiation Delivered?
> III. Side Effects of Radiation
> IV. Erectile Function Outcomes after Radiation

I. How Does Radiation Work?

Radiation therapy using x-rays was first discovered by the German physicist, Dr. William Roentgen, in 1895. Very rapidly, these x-rays were used for imaging the body, and Dr. Roentgen was awarded the Nobel Prize in Physics in 1901. His research was furthered by Dr. Marie Curie, who, working with her husband Pierre, discovered radium. Madame Curie went on to win the Nobel Prize on not one, but two occasions.

The first radiation therapy for prostate cancer in men was performed at Johns Hopkins University by Dr. Hugh Hampton Young, who was also involved in the development of radical prostatectomy for prostate cancer. Dr. Young inserted a radiation pellet into the prostate. Although there were some benefits seen, oftentimes this was associated with significant side effects. Seed implantation in its original form was not very precise. Doctors would open the area around the prostate surgically and insert radioactive pellets into the prostate. Given the lack of precision, some areas of the prostate would receive less than adequate radiation, and then other areas would receive too large a dose.

External beam therapy, that is, the use of external x-rays that penetrate the body wall to reach the prostate, was developed in the 1940s using Cobalt. Cobalt was a highly effective form of radiation for tumors requiring low radiation doses, such as certain types of testicular cancer. For prostate cancer, which requires higher radiation doses to kill tumor cells, it proved to be relatively ineffective largely because of inadequate penetration of x-ray beams into the body. The development of the linear accelerator in the 1950s allowed radiation oncologists to deliver higher-energy radiation with more beam penetration and greater safety and precision than was previously possible. The use of the linear accelerator with external beam therapy resulted in a significant improvement in cure rates of prostate cancer. However, since the optimal radiation dose was still unknown, they fell far short of our current cure rates.

There was a revival of interest in seed implantation in the 1970s. Seed implantation got a new name, brachytherapy. Using more modern radiation techniques and improved computer technology, it was possible to deliver very high doses of radiation to the prostate. One of the keys to understanding radiation therapy is that higher radiation doses to the prostate lead to greater cure rates for prostate cancer. Unfortunately, the higher the dose to the prostate the more likely one is to damage the surrounding tissues, such as the bladder, the rectum, the erectile nerves, and erectile tissue. With the development of sophisticated computer programs, multi-dimensional imaging, and better radiation delivery techniques, radiation oncologists can now deliver high doses of radiation with high precision. As you read earlier in this book, as with surgery, choosing an expert is critical to the successful treatment of your prostate cancer.

Radiation therapy works by killing cells. It kills not just cancer cells but also kills normal cells. However, those cells that are most rapidly dividing are the most sensitive to radiation (as is true for chemotherapy). Fortunately, most cancers have cells that are dividing more rapidly than normal tissue cells.

Radiation attacks the DNA in our cells. It causes breakages in the DNA, and when this occurs, the cells commit suicide, a process known as apoptosis. Normal cells also have better repair machinery to fix some radiation damage, whereas cancer cells do not. As well as killing off the actual prostate cancer cells, radiation causes injury to the blood vessels that supply the cancer.

The key to the effective treatment of prostate cancer by radiation is giving enough of a dose, precisely enough, to kill the prostate cancer and minimize the side effects.

II. How Is Radiation Delivered?

Modern radiation can be delivered in two ways, either external beam therapy or radioactive seed implants (brachytherapy). There are certain circumstances where a physician may advocate a combination of these two. Radiation is delivered in units known as Gray (Gy), named after an English radiologist, Louis Gray. Previously, the unit used was called a rad, and fortunately, translating one to the other is relatively easy, as 100 rads is equivalent to 1 Gy. Using external beam therapy, minimum doses of 75 to 80 Gy (and sometimes higher) are typically necessary. Using Brachytherapy, doses of 140 to 160 Gy are achievable.

External beam radiation therapy can be delivered in three different ways: firstly, conventional external beam; secondly, three-dimensional conformal radiation therapy (3D-CRT); and finally, the most modern approach known as intensity-modulated radiation therapy (IMRT). Conventional external beam radiation therapy involves the administration of radiation to an area around the prostate gland based on bone landmarks. This approach is not commonly used by larger centers, as they now use one of the other two forms of external beam therapy. As previously mentioned, the prostate is in very close contact with the rectum, the bladder and the urethra, and with conventional external beam therapy, these organs will generally fall within the radiation field.

3D-CRT was developed in the late 1980s and uses computer technology linked to a CT or a MRI scanner. The prostate gland is outlined very accurately in three dimensions, which allows better definition of the prostate gland and surrounding tissue. There is a significant reduction in the amount of radiation that is delivered to the surrounding tissues and a dramatic reduction in serious side effects with 3D-CRT. Radiation oncologists soon increased the dose prescribed up to 75 Gy with even better cure rates. An increase in radiation dose from 70 Gy to 75 Gy results in a 50% increase in the success of prostate radiation. When delivering 65 Gy, half of men have prostate cancer present if the prostate is biopsied three years after treatment. This figure is 30% after 70 Gy and, with the use of 81 Gy, less than 10% of men have prostate cancer present on prostate biopsy at this point. Thus, when the accuracy of radiation delivery increases, this allows more radiation to be given, as less of it gets to the surrounding (non-prostate) tissues, and so, severe side effects are limited. While the technology for 3D-CRT is not available at every institution, it is widely available nationally and internationally. In general, the higher the dose, the better the rates of killing the cancer but the higher the rates of side effects.

Taking technological advances to an even higher level, IMRT was developed within the last decade using highly sophisticated computer programs. This technique delivers the radiation dose at various intensities throughout the field of radiation. Because of this, higher doses of radiation can be used (80 to 90 Gy), while keeping the side effects incidence to a low level.

Just as there have been significant advances in the delivery of external radiation beam, there have also been significant advances in the use of brachytherapy for prostate cancer. The radioactive seeds that are used currently for prostate cancer brachytherapy are made of either palladium or iodine in a titanium casing. Other less commonly used seeds are made of cesium and iridium. A radioactive core is contained within the seed, which is approximately the size of a grain of uncooked rice. These seeds emit low doses of radiation over time. Prescription doses are about 140 Gy with iodine and 125 Gy with palladium. There are other forms of radiation therapy, including proton beam and neutron beam radiation, which are available at select centers, but given that they are used so infrequently, a discussion of their advantages and disadvantages are beyond the scope of this book.

The precise delivery of external beam radiation relies heavily upon mapping out the prostate size and shape using a CT scan or MRI. Over the weeks preceding the start of your radiation therapy, you will have what is known as "simulation," where the prostate is imaged using a CT scan in an effort to ensure the most precise delivery of the radiation. In order to be sure that you are in the same position each and every day, you have your radiation treatments, a mold of your pelvis is made and fixed to the treatment table (Figure 1). You will also have permanent tattoo marks placed on the skin, again to help the precise targeting of the prostate with the radiation. Sometimes, gold marker seeds that are not radioactive but can be seen on x-ray film are placed into the prostate before simulation. These seeds can be seen daily and matched up to make sure your prostate is in the same position every day. External beam is typically delivered every weekday over the period of 9 to 10 weeks. The x-ray beam is only on for a few minutes, but it can take some time to make sure you are in the proper position. Most patients spend

PROSTATE RADIATION AND SEXUAL FUNCTION

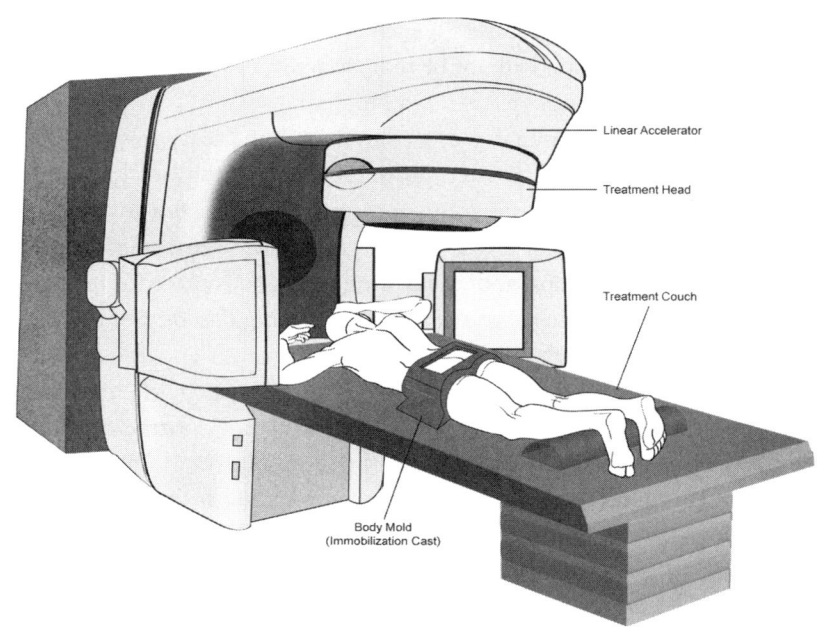

Figure 1 • Set up for external beam radiation therapy.

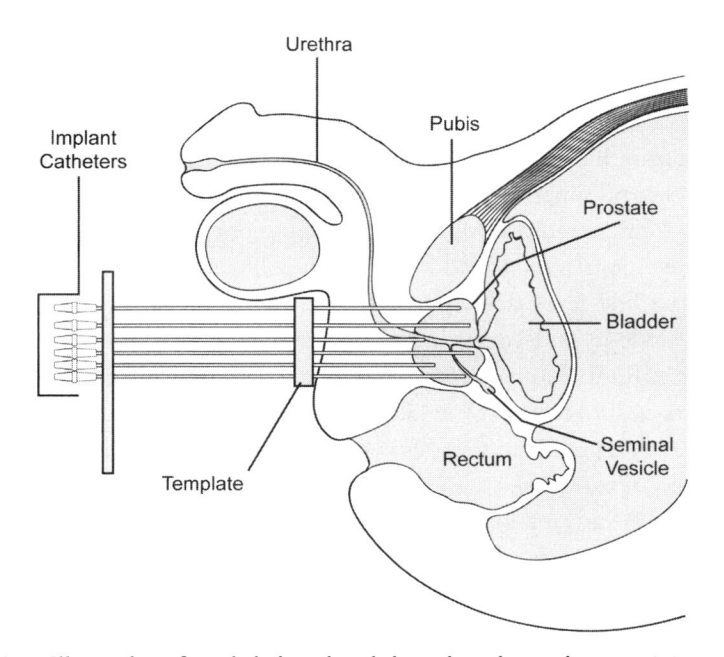

Figure 2 • : Illustration of seeds being placed through perineum into prostate.

less than one hour in the hospital for each of the radiation visits. It is important to remember that you will not be radioactive during your treatment, and close contact with other people is not a problem.

Brachytherapy is a same day procedure (enter and leave hospital on the same day). As with any operative procedure, before the brachytherapy is conducted, you will require preadmission testing, which will involve blood tests, a chest x-ray, and an EKG. Using general or spinal anesthesia, the patient is placed in stirrups, and an ultrasound probe is placed into the rectum and used to take images of the prostate and help guide needles placed through the perineum (that area between the scrotum and the anus) and into the prostate. A special template is used to accurately guide needles into the prostate for the delivery of the seeds and help guide treatment planning. The prostate, urethra, and rectum are outlined on ultrasound images, and a specialized computer program is used in the operating room to achieve the best positioning of the seed. A special applicator is used to deposit anywhere from 80 to 100 seeds within the prostate gland. Once the seeds are placed, a CT scan will be performed to make sure that the seeds have been correctly placed and the radiation dose is appropriate.

It is important for you to speak to your radiation oncologist about radiation safety precautions once you are finished with your procedure. In contrast to external beam therapy, you will have active radiation inside your body, and precautions for other people, particularly children and pregnant women, are necessary for some months after the implant procedure. Fortunately, the radiation from the seeds does not travel very far. Therefore, to pass radiation onto another person, they need to be sitting close to you (almost in your lap, actually). You are radioactive for about nine months with iodine seeds and about three months for palladium seeds. It is likely that you will be advised to have the first few ejaculations after brachytherapy without a partner or using a condom, and you will be instructed how long your should avoid intercourse. Radiation has a profound damaging effect on the DNA within the sperm, and therefore, if you have a partner who may become pregnant, it is essential that protected sex occurs for a period of 6 to 12 months after the completion of radiation.

One of the advantages of seed implants is its convenience. Seeds can be implanted, and you can be home the same day and back on your feet and back to regular activities in a very short period of time. Generally patients do not need a catheter and most patients experience no pain other than mild discomfort in their perineums, where the needles were placed for the placement of the seeds. If necessary, most patients will require only acetaminophen (Tylenol) or ibuprofen (Motrin, Advil). The seeds are permanent and are not removed at a later date.

III. Side Effects of Radiation

During external beam radiation, it is not uncommon for some patients to complain of reduced energy level and general fatigue. While the majority of patients have no such problems, some patients are bothered by this. The major complaints that occur after radiation therapy are urinary problems, bowel problems, and sexual problems.

Basically, radiation causes inflammation changes in tissues. Inflammation in the prostate, urethra, and bladder cause irritation-like symptoms during radiation therapy in the majority of patients, such as frequent urination, getting up at night to urinate, and mild burning upon urination. These symptoms typically reduce or resolve over time after treatment. Long-term changes in the bladder may result in a condition known as radiation cystitis, which is caused by fragile blood vessels in the bladder wall which may tear and you may see blood in the urine (hematuria) on occasion. It is often not dangerous and does not require treatment. Some side effects such as erection problems occur in a very delayed way, between one and three years after the completion of radiation. Significant blood loss requiring transfusion is rare, occurring in less than 1% of patients. The use of IMRT dramatically reduces the risk of serious urinary side effects due to radiation to the bladder.

As you can imagine, the placement of needles into the prostate and delivery of the seeds itself, never mind the radiation, result in swelling of the prostate. This can lead to symptoms such as frequent urination and urgency to urinate. While uncommon, about 5% of men experience urinary retention where they are completely unable to pass urine. In this case, they will need catheters in their bladders until the swelling subsides. This is most often seen in men with large prostate glands and sometimes it is recommended to take a short course of hormone therapy to reduce the prostate size before implantation. Many patients are placed on alpha-blocking drugs such as terazosin (Hytrin), doxazosin (Cardura), tamsulosin (Flomax), and alfuzosin (Uroxatral) after brachytherapy to try to minimize the risk of acute urinary retention and try to maximize urinary flow.

Because the rectum is close to the prostate and because radiation is typically delivered to the prostate and a 1cm margin around the prostate, the rectal wall immediately behind the prostate may be included in the radiation field. Modern approaches using IMRT and ultra-precise placement of brachytherapy seeds have minimized these problems. However, some men experience radiation injury to the rectum, which is known as radiation proctitis. During radiation, this can cause bowel movement changes and a pressure-like sensation with urgency to defecate without there being stool present in the rectum (a condition known as tenesmus). Rarely, diarrhea may develop. Similar to changes seen in the bladder, new blood vessels can form in the rectal wall which may bleed with trauma, such as straining during a bowel movement. Often, this is simply results in spotting of blood on the toilet tissue (just like hemorrhoids) but can be more significant. It is estimated that the incidence of bowel problems with 3D-CRT is around 15% and this drops down to less than 5% with IMRT.

Radiation therapy results in reduced ejaculate volume as the function of the prostate and seminal vesicles is to produce ejaculatory fluid and, in most men, will result in loss of ejaculation completely. Despite this change, normal orgasmic sensation is still possible. If fertility is of concern to you, then you should bank sperm before your radiation treatments just as you would before surgery. Radiation therapy can cause painful ejaculation, although less often than surgery. The exact cause of this is not clear, but it appears that it may be related to spasm in the muscles at the level of the bladder neck or the pelvic floor. Research that I have conducted has also shown that this condition is sensitive to the alpha-blocking drugs listed above. This research has shown that 68% of men have significant reduction in their ejaculatory pain with the use of tamsulosin (Flomax).

IV. Erectile Function Outcomes after Radiation (Tables 1 and 2)

As previously discussed, the erection nerves are pasted onto the surface of the prostate, and even with the most precise delivery of radiation, some of this radiation will get to the erection nerves. Furthermore, the back portion of the penis (the part that is housed inside the body) sits at a distance of no more than 1 to 2 cm below the prostate. My research has shown that with 3D-CRT, up to 40% of the radiation dose is actually delivered to the back one inch of the penis. Further research has also shown that the dose delivered to the penis is reduced by 40% when IMRT is used. While there is no data at this time comparing erectile function recovery with 3D-CRT and

Table 1 • **Incidence Of Erectile Dysfunction After External Beam Radiation Therapy (Adapted from Incrocci)**

Author	Year	Number of patients	Average age (years)	Potent prior to radiation therapy (%)	Average Total dose (Gy)	Average follow-up (months)	Incidence of erectile problems
Bown	2007	32	68	NR	NR	37	75%*
Chen	2001	144	NR	NR	70	21	42% @ 1 year
Wilder	2000	51	68	69	74	15	37% @ 3 years
Johnstone	2000	46	80	NR	67	167	76%
Fransson	1999	83	73	NR	65	96	65% @ 8 years
Zelefsky	1999	743	69	73	NR	42	39%
Turner	1999	290	69	182	66	23	59% @ 3 years
Nguyen	1998	101	NR	81	NR	24	49%
Borghede	1997	290	69	182	66	23	59% @ 3 years
Beard	1997	121	NR	69	NR	NR	64% @ 1 year
Fossa	1997	114	69	22	NR	NR	61%

* SHIM >21
NR: not reported

IMRT, I believe it is likely that we will see in the future that IMRT results in lower erectile dysfunction rates than 3D-CRT.

Interestingly, radiation therapy causes erectile dysfunction in an identical way to that of surgery. Remember that surgery causes problems with the erection nerves, that there is a possibility for artery damage, and that erection tissue can degenerate in response to nerve injury and in response to the absence of erection after surgery. In radiation therapy, the radiation damages the erection nerve. It is delivered to erection tissue and one of the primary ways that radiation causes side effects is by damaging blood vessels. Indeed,

Table 2 • Incidence Of Erectile Dysfunction After Seed Implantation

Author	Year	Seed type	External beam also	Number of patients	Average age	Patients potent prior to seeds	Average radiation dose	Average follow-up (months)	Incidence of Erectile Problems
Cesaretti	2007	I	No	233	66	59%	NR	96	42%*
Potters	2001	I	Yes	482	NR	NR	NR	34	47% @ 5 years
Zelefsky	2000	I	No	248	65	89	160	48	29%
Sharkey	2000	Pd	No	299	73	NR	NR	NR	15%
Sanchez-Ortiz	2000	I	No	114	69	81	115	23	51%
Kesrin	2000	Ir	Yes	161	69	NR	NR	34	29%
Joly	1998	Ir	Yes	71	68	NR	NR	NR	89%

* SHIM score of >16
I: iodine; Ir: Iridium; PD: Palladium
NR: not reported

the radiation has a damaging effect on the endothelium (the lining of the blood vessels), and much of the toxicity associated with radiation is related to endothelial dysfunction. What is very interesting is that the amount of radiation required to cause endothelial damage is tiny, ranging from 0.1 to 1 Gy. It is estimated between 15 to 20 Gy is required to injure large blood vessels (when given in a single dose). This damage to blood vessels is known as endarteritis obliterans and may take up to a decade to manifest itself maximally. It is likely that radiation injury to the nerves is not the most important factor in the development of erection problems. I say this because we know that many patients in the first three years after radiation respond very well to Viagra, Levitra, and Cialis, which would imply that the erection nerves are functional.

The average time for a man to develop erectile problems after radiation is approximately one year. This will depend to a large extent on his baseline erectile function as well as his age at the time of radiation and other factors affecting erectile function, just as it does with surgery. However, we do see men presenting with erectile dysfunction very early after radiation, from three to six months after it finishes. This is likely to be due not to nerve injury or to blood vessel injury but to the erection tissue damage. We talked previously about the concept of the penis being like a tire with a hose (in fact there are two hoses) and a valve. When the valve is leaky, the patient has a condition known as venous leak. Erection tissue damage leads to venous leak and my research has shown that men who have erection problems early after surgery frequently have venous leak. The problem with venous leak is that it is irreversible and means most men will not have recovery of their own erections and will struggle to respond well to Viagra-like pills.

I see many patients who have not yet been treated for their prostate cancer who are wondering if they should have radiation or surgery. I tell all of them the same thing: "You should never base your decision on surgery versus radiation on sexual function outcomes." The reason for this is that, in the current literature, the incidence of erectile dysfunction after three years after radiation versus the incidence of erectile dysfunction three years after surgery appears to be approximately the same. It is important to understand that the literature is not comparative, meaning that there is no study that has directly compared radiation to surgery. So, in the absence of comparative studies, drawing conclusions as to which treatment has the lower incidence of sexual side effects is impossible.

As with the surgery literature, there are significant flaws in the radiation literature as it pertains to erectile function outcomes. The most glaring of these deficiencies is that is it common for radiation oncologists to talk about erectile function rates 12 months after radiation. I have already alluded to the idea that the peak negative erection effects of radiation occur probably three to five years after the completion of radiation. Any study looking at erectile function outcomes should really assess these outcomes at no sooner than 24 months, if not 36 months, after the completion of radiation.

In Tables 1 and 2, you will see a list of erectile dysfunction rates after radiation treatment with both external beam and brachytherapy. You will see a wide variation in the number of patients studied, the duration of follow-up, and the incidence of erectile dysfunction after treatment. As with surgery, a man's erectile function level before radiation treatment and his age are significant predictors of whether he will develop erection problems after radiation treatment. Besides these two factors, of course, the dose of the radiation and the modality of delivery of the radiation are critical components in deciding whether a man will have erection problems after treatment or not. As with surgery, choosing an expert in the field of radiation oncology is important to minimizing any side effects, particularly erectile dysfunction.

I frequently hear from patients that they were told that erectile dysfunction is not a significant concern after radiation and this is a grossly untrue statement (and unfair to the patient). I am a great believer in realistic expectations for a patient and that patients should be allowed to make informed decisions about the right option for them. Without having an honest, fair and balanced discussion regarding the side effects of radiation or surgery, then the patient is at a disadvantage in his effort to make a truly informed decision. Erectile function preservation after radiation therapy is a novel concept and is discussed in detail in Chapter 7.

CHAPTER 6

THE EFFECT OF HORMONE THERAPY ON SEXUAL FUNCTION

> I. What Is Androgen Deprivation Therapy?
> II. Side Effects of Hormone Therapy
> III. The Effect of Hormone Therapy on Sexual Function

I. What Is Androgen Deprivation Therapy?

In general hormone therapy, also known as androgen deprivation or ablation, is used in at least three scenarios with prostate cancer patients including in combination with radiation therapy for the primary treatment of prostate cancer, in patients who have very high-risk disease (those who, on prostate exam or CT/MRI, have disease spread outside of the prostate and have very high Gleason scores, such as 9 or 10), and for men with PSA or cancer recurrence outside of the prostate after surgery or radiation.

In combination with radiation, androgen deprivation therapy (let's call it ADT) results in higher survival rates for large cancers or for high-grade cancers. In most cases, ADT is started several months prior to the commencement of radiation and continues until the last day of radiation treatment. In patients with more aggressive prostate cancer, hormones may be continued for up to two to three years to get the best results. Men who present with prostate cancer, whose prostate biopsy shows large tumors, and who have

Gleason scores of 9 or 10, are often considered candidates for early hormone therapy since the risk of them having extra-prostatic disease and metastatic disease is far greater than for men with Gleason scores of 6 or 7.

ADT is the process where physicians either surgically or chemically prevent testosterone from being produced. Historically, the approach to androgen deprivation was to remove both testicles, an operation known as orchiectomy. In fact, in the 1940s, Charles Huggins, a urologist at the University of Chicago, showed that the use of orchiectomy in men with metastatic prostate cancer dramatically changed the biology of the prostate cancer and resulted in regression of the cancer. He is one of only two urologists who have won the Nobel Prize for their research.

The advantage of orchiectomy is that it is a very simple and significantly less expensive treatment than the use of prolonged medication for androgen deprivation. Of note, the side effects of ADT, whether surgical or chemical, are nearly identical. On the downside, for more men, there is a significant psychological burden associated with having one's testicles removed, although if a man wishes to retain the normal appearance of the scrotum, he may ask the surgeon to place prosthetic (silicone) testicles into the scrotum at the time of the orchiectomy.

A more modern approach to ADT is using medications to achieve the same goal. This is sometimes referred to as chemical castration. Remember, as I previously mentioned, testosterone is produced predominantly by the testicles (95%), while 5% comes from the adrenal glands. Therefore, there are two approaches to reducing testosterone levels in men with prostate cancer. As previously mentioned, one is to perform an orchiectomy and the other is to block the hormones that come from the brain which stimulate the production of testosterone. Testosterone is produced in the testicle by cells known as Leydig cells inside the testicle. Leydig cells' production of testosterone is controlled by a hormone that comes from the brain (pituitary gland), called luteinizing hormone (LH). LH is further stimulated by another hormone known as luteinizing hormone releasing hormone (LHRH). If we can block the production of luteinizing hormone, then this will, in effect, starve the Leydig cells of the stimulus needed for the production of testosterone and the testosterone level drops dramatically. With chemical or surgical castration, testosterone levels will never drop to zero as the adrenal glands continue to produce some level of testosterone (Figure 1).

One of the advantages of medication-induced ADT is that it may be reversible, as long as the duration of ADT is short (maybe less than 6

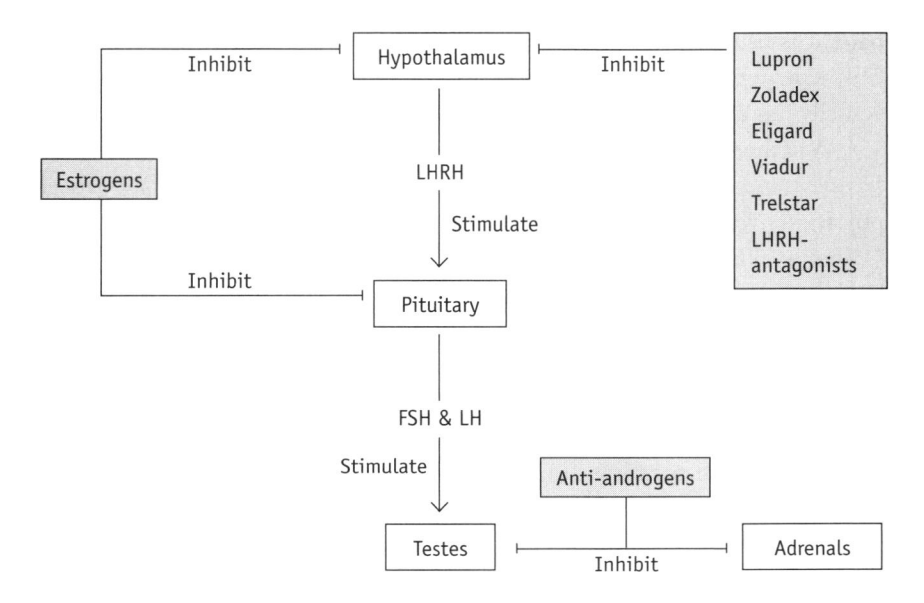

THE EFFECT OF HORMONE THERAPY ON SEXUAL FUNCTION

Figure 1 • Diagram demonstrating the means by which hormone therapy affects testosterone production and function.

months). If a man is on hormone therapy for a short period of time, then it is likely that he will have recovery of his testosterone production after he stops the medication. The disadvantage is that it is expensive and it does require injections of medication periodically. There are a number of LHRH stimulators (called agonists in the medical field) available at the moment, including Leuprolide (Lupron, Eligard, Viadur) and goserlin (Zoladex). These two medications can be administered as injections at different time intervals, depending on their strength: once a month, every three months, every four months, every six months (Eligard) or once a year (Viadur). They result in testosterone levels below 30 nanograms per ml compared to the normal testosterone level, which ranges significantly between 300 and 800 ng/ml.

A second class of drugs, known as anti-androgens, have been developed to block the effects of any remaining testosterone on cancer cells. Examples of anti-androgens include flutamide (Eulexin), bicalutamide (Casodex), and nilutamide (Nilandron). These can be taken in conjunction with LHRH agonists in a treatment known as total androgen blockade. Because LHRH agonists initially promote the production of LHRH, they actually may cause a short-lived increase in testosterone levels. This is known as testosterone flare. Therefore, in the initial two weeks of LHRH agonist therapy, the patient is usually prescribed an anti-androgen as well to limit this. Beyond this, it is unclear whether the addition of Eulexin, Casodex, or Nilandron actually has any further benefit to men when used long term.

Whether androgen deprivation therapy is used for you in your particular setting requires a detailed and honest discussion with your prostate cancer physician. My suggestion to you is that you ask your physician the question, "What are the benefits to the use of androgen deprivation for me?" If the benefits from androgen deprivation (improved survival, reduced failure after radiation therapy, improvement of symptoms due to metastases) outweigh the side effects and its negative impact on quality of life which you will experience, then, of course, there is a value. However, if the survival advantage is minimal, there may be an argument made to avoid ADT so that you can retain your current quality of life. It is important for those of you who have not yet had your prostatectomy to know that there is no evidence to demonstrate any benefit to the use of hormone therapy before surgery. It is not uncommon for me to see a man in my clinic who had prostate cancer diagnosed, opted for surgery, but wanted to go away on vacation for a period of time before having his operation. Because the surgery was postponed for, let's say, three months, the surgeon decided that the patient should have a shot of Lupron to prevent spread of the disease. This has no scientific basis whatsoever. The ability for most prostate cancers to increase in size occurs very slowly and, in the vast majority of cases, a three-month delay in surgery is not going to impact the cancer or cause it to spread outside of the prostate.

Whether ADT is used early on or later is another issue that needs to be discussed with the physician. If you had a prostatectomy and your PSA has started to increase, then there are arguments in favor of using hormone therapy immediately and arguments in favor of delaying it until the PSA rises to a significantly elevated level. The pros and cons of this argument are beyond the scope of this book and I encourage you to go to Dr. Peter Scardino's *Prostate Book* to get a better sense of the arguments. Likewise, there are some physicians who offer intermittent ADT. This is a treatment strategy where the testosterone-suppressing drugs are given until the PSA drops to an undetectable level. When it does, the medications are stopped and the PSA is monitored frequently. As the PSA rises to a certain predetermined level, ADT is restarted. It remains unclear exactly whether intermittent hormone therapy is as effective as continuous hormone therapy from a survival standpoint. However, when patients are off ADT, they frequently have improvement in the side effects that occur with ADT (see next section).

THE EFFECT OF HORMONE THERAPY ON SEXUAL FUNCTION

Table 1 • **Side effects of Hormone therapy**

- Hot flashes
- Decreased energy
- Decreased motivation
- Difficulty concentrating
- Loss of bone density
- Loss of libido
- Erection problems
- Problems with sugar control
- Weight gain
- Breast enlargement
- Anemia

When hormone therapy stops working, then the cancer is known as hormone refractory prostate cancer and treatments such as second-line hormone therapy, chemotherapy, and experimental vaccines may be used. These treatments are actively being studied in trials at this time (www.clinicaltrials.gov).

II. Side Effects of Hormone Therapy (Table 1)

Testosterone is a vitally important hormone for men and, indeed, for women. It is the primary libido hormone in men and women, and therefore, most menopausal women whose ovaries stop functioning have a significant (approximately 60%) drop in the testosterone levels in their blood. This is a contributor, but likely not the only cause, for postmenopausal women having lower libidos compared to premenopausal women.

Testosterone is vital for bone density, muscle integrity, body fat composition, motivation, energy, and sex drive. Some testosterone is also required for erectile function. ADT is associated with libido problems and erectile dysfunction, and we will talk about both of these in the next section. However, there are other side effects that are important to understand. Firstly, it is common for men using LHRH agonists, anti-androgens, or combination therapy to suffer hot flashes. This results from the dramatic reduction in testosterone levels and, essentially, men experience hot flashes identical to those of women going through during menopause (change of life). These can range from mildly annoying to debilitating in their severity.

Withdrawal of testosterone to the level that occurs with ADT results in loss of muscle mass and deposition of fat, and men tend not to respond as rapidly to working out as they did when their testosterone levels were normal. It is not uncommon for men to experience enlargement of their breasts (gynecomastia), sometimes associated with tenderness. They may also experience a drop in their red blood cell counts, leading to anemia and changes in cognitive function (memory, concentration) and motivation. It is not uncommon for me to see a man on two years of ADT who has some reduction in his memory and general life motivation. As previously stated, it is important that you and your physician balance the benefits versus the risks of androgen deprivation to decide if this form of treatment is right for you.

Dr. Peter Scardino in his book states that he "recommends a cautious approach to hormone therapy for metastatic prostate cancer." While it can be comforting to have your PSA fall dramatically or become undetectable, the relevant issue is what is really happening to your cancer and how you can enjoy the best quality of life for as long as possible. This is an excellent philosophy and one to which I subscribe. I discuss this with my patients when I see them.

One of the most concerning side effects of androgen deprivation is osteoporosis, the softening of the bones. The step that precedes osteoporosis, known as osteopenia, is common in men on ADT and both of these increase the risk of hip fracture as well as vertebral compression fractures, which result in loss of height.

While on ADT, it is recommended that a man have a bone density test every one to two years and to continue this as long as his testosterone level has not returned to normal. I recommend that all men undergoing hormone therapy have a baseline bone density test (also known as bone densitometry or DEXA scan) to define what the pretreatment bone status is. Bone density assessment simply involves having an X-ray and, unlike the bone scan, which is used to detect metastatic prostate cancer, does not require administration of any radioactive agent. A bone density test simply assesses the quality and density of the minerals within the bones of the hip, the forearm, and the lumbar spine. For men who have baseline osteopenia or osteoporosis, or who develop bone loss while on ADT, there are a number of options, including drugs (known as bisphosphonates) such as Fosamax, Actonel, Forteo, and

Boniva. Some lifestyle modifications may also help in the prevention of loss of bone density, including exercise, good diet with calcium intake, avoidance of cigarette smoking, and, if you are white, making sure you have some sun exposure (as this produces Vitamin D in our bodies). Finally, it is my recommendation that all men undergoing ADT have a early morning total testosterone levels checked prior to starting ADT and to have testosterone levels repeated every three months once ADT is stopped until their testosterone levels returns to normal.

III. The Effect of Hormone Therapy on Sexual Function

ADT results in reduced libido, reduction in erectile function, and loss of ejaculation. If the patient has had a radical prostatectomy or if he is more than three to five years after radiation therapy, he is unlikely to be ejaculating anyway, but for patients who are pre-radiation and for patients who have not been exposed to surgery or radiation, ADT will result in the failure to produce any semen. Testosterone is required for the production of semen and when there is a very low level of testosterone, very little or no semen can be produced. However, this is not the same as loss of orgasm, although it is my experience that more men on ADT struggle to have an orgasm compared to men not using ADT.

Testosterone is the primary libido hormone and reduction of testosterone to the levels that occur with orchiectomy or the medications listed above results in dramatic loss of libido for the vast majority of men. We ask patients to grade their libido on a 10–point scale, where 0 is no interest in sex and 10 is the same level of libido that they had at 18 years of age. Most men in their 60s not using ADT say that their libido ranges somewhere between 5 and 7. Most men on ADT (approximately 90% in my practice) have libido levels of 0 to 2 on that scale. Surprisingly, there is a small group of men (approximately 10%) who continue to have significant libido and, when questioned, these are typically men who have always had high levels of libido in their lives. They appear to be constitutionally sexual and even though there is no testosterone, they retain some of this libido.

For the man who has had significant reduction in his libido due to low testosterone, there are relatively few options for him to improve his libido. Interestingly, men on ADT are very similar in their sexuality to women who are postmenopausal. The state in which most postmenopausal women exist is called sexual neutrality, and this is what men on androgen deprivation generally experience. That is, they rarely think about having sexual activity, but when they have sex they actually enjoy it.

There are two strategies that I use in my practice to try to improve sexual activity frequency in men who are on ADT. The first is intellectualization, where the couple will need to keep an eye on the calendar so that they can see how long it has been since they have had sex. The second approach is to encourage the partner to be more proactive in her or his initiating sexual relations. Particularly with postmenopausal women, who tend to have very low levels of sexual assertion, I make an effort to encourage them to increase this assertive behavior in an effort to increase sexual activity frequency. Now you may ask, "Why is continuing to have sex important?" For the couple who has previously been sexually active, such a hiatus from activity can introduce yet another stressor into the relationship. Furthermore, sexual activity may be the only cardiovascular exercise that a man obtains and continued sexual intercourse will help keep the vagina healthy, which in turn may reduce urinary tract infections for women.

The amount of testosterone that is required for normal erectile function is not well known. As I previously mentioned, the normal testosterone level ranges between 300 and 800 ng/ml. However, it is extremely likely that levels below 300 are more than adequate for normal erectile function. Those levels may not be adequate for normal libido. However, when testosterone levels drop below 100, and certainly at the levels that occur with ADT, there are significant negative effects on erectile tissue.

Remember, erectile tissue is a complex mixture of muscle, elastic fibers, as well as tissue known as endothelium, which lines the erection spaces itself. It is well documented that withdrawal of testosterone through castration in a rat results in profound structural changes to the erection tissue. The erection tissue, in fact, undergoes scarring, as well as fat deposition within the erection chamber. Once this smooth muscle content decreases to be replaced by scar or fat, then erectile function is dramatically reduced. In a rat, it takes no more than seven days after castration to see these negative effects. Seven days in a rat approximates to six months in a human. Thus, for men who are on androgen deprivation for longer than six to twelve months, there is significant risk for irreversible structural damage to erectile tissue. I will say this once again: this information is in no way designed to encourage you to avoid ADT. If this therapy is appropriate for you and results in improved survival, then I think that this is a risk that you should consider taking.

As mentioned in Chapter 1, once erection tissue undergoes degeneration, then it is irreversibly damaged and this leads to venous leak, where the valve inside the erection chambers no longer functions properly and blood leaks out of the erection spaces back into the veins of the pelvis. Most men with venous leak will not recover their natural erections and will struggle to be Viagra, Levitra or Cialis responders. These patients will most likely require either penile injection therapy for the rest of their lives or penile implant surgery. There are men who are more at risk for having these changes: older men and men with small testicles before treatment. There are no studies in humans looking at ways to prevent these structural changes related to hormone therapy. However, in an animal model in my laboratory, we have shown that the regular use of Viagra in a rat that has been castrated reduces the amount of damage to the erection tissue.

Whether this approach is useful in humans at this time is not known. Therefore, when patients are being placed on hormone therapy in my practice, we start low-dose Viagra, Levitra, or Cialis in the weeks leading up to the initiation of ADT and for at least as long as the patient is on ADT. Indeed, I recommend that patients continue to use the low-dose Viagra therapy for as long as the testosterone level remains abnormal. Saying this, a large, randomized study is needed to answer this question and is awaited.

This is a nice segue into a discussion about testosterone recovery after cessation of ADT. Eighty-five percent of these men on ADT for four to six months, will have normalized their testosterone levels by 12 months after stopping the medication. This, however, means that 15% do not have normal testosterone levels by this time. This indicates that, in some men, the recovery of testosterone after stopping these medications is very slow and, indeed, a small number of men never return to normal testosterone levels. The older the man is and/or the smaller his testicles are at the time of starting the medication, the less likely he is to have recovery of a normal testosterone level. Thus, a four- to six-month treatment phase with an LHRH agonist may result in a life-long reduction in testosterone level. We await a trial looking at the use of PDE5 inhibitors in men on ADT.

CHAPTER 7

PENILE REHABILITATION AND PRESERVATION

> I. Introduction
> II. What is Penile Rehabilitation?
> III. Structure of the Penile Rehabilitation Program
> IV. Other Strategies for Rehabilitation

I. Introduction

I previously mentioned the way erectile dysfunction (ED) occurs after radical prostatectomy and radiation therapy. ED after both surgery and radiation is common. In 1997, Francesco Montorsi MD from Milan presented and published evidence that the early use of penile injection therapy after radical prostatectomy to promote erections may, in fact, improve long-term erectile function recovery. He studied a very small number of patients (only 30); divided into two groups, where one group received penile injection three times a week and the other group received no treatment. He showed that the patients who were receiving injections were three times more likely to recover erectile function between six and twelve months after surgery. This finding was the start of the concept of penile rehabilitation. These days, using only 30 patients in any study would not be acceptable, but in his data, there is a clear suggestion that

Table 1 • **Recovery of erectile function in men using penile rehabilitation compared to men who did not use rehabilitation. (Adapted from Mulhall, et. al.)**

	Rehabilitation group	No-rehabilitation group
Patients with functional erections without medication	52%	19%
Patients responding to Viagra	64%	24%
Patients responding to penile injections	95%	76%

there is a benefit to getting erections early after surgery. This should not be at all surprising given the fact that the average man, prior to surgery, experiences three to six erections every night of his life (approximately 70% rigidity and 10 to 15 minutes in duration). It is believed that these nocturnal erections are to protect erectile tissue during periods of sexual abstinence.

In 2005, I published data from Dr. Robert Flanigan's database at Loyola University in Chicago (where I was formerly a faculty member), which was based on patients being instructed to obtain three erections per week (with or without a partner) after surgery, as part of a rehabilitation program (Figure 1). While this was not a randomized trial (patients were not randomly assigned to a treatment group or a no-treatment group), it studied a large number of men, some of whom did the rehabilitation protocol and others who did not. All were followed about every four months for at least 18 months after surgery. 58 patients did rehabilitation and 74 patients received no rehabilitation by their own choice. Interestingly, while penile injection therapy was the most commonly used means of obtaining erections, there were some patients who responded to Viagra (as this was the only medication available at that time), although the number of responders was small. The rehabilitation group had higher rates of recovery of natural erections, 52% versus 19% in the no-rehabilitation group. They had a higher rate of response to Viagra, 64% versus 24% in the no-rehabilitation group, and, interestingly, also had a higher rate of response to penile injections, 95% versus 76% in the no-rehabilitation group. Again, even though this is a non-randomized control trial, there is evidence in this paper that there is a benefit to early erections post-prostatectomy.

I previously mentioned that men develop erectile tissue damage with time after radical prostatectomy. I also discussed how the old approach to the treatment of erectile dysfunction after radical prostatectomy has been to allow men to go 12 months or more using Viagra only for sexual relations and to talk about penile injections or other treatments only after 12 months postoperatively. This exposes the patient to the risk of erection tissue damage. Even when there is complete nerve recovery, if the erectile tissue is damaged, it will be unresponsive to the nerves, and therefore, the patient will have permanent erectile dysfunction. The means by which erectile dysfunction occurs after radical prostatectomy, including nerve injury, artery injury, and erection tissue damage, are the same mechanisms by which radiation therapy to the prostate causes erectile dysfunction, albeit these factors are weighted slightly differently (nerve injury being the biggest factor in surgery, and blood vessel damage and erectile tissue damage being the most significant causes in the radiation patient). However, given the similarities between surgery and radiation in the development of erectile dysfunction, recently a lot of interest has been generated in the concept of penile rehabilitation in the radiation patient. It is probably more appropriately termed penile preservation because in contrast to patients post-prostatectomy who routinely have problems in the early months, most men in the first year after radiation have few erectile problems, and so we are really trying to preserve the erectile function rather than rehabilitate the tissue. There is currently no data on post-radiation therapy penile preservation strategies, although there are trials in progress, one of which is being conducted by Dr. Michael Zelefsky and me at Memorial Sloan-Kettering Cancer Center.

II. What is Penile Rehabilitation?

This concept simply revolves around the idea that we give men medications to give them erections, to protect erectile tissue (which is predominantly a muscle), to maximize the ability of the patient to recover his preoperative erectile function (if the patient has had radical prostatectomy), or if the patient has had radiation therapy, to maximize the chances of him preserving his pretreatment erectile function. It is important for patients to understand that any treatment we institute is aimed at getting the patient off treatment. For example, when we suggest penile injections to men, we tell them that the idea behind us putting them on injections is to maximize the chances of getting them off injections and onto pills, and then, hopefully, off pills and onto nothing.

Secondly, recovery of erectile function after prostatectomy is approximately 18 to 24 months after surgery (Figure 1). Yes, there are men who have

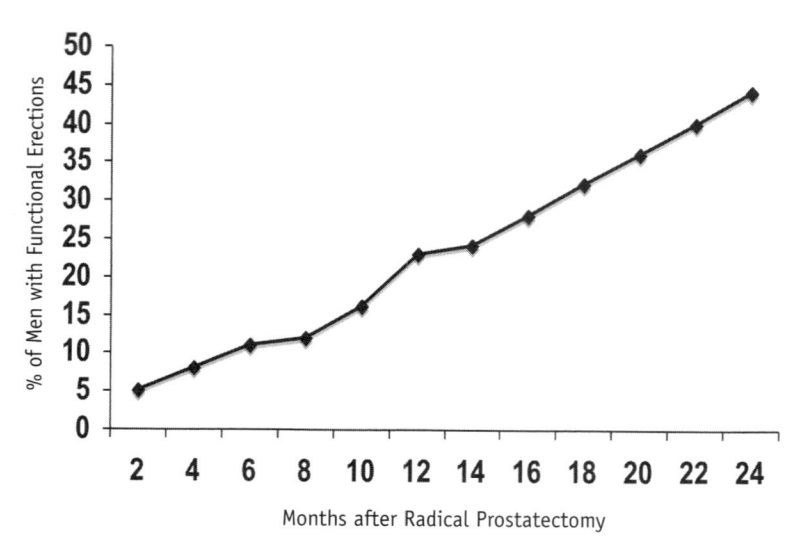

Figure 1 • Diagram showing the continued recovery of erectile function after radical prostatectomy up to 24 months after surgery

fully functional erections at six months, but if you look at the general prostatectomy population, the vast majority of men experience erectile function recovery in the second year and many between 18 and 24 months postoperatively. This is important because many patients, if not given these realistic expectations, between six and 12 months will get significantly depressed because of failure of erections to recover.

Thirdly, the longer a man goes after surgery without erections, the more likely he is to suffer permanent erectile tissue damage. The damaged is called "atrophy," but, in fact, it is scarring of the erectile tissue, and if the erectile tissue scars, the patient will never get his own erection back and will always struggle to respond to a medication. There is evidence to suggest that the incidence of erectile tissue damage, as measured by the presence of venous leak (remember the leaky valve I have previously discussed), is very uncommon before the fourth month after surgery. However, at eight months after surgery, it occurs in approximately 30% of men, and at one year, 50% of men have permanent erectile tissue damage. It is believed that this damage results from two main factors: erection nerve injury and the absence of blood (and therefore oxygen) getting into the penis. This is the "if you don't use it you lose it" phenomenon. The aim of penile rehabilitation is to keep the erectile tissue healthy while we are waiting for the nerves to recover from the trauma of surgery.

Finally, rehabilitation in the current era involves two approaches used side-by-side. The first and probably more important of the two approaches is that the patient should be getting erections. I mentioned before that the average man gets three to six erections every night of his life and this is not the case after radical prostatectomy because of nerve injury. We encourage men to get erections two to three times per week (in our practice, this is defined as a penetration hardness of 6/10 on the hardness scale). This erection does NOT have to be combined with orgasm or even sexual intercourse. The erections bring blood and oxygen into the erectile bodies, thus protecting erectile tissue. If a patient gets a good rigid erection in response to a Viagra-like mediation in the first few months, he continues to use this for the two to three erections a week. It is worth noting that, in my experience, only 15% of our patients respond to these pills in the early stages after surgery. If the patient fails to respond to one of the PDE5 inhibitors (Viagra, Levitra, Cialis), then I suggest to the patient as early as four weeks after surgery that he moves on and does penile injections.

The second strategy, which is a newer approach, is the use of regular PDE5 inhibitors in low dose on the non-erection days. I encourage my patients to use either Viagra or Levitra going to bed at night in low dose, 25 or 50 mg of Viagra, or 5 or 10 mg of Levitra. We encourage our patients to split the Viagra 100 mg pills in four and the Levitra 20 mg pills in two or four if the patient can manage that (the Levitra pill is very tiny). If the patient is using penile injections regularly (as I suggest patients do), I avoid using Cialis in this penile rehabilitation strategy as the medication lasts a long time (up to five days) in the blood. This means men will likely have Cialis in their blood at the time of a penile injection, thus increasing the risk of a prolonged erection occurring if an injection is used.

With regard to penile preservation in post-prostate radiation, I apply the same concepts, although there is no human evidence to prove this at this time. I encourage patients to obtain erections on a regular basis in the early stages after radiation, and we also encourage them to use low-dose Viagra or Levitra when going to bed every night for the first 12 months after the completion of radiation. This is an identical time frame to that for the radical prostatectomy patients. We encourage patients to get two to three erections a week because the data that is published suggests this frequency has some benefits. However, it is unknown to us whether one erection every two weeks or five erections every week is better for erectile tissue health. Most patients post-radiation who have good function before radiation do not need to use a Viagra-like medication in the first year after radiation, although the frequency with which they will need to use PDE5 inhibitors increases in the following three years.

III. Structure of the Penile Rehabilitation Program

While I am urologist, I do not perform prostatectomies nor do I coordinate radiation therapy, so my entire focus is a man's (and in turn a couple's) sexual and reproductive health. My role in the care of patients with prostate cancer who have undergone or are about to undergo treatment is to educate them about the potential consequences, to give them realistic expectations, to inform them of strategies they can use to minimize the negative effects of treatment on their sexual function and to treat them effectively when they experience sexual problems.

While I like to see patients before their surgery, less than 10% of our patients ever come in for a discussion prior to their operations. The patients most likely to come to see me before surgery are the younger ones as well as those most concerned about their sexual function. There are likely two main reasons why a minority of patients see me preoperatively. Firstly, the physician is focused on the treatment and curing the cancer, so little focus is aimed at the sexual consequences of surgery or radiation. Secondly, the patient's stress level is usually high due to coping with the cancer, and his focus is generally not sexual function. The people who are most likely to see me before treatment are young patients and patients with a high frequency of sexual intercourse, for whom sexual intercourse is usually important.

When a patient does come in prior to his operation, we currently treat him with a low-dose PDE5 inhibitor for the two weeks prior to the radical prostatectomy. This is a novel concept called endothelial preconditioning, whereby the endothelium (which is the lining of the erection spaces) is in some way protected by pre-treatment. There is evidence from animal studies in my laboratory to support this idea.

However, most patients that I see come to see me after their surgeries. I like to see them as soon as possible after the operation, which usually means four to six weeks after the operation. The patient will get a prescription for a PDE5 inhibitor the day the catheter comes out, which is usually one to two weeks after surgery, and he is told that over the following four weeks, before he sees me in clinic, to do two things. Firstly, on one occasion per week, he is told to take a full dose of a pill (Viagra 100mg or Levitra 20mg) with stimulation to see if he obtains a good erection or not (6/10 on the hardness scale or better). Secondly, on the other six nights he is told to take a low-dose pill (Viagra 50mg or 25mg, or Levitra 10mg or 5mg) just before going to bed at night, just like one would take a vitamin. If he prefers to use Cialis, then I tell him to take a half dose (10mg) twice a week (let's say Monday and Wednesday) and then take a full dose once a week (let's say Friday) with sexual stimulation. This regimen is probably equivalent to the Viagra/Levitra approach outlined above.

The patient is encouraged to come to see me in the office four to six weeks postoperatively. However, some men fail to come in for more than a year. These men are often those most anxious about their PSA and cancer recurrence or those that have severe incontinence after surgery, situations where sex is not the most important thing on their minds. The problem for these men, as I have stated before, is that the longer a man goes after surgery without erections, the more likely he is to experience permanent damage to his erectile tissue. The same is almost certainly true for radiation patients also. At six weeks after surgery, if the patient has not responded to a full-dose pill with a penetration-hardness erection (6/10), then we tell him that he will need to consider using penile injections to get erections. It is likely in the future that we will be treating men with these low-dose PDE5 inhibitor medications sooner after surgery, maybe even the day of the operation, but historically we have avoided giving these pills to men when they have a catheter in place (Figure 2).

There is much controversy regarding the role of regular pill use in penile rehabilitation. There is a recent suggestion from Dr. Montorsi in Milan that there is no difference in recovery of erections between men who have used Viagra on a daily basis versus those who have used it as required for sexual relations. While the study has some limitations, it does suggest that perhaps daily dosing is not required. Indeed, we know that the effects of medications on the endothelium like Viagra and Cialis are long lasting, well beyond the presence of the medication in the blood. Therefore, it is unlikely that the medications have to be used on a daily basis, although I believe that optimization of erectile tissue health is maximized by regular use of the medication. The concept of optimization I believe is important. Simply put, this is the difference between men being able to have sex without having rigid erections versus men being able to get the same level of hardness back after surgery

```
                    ┌─────────────────────────┐
                    │ Preoperative evaluation │
                    │     and counseling      │
                    └─────────────────────────┘
              ┌──────────────┴──────────────┐
   ┌──────────────────────┐      ┌──────────────────────┐
   │  PDE5i prescription  │      │  PDE5i prescription  │
   │ for 2 weeks before   │      │  at time of catheter │
   │       surgery        │      │       removal        │
   └──────────────────────┘      └──────────────────────┘
```

4 doses at maximum-dose PDE5i 2–4 weeks PLUS low-dose PDE5i on non-maximum-dose nights	4 doses at maximum-dose PDE5i for 2–4 weeks PLUS Low-dose PDE5i on non-maximum-dose nights

Patient seen at 6 weeks after surgery

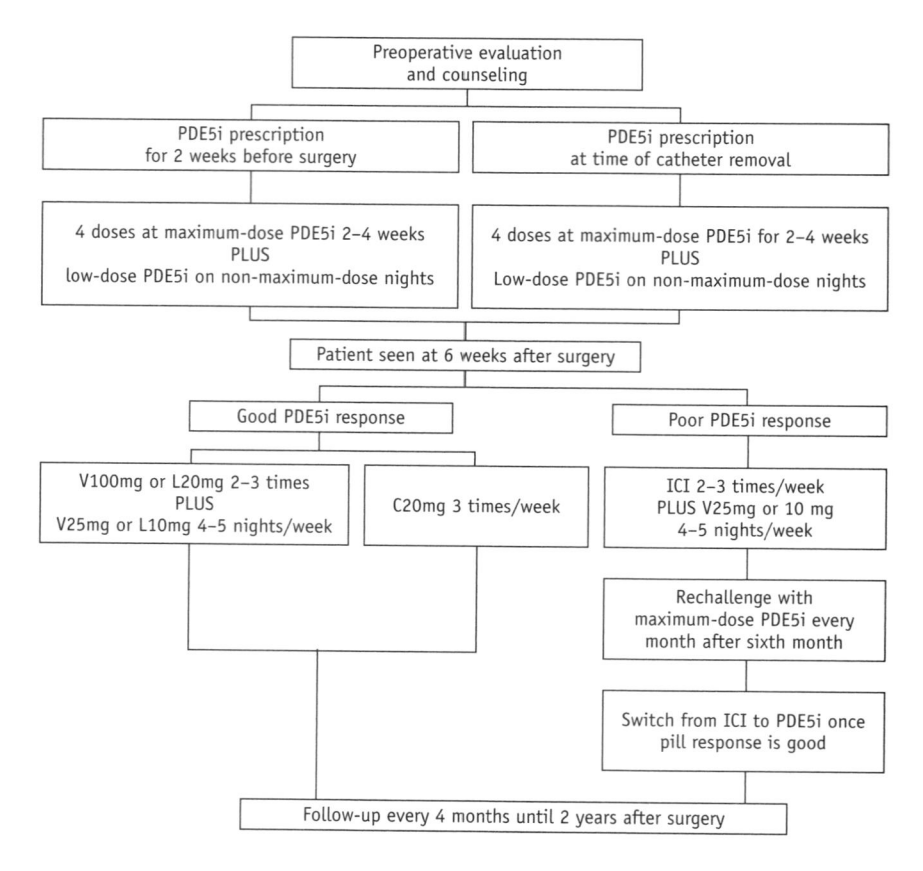

Good PDE5i response	Poor PDE5i response
V100mg or L20mg 2–3 times PLUS V25mg or L10mg 4–5 nights/week · C20mg 3 times/week	ICI 2–3 times/week PLUS V25mg or 10 mg 4–5 nights/week
	Rechallenge with maximum-dose PDE5i every month after sixth month
	Switch from ICI to PDE5i once pill response is good

Follow-up every 4 months until 2 years after surgery

Figure 2 • **Current treatment plan for penile rehabilitation after radical prostatectomy at Memorial Sloan-Kettering Cancer Center. V: Viagra; L: Levitra; C: Cialis; PDE5i: PDE5 inhibitors; ICI: penile injections.**

that they had before the operation.

There is great debate about this topic, and what many physicians (even urologists) and patients do not understand is that there is excellent animal and some interesting human data to support the use of these medications. There is evidence from rats with penis nerve injury that the use of Viagra, Levitra and Cialis (at doses that give the same blood levels that we see in humans) protects erectile tissue from degeneration and also protects the endothelium. There is also suggestion in one medical paper that Viagra used in animals that have had a stroke may help the nerves regenerate, although this has not been corroborated by other centers.

There are two human studies suggesting that there is a value to using

PDE5 inhibitors, both of which have studied Viagra. The first was conducted by Pfizer (the manufacturer of Viagra) and this was a randomized, controlled trial of men receiving placebo, 50 mg or 100 mg of Viagra nightly starting at one month after surgery and ending at 10 months after surgery. Thus, the patients were on treatment for nine months. The medication was stopped at 40 weeks after surgery, and eight weeks later, the patients had their natural erection function assessed. Forty-seven percent of the patients in the Viagra groups (no difference between 50 and 100 mg) versus only 4% of the patients in the placebo group had recovery of erectile function back at the level they experienced preoperatively. Now, if we look at the figures on the recovery of the same erection hardness after surgery that was present preoperatively, this figure is probably in the 10% to 15% range. So again, in this study, there is a sign that there is a value to a patient's regular use of PDE5 inhibitors.

The other piece of evidence is from a study that biopsied men's penes before surgery and six months after surgery. They studied the smooth muscle in the erectile tissue. This was a study involving two groups of patients, one receiving 50 mg daily and the other 100 mg daily, but there was no placebo group in this study. What the researchers were looking at was whether the use of Viagra over a six-month period protected the erectile tissue from degeneration. Much to everyone's surprise, the use of these medications at these doses preserved the amount of smooth muscle that was present in the biopsy specimen six months after surgery.

Even though the Pfizer study used 50 mg of Viagra as its lowest dose, I am comfortable with patients using 25 mg for two reasons. First of all, it is more cost effective and I would much prefer to see a patient use some dose of Viagra for the first twelve months rather than not be able to afford it after the sixth month after surgery. Secondly, there is excellent evidence in diabetics that blood vessel health (actually endothelial function) is improved when 25 mg of Viagra is used on a daily basis.

As previously stated, the approach for radiation is very similar, the difference being that most of these men (if they had good erections before radiation started) in the early stages after radiation are able to get their own erections or may have to use a small-dose pill to generate a good erection. However, besides these erections, we encourage patients to use low-dose Viagra or Levitra before going to bed at night or Cialis three times a week for the first 12 months after the completion of radiation. While we have no data currently, I believe that it is likely that we will see a significant benefit to this approach, very similar to the benefit that appears to be derived in the prostatectomy patients.

IV. Other Strategies for Rehabilitation

While penile rehabilitation currently revolves around men getting erections, whether it be a response to a pill or penile injection and the regular use of a PDE5 inhibitor nocturnally, there are two other approaches that have been employed and are currently under investigation. MUSE, as I will discuss in Chapter 13, is a suppository about the size of a grain of rice, which is placed into the urine channel approximately an inch from the tip of the penis. This is a pure prostaglandin erection medication and at maximum doses is associated with a significant likelihood of burning penile pain because of the hypersensitivity of the penile nerves to prostaglandin in the early stages after radical prostatectomy. However, there are a number of medical centers that are interested in using very low-dose MUSE, very much in the same way as we now use low-dose Viagra, before going to bed at night. Patients are given the lowest dose of MUSE (125 mcg) into the urethra either nightly or three times a week. There is a suggestion from some preliminary research that there is a benefit to this. If the patients tolerate 125 mcg, then the dose can be increased to 250 mcg, and if pain occurs then, the dose can be dropped back down to 125 mcg. The bottom line is that it is too early to answer whether MUSE is worthwhile or not, although in a year to two we tell have that answer.

Finally, there is a lot of interest in the use of a vacuum device for penile rehabilitation. I will discuss vacuum devices in Chapter 16 in more detail. There is currently no human or animal evidence to show that vacuum devices are of any benefit in the post-prostatectomy patient. However, there may indeed be an intrinsic value to penile stretching. Vacuum devices do not bring much fresh blood into the penis and, therefore, the oxygen content is not very high compared to what a pill- or injection-induced erection achieves. I suggest to patients that if they are truly interested in trying vacuum device therapy, that they use it in conjunction with our standard approach (low-dose pill and two to three erections a week), but I do not believe that patients should be using the vacuum device as a single therapy. It is likely that in the near future, we will have evidence to answer the question about the role of vacuum devices in prostatectomy and radiation patients, but at this time, it is lacking.

CHAPTER 8

MISCELLANEOUS SEXUAL PROBLEMS IN THE PROSTATE CANCER PATIENT

> I. Urine Leakage during Sex
> II. Changes in Orgasm
> III. Penile Length Changes
> IV. Penile Curvature
> V. Fertility Options

While erectile dysfunction has received most of the attention in the medical literature and the press, there are a number of other sexual problems that can occur after radical prostatectomy or radiation therapy. These include urine leakage during sex, orgasm problems, changes in penile length, curving of the penis, ejaculation problems, and fertility problems. Also men who have been exposed to hormone therapy may have permanent loss of libido.

I. Urine Leakage during Sex

Urine leakage can occur at two times during sex, the first being leakage during foreplay and the second being that which occurs at the time of orgasm. To understand the leakage during sex phenomenon, it is important to have an appreciation for how continence is achieved. In a normal healthy male, there are two sphincters. The inner sphincter is the bladder neck, that portion of the bladder that joins the urine channel at the level of the prostate. The second is the external sphincter and this is the muscle that we use to stop and start our urine stream. When this sphincter is contracted, we cannot urinate; when it is relaxed, we can urinate. The bladder neck typically closes at the time of orgasm. Semen is deposited into the urethra inside the prostate, and after pressure builds up, the external sphincter opens and muscles around the urethra contract rhythmically to force semen out of the penis. Because the bladder neck closes, the semen does not go back into the bladder. There are certain medical conditions and medications which cause paralysis of the bladder neck and result in retrograde ejaculation (semen traveling back into the bladder rather than out of the penis), the most well known being drugs used for benign enlargement of the prostate, such as terazosin, doxazosin, tamsulosin, and alfuzosin.

After radical prostatectomy, the external sphincter, at least in the early stages after surgery, does not function properly. It fails to contract efficiently and, therefore, most men have some degree of incontinence early on after surgery. This incontinence is called stress incontinence, as it is most likely to occur when a man increases his abdominal pressure, for example, when he stands up, coughs or sneezes. The degree of incontinence and the duration of this incontinence are tremendously variable from patient to patient and it may take up to 12 months to fully resolve. Therefore, something in the range of 2% of men will have permanent significant incontinence after radical prostatectomy surgery.

After radiation, the bladder gets tremendously irritated from the radiation and this translates into incontinence that is slightly different in nature to that after surgery, but is still sometimes problematic. It results from irritability of the bladder (men complain of having to go to the bathroom frequently and having urgency) and is not the stress type of leakage (leaking with coughing and sneezing, for example) that occurs after radical prostatectomy. Incontinence is most prevalent in the early stages after radiation and tends to settle down within a few months. For men who have seed implantation into the prostate, this often results in prostate swelling, which can cause difficulty with urination. Often, these men are placed on alpha-blocker medications, which may help them urinate with greater ease. Once again, the use of these medications is usually temporary.

Men in the early stages after surgery, when the external sphincter is not functioning fully during sexual relations, particularly when the bladder is

MISCELLANEOUS SEXUAL PROBLEMS . . .

CASE HISTORY 2
Orgasm-Associated Incontinence

Michael is a 62-year-old man who is married to Maria, a 62-year-old woman. He is four months after his radical prostatectomy, which was performed for a Gleason 6 prostate cancer, which, on examination by the pathologist, was completely confined to the prostate. When he sees me for the first time, he has excellent continence, although he wears one pad per day for fear of leaking urine. He had excellent erectile function prior to his surgery. At four months after surgery, his erections are poor; he grades it as 2/10 on the hardness scale using maximum-dose Levitra. He is not concerned as his surgeon had forewarned him that his erectile function might take 12 to 24 months to recover completely. His biggest complaint is that he leaks urine every time he has an orgasm. This is a turnoff for his wife and because of this, he avoids sexual relations. His local urologist tells them to make sure he empties his bladder prior to sex, which he has done, but this has not resulted in any improvement. He has used penile injections with great success, but has not injected in over a month because of fear of leaking urine on his wife. He sees me, and I explain to him why he is leaking urine at orgasm and suggested to him that he use the ACTIS™ band. He is told to apply this rubber constriction band to the base of his penis once he has obtained an erection after a penile injection and that this will likely stop his orgasm-associated incontinence. When he sees me eight months after surgery, he no longer has to use the band as his orgasm-associated incontinence has resolved. At this time, he is responding to maximum-dose Levitra with a 4/10 erection and continues to inject successfully.

This case history illustrates the impact of leakage of urine during sex on a man's interest in having relations. While sometimes a turn-off for a man, this is often a turnoff for his partner. The biggest concern for patients and partners about the presence of orgasm-associated incontinence is that it may harm the partner. Urine is generally sterile and will not result in a woman getting a urine infection or a yeast infection. Indeed, a woman's vagina is exposed to urine every day of her life at the time of urination. From a penile rehabilitation standpoint, the concern about this problem in the early stages after surgery is that it will interfere with a man's interest in trying to get

continued on the next page

continued from the previous page

> erections. As rehabilitation is largely dependent upon getting erections, this will result in poorer post-prostatectomy rehabilitation. The case history also illustrates the benefit of using the ACTIS band in addressing this problem and that orgasm-associated incontinence is a short-term problem usually resolved by the second year after radical prostatectomy.

full, may leak small amounts of urine. Firstly, urine is not a toxic substance and, in the vast majority of circumstances, it is totally sterile. It will not cause a yeast infection or a urinary tract infection in a patient's partner. Indeed, the vagina is exposed to urine every day of a woman's life as she sits on the toilet urinating. The vagina is a very hardy organ with a lining that makes it resistant to urine. However, the leakage of urine during sex is a cosmetic issue which is distressing for some men and their partners.

In effect, continence in the early stages after surgery is based on the patient's ability consciously or subconsciously to contract the muscles in the pelvic floor. There are typically three circumstances which interfere with this. One is fatigue; men often complain of worsening incontinence at the end of the day compared to earlier in the day. The second is alcohol. Alcohol is not just a diuretic (urine producer); it is also somewhat of a bladder irritant and it will go some way toward relaxing those muscles which need to be contracted for continence. The third factor is sexual stimulation. Sexual stimulation results in relaxation of the pelvic floor musculature, which will cause leakage of urine.

Most men who have what is called foreplay incontinence tend to have a very small amount of leakage, and when the bladder is emptied prior to sexual relations, this is usually not a problem. This kind of incontinence is directly related to daytime urine control and as the urine control during the day improves over the course of the first several months after surgery, then too does the foreplay incontinence improve.

Another concern is orgasm-associated incontinence (OAI), also known as climacturia (Table 1). As I mentioned before, the bladder neck is supposed to close fully at the time of orgasm so that urine does not leak out and semen does not pass into the bladder. However, in the early stages after surgery and in rare cases after radiation therapy, the bladder neck does not function properly. It fails to close fully and thus urine can leak out of the penis at the

Table 1 • **Orgasm Associated Incontinence After Radical Prostatectomy**

Author	Year	Number of Patients	Orgasmic dysfunction type and rate
Choi	2007	475	20% orgasmic incontinence (climacturia)
Lee	2006	42	45% orgasmic incontinence (climacturia)
Barnas	2004	239	22% no change in orgasm intensity
			37% complete absence of orgasm
			37% decreased orgasm intensity
			4% increased orgasm intensity
			14% orgasmic pain (dysorgasmia)
Koheman	1996	17	64% orgasmic incontinence (climacturia)
			82% decreased orgasmic intensity
			14% orgasmic pain (dysorgasmia)

time of orgasm. Furthermore, the bladder routinely contracts at the time of orgasm, which compounds this problem. Even in men who empty their bladders immediately prior to sexual relations, over the 15 to 30 minutes after sexual relations begin, the bladder refills and, at the time of orgasm, they may leak urine. This is a very common occurrence in the early stages after surgery and occurs on at least one occasion in up to 90% of men when questioned after surgery. However, about 20% of men have it on a consistent basis after prostatectomy. Of note, our research at MSKCC indicates that this problem is just as common after laparoscopy as it is after open radical prostatectomy. While men do not ejaculate semen after radical prostatectomy, they may ejaculate urine, sometimes several ounces. This amount of urine leak may be distressing for some men and partners.

Historically, the treatment of patients with foreplay or orgasm-associated incontinence was to use a condom to collect the urine at orgasm. The problem with this strategy is, of course, that most men in the early stages of post-prostatectomy are not obtaining good erections and the use of a condom is difficult for them. Furthermore, many men in their 60s have spent many years without ever having to use condoms and having to start using condoms again after so many years is sometimes just as distressing as the urine leakage itself.

There is a medication that helps the bladder neck contract, although these are less effective in men who have had radical prostatectomy. This drug is called imipramine and while classically used for the treatment of depression, it has as a peculiar side effect—relaxing the bladder and causing the bladder neck to contract more efficiently. It is our experience in men with orgasm-associated incontinence that imipramine is minimally effective in most men, although we have had some men who have had significant improvement. The way we use this drug is to administer 25 mg every night when going to bed, consistently for a month, ensuring that there are attempts at sexual relations over this period of time to find out if the medication is effective or not. If it is effective, then we will allow patients to stop using the medication on a nightly basis and use it four hours before sexual relations. It has been our experience that men who are responders to imipramine when using it daily tend to do more poorly when using it on an on-demand basis.

The cornerstone of treatment for sex-associated incontinence is now the use of a constriction band. The band that we use is called the ACTIS band, which is a band whose tightness can be varied by the patient, and is applied around the base of the penis once an erection occurs. It is very effective at controlling foreplay and orgasm-associated incontinence as it compresses the urethra in such a way as to prevent urine leakage. It does, however, require the use of a band, and for some men this is unacceptable as it may be somewhat uncomfortable and some say it interferes with the naturalness of sex. The good news is that the incidence of sex-associated incontinence is lower in the second year than it is in the first year, and even lower in the third year compared to the second year after surgery. Sex-associated incontinence is far less common with radiation therapy. However, these men, as mentioned before, often have significant urge incontinence where they have intense urges to go to the bathroom and need to get to the bathroom quickly or they will leak urine.

II. Changes in Orgasm

It is often surprising to patients that in the complete absence of any erection hardness whatsoever, they can achieve an orgasm. Orgasm, considered the ultimate height of the sexual experience, is still one of the least understood phases of the sexual response cycle. Although researchers have made important strides in understanding many of the aspects of orgasm, our knowledge of this phase does not yet equal the amount of information and understanding regarding erectile function. At the present time, the nature of orgasm and the presence of orgasmic disorders are directly related to a person's quality of life. The reliability, quality and pleasure of an orgasm are all associated with relationship stability and happiness. Likewise, orgasm disorders are related to a reduction in emotional and physical satisfaction during sexual intimacy, which can lead to avoidance of sexual contact by men and secondarily to relationship discord.

It is believed that orgasm is a brain event. That is, an event that occurs in the brain within the pleasure center in the frontal lobe. Men, when asked what an orgasm is, will often describe it as a throbbing sensation in the perineum, and this is not surprising because, while the pleasure comes from the brain, this throbbing sensation is related to the rhythmic contraction of the muscles around the urethra. What is interesting is that it appears these muscles continue to contract even in the absence of semen, such as what occurs after radical prostatectomy. It is likely that there is some pleasure benefit to semen passing through the urethra and the urethra distending at that time. However, most men after radical prostatectomy are going to obtain some form of orgasm.

In a study of more than 200 men who underwent radical prostatectomy, more than 12 months after radical prostatectomy, one-third of these men still reported a complete absence of orgasm. Secondary anorgasmia, that is, when a man has difficulty achieving an orgasm but has previously had no problem, is generally psychologically based, if not related to medications such as Prozac, Zoloft, or Paxil (which are well known to prolong the time to orgasm and sometimes cause failure to achieve orgasm). In the same study, one-fifth of men had no change in orgasm intensity, one-third had a decrease in orgasm intensity and about 5% reported more intense orgasms after prostatectomy compared to before surgery. There are many reasons why men after radical prostatectomy may not obtain orgasms, including post-operative pain, anxiety about follow-up PSA levels, and general anxiety regarding coping with the diagnosis of prostate cancer. More specific causes include the use of antidepressant drugs as outlined above, such as Zoloft, Prozac, Paxil, Celexa, Luvox, Zyprexa, Lexapro and Effexor. These drugs affect serotonin levels in the brain and spinal cord, and this may negatively affect the ability to obtain an orgasm.

The other major cause of this is sensation problems in the penis, which do not typically occur after radical prostatectomy. In the diabetic popula-

Table 2 • **Penile Length Changes after Radical Prostatectomy**

Author	Year	Number of Patients	Follow-up Interval after Surgery	Main Outcomes
Gontero	2007	126	1 year	1.3 cm shortening—flaccid length 2.3 cm shortening—stretched length
Briganti	2007	33	6 months	No statistically significant length changes, both flaccid and erect states
Savoie	2003	63	3 months	19% had ≥15% shortening stretched length 1.2 cm shortening—flaccid length 1.1 cm shortening—stretched length
Munding	2001	31	3 months	13% increased stretched length 16% no change in stretched length 71% had decreased stretched length: 23% - up to 0.5 cm 35% - 1–2 cm 13% - more than 2 cm
Fraiman	1999	100	2–28 months	8% decrease in flaccid length 9% decrease in erect length Greatest change at 4–8 months

tion that has penile sensation nerve injury, the sensation reduces and this significantly negatively impacts upon the ability to achieve an orgasm. The nerves that are traumatized during radical prostatectomy run right alongside the prostate as previously mentioned, and these nerves supply erection only. The sensation nerves are nowhere near the prostate and cannot be injured at the time of surgery, and therefore, there is no change in sensation in the penis after the operation. Thus, most men who have an inability to obtain an orgasm after radical prostatectomy or radiation therapy, in fact, have psychogenic anorgasmia. My discussion with the patient will often highlight a cause of this, whether it is interpersonal conflict with his partner, anxiety related to his cancer diagnosis or treatment, or whether it is due to low levels of arousal. Men who have recurrent erection problems will often have difficulty in obtaining an orgasm. This is likely, in part at least, related to their lack of confidence in their erection ability. Most men who have secondary anorgasmia are potentially curable, that is, we can get them back to having normal orgasm capacity at some point in time. This is best achieved using a combination of sex therapy with a certified sex therapist as well as treatment of any underlying problem, such as erectile dysfunction, and in certain cases, the use of penile vibrators to allow a man to achieve an orgasm while we are trying to resolve the primary underlying problem.

Another problem that occurs in men both after radical prostatectomy and radiation therapy is orgasmic pain known as dysorgasmia. This is a peculiar problem which is seen more commonly after surgery than radiation, but is seen in both cases and believed to be related to spasms of the muscles of the pelvic floor at the time of orgasm. As mentioned previously, the bladder neck is supposed to close at the time of orgasm, and the belief is that the bladder neck muscle and the muscle surrounding this in the pelvis floor may in some men go into spasm at the time of orgasm with pain referred to the penis, testicles, lower abdomen, or rectum area. Most men who experience this kind of pain say it is very mild in nature (on a 10–point pain scale, perhaps a 3 to a 4), but we do occasionally see men who have profound pain which causes complete avoidance of sexual activity in the future. The pain usually lasts from seconds to a minute, but we do have men who have lingering pain for several hours after orgasm, and of course, this will interfere with a man's interest in sexual activity. Two pieces of good news: firstly, the pain tends to improve with time after both surgery and radiation; secondly, if the pain is significant, this pain is very responsive to medications, such as tamsulosin and alfuzosin. In one of my research studies, 68% of men with orgasmic pain after prostatectomy surgery who used tamsulosin (Flomax) had a significant reduction in the intensity of the pain as well as its duration.

Oftentimes, the average physician will not ask you about these problems. It is extremely important that you raise these issues with your physician. There is tremendous discomfort among most physicians, male and female, general and specialist, to talk about a man's orgasm. One of the major reasons for this is that most physicians are not trained in how to hold this discussion. It is estimated that the average medical student receives less than two hours of sexual medicine training during their four years in medical school. Thus, being proactive is important to getting these problems treated.

Table 3 • **Treatments for Peyronie's Disease**

Oral

Vitamin E
Potassium paraminobenozoate
Tamoxifen
Carnitine
L-arginine
Pentoxifylline

Gels

Transdermal verapamil
Iontophoretic* verapamil/steroids

Intralesional injections

Verapamil
Interferon
Steroids
Collagenase**

Shock wave therapy*

Penile extender therapy^

   * Iontophoresis uses low-level electrical current to drive medication across skin into the plaque
 ** Formal trials of this agent are awaited
*** There is now a randomized, controlled trial demonstrating no benefit to this therapy
  ^ Only a single small trial has suggested a benefit to this treatment. A larger trial is awaited

III. Penile Length Changes

It is common for men to come to see me after surgery complaining of loss of penile length. Penile length problems are broken down into two types. The first scenario involves those men who come in the very early stages after surgery (let's say less than three months after surgery), who complain of their penes "being sucked back into their bodies." We know that this is true as we see many men who were circumcised at birth and when they are examined in the office their penes look uncircumcised! The penis has been sucked back in and the skin advances over the head of the penis. There is a very simple explanation for this: when erection nerves are injured even temporarily, then the contraction nerves (remember that these erection nerves have both contraction and relaxation nerve fibers) have the upper hand, which means that they overgrow the areas that are supplied by the relaxation nerves. This condition is known as competitive sprouting. When this happens, the penis is in a state of high contraction. Remember the Seinfeld episode where George has just come out of the swimming pool and is seen naked by a woman who marvels at the "shrinkage factor." The shrinkage factor is genuine. The penis is a muscle that is under adrenaline control. Under very cold conditions or conditions of anxiety, or in the presence of competitive sprouting, hypercontraction of the penis occurs. When the man with early penile shortening is examined and the penis is stretched gently, it stretches perfectly, indicating that there is no permanent erectile tissue damage. Competitive sprouting improves as the nerves recover from the trauma from during surgery.

The second and more alarming kind of penile length change occurs in a more chronic fashion, that is, when men are six months plus after surgery. The belief is that these permanent penile length changes are related to damage to the erection tissue that occurs after nerve injury and with the chronic absence of erection. Once a man has had permanent structural damage to his erection tissue, we believe that this is permanent and can never be fixed. Of note, there is a lot of interest in looking at treatments that may reverse this scarring phenomenon but as of yet, none are available. (See Chapter 14 for information on stem cell therapy.)

There are currently five medical papers published on penile length changes after surgery. Three of them show very clear evidence that there is length loss; approximately 70% of men have documentable loss of penile length with the average loss of length being about 1 cm. It is very common for a patient to see me who has been told that the reason his penis is shorter after surgery is because the prostate was removed and since the prostate is 2 cm long, he should lose 2 cm of penile length. This is an untrue statement. When the prostate is removed, the bladder is brought down to the urethra and the urethra is fixed at the level of the pelvic floor muscle, so it cannot be pulled inwards. So, removing the prostate does not cause any penile shortening. While there is no evidence that penile rehabilitation as we have alluded to in Chapter 7 can lead to improved penile length or preservation of penile length, there is a suspicion that this will be shown to be the case in the future, particularly given the fact that we believe, based on animal and human studies, that the erection tissue can be protected by the use of PDE5 inhibitor drugs (Viagra, Levitra, Cialis) and obtaining erections in the early stages after surgery.

IV. Penile Curvature

Acquired penile curvature, that is, when a man who has had a straight penis for most of his life develops penile curving, is known as Peyronie's disease (Figures 1 and 2). Actually, it is better described as a condition rather than a disease. It is named after Baron Francois Gigot de la Peyronie, the surgeon to Louis XV, as he was the first physician to describe it in the medical literature in 1743. This is a poorly understood condition that is believed to occur in around 3% of the male population. It is worth noting that the more recent literature has higher rates of occurrence of this condition (up to 9%). The vast majority of men with Peyronie's disease have not had irradiation therapy nor have they had radical prostatectomy surgery. However, there is an indication that radical prostatectomy may result in a higher incidence of Peyronie's disease. Ongoing research at MSKCC indicates that approximately 15% of patients after radical prostatectomy will develop penile curvature within three years after surgery. Despite the fact that we have known of Peyronie's disease for more than 250 years, it is still unclear as to why this occurs.

There are many centers that have done excellent research looking at various factors involved in the cause of Peyronie's disease, but the bottom line is that the cause is not clear. It is likely that there is some genetic susceptibility to development of this problem. We know this because the incidence of Peyronie's disease in Caucasians is far higher than that in African-Americans and Peyronie's disease is practically unheard of in the Asian population. The belief is that in a genetically susceptible man, repetitive minor trauma to the penis over months or years translates into small cracks developing in the outer lining of the erection chamber (the tunica) and, in these men, such small cracks lead to scar formation. This scar formation results in decreased penile stretch and angulation of the penis towards the side of the scar (known as a plaque). In cases where Peyronie's disease is not related to radical prostatectomy, we know that approximately 50% of these men will worsen over the course of the first 12 months after its onset, 30% will stay the same, and about 10% will actually have improvement of their curvatures without pursuing any treatment. While there is a presumption that the natural course of Peyronie's disease after prostatectomy is the same as that of the general

CASE HISTORY 3
Peyronie's Disease

Carlos is a 46-year-old divorced male who has a 40-year-old girlfriend. He is four months after radical prostatectomy for a Gleason 7 organ-confined prostate cancer. He failed maximum-dose PDE5 inhibitor early after surgery and is currently on rehabilitation using a quarter Viagra pill (25 mg) every night. His most recent attempt at Viagra 100 mg resulted in a 3/10 erection. At this stage after surgery, he is frustrated by his inability to have sexual intercourse. He calls wanting to try penile injection therapy. He comes in for his first office visit, and an injection of a standard dose of trimix is given. He has a 9/10 erection. However, he also has noted an upward curvature of his penis, measuring approximately 20 degrees. There is no prior history of penile curvature and on examination, he has a well-defined plaque (scar) on the upper aspect of his penile shaft. I discuss intralesional verapamil therapy with him as a form of prevention of progression and he proceeds with a six-injection, 12-week course. Six months later, he has had no worsening of his curvature, although on re-measuring, it is still approximately 20 degrees.

This case history highlights the link between radical prostatectomy and Peyronie's (acquired penile curvature) disease. This is a very recent observation with very little medical literature published on this topic. It appears that radical prostatectomy may accelerate the onset of Peyronie's disease in men who are predisposed to this condition. The exact link between the two is unknown. While there does not appear to be a similar link with radiation therapy, I have seen cases of Peyronie's disease after radiation therapy, although whether they are related to the radiation therapy or not is unclear at this time. The curvature that occurs in this condition is seen only during a good erection, so he did not see it when using Viagra but only when he received his first penile injection in the office. There is no evidence to prove that penile injections cause Peyronie's disease.

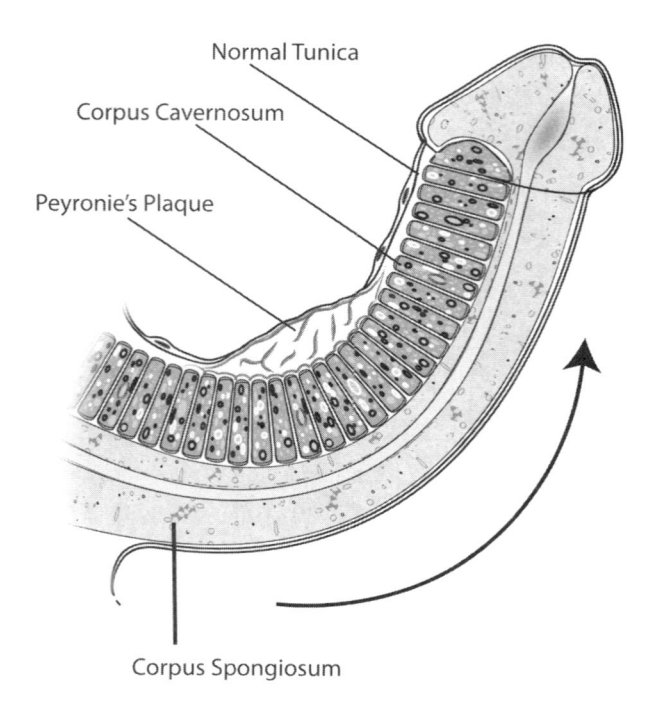

Figure 1 • Illustration of the location of Peyronie's disease plaque within the tunica albuginea. Most plaques occur on the top surface and cause upward curvature.

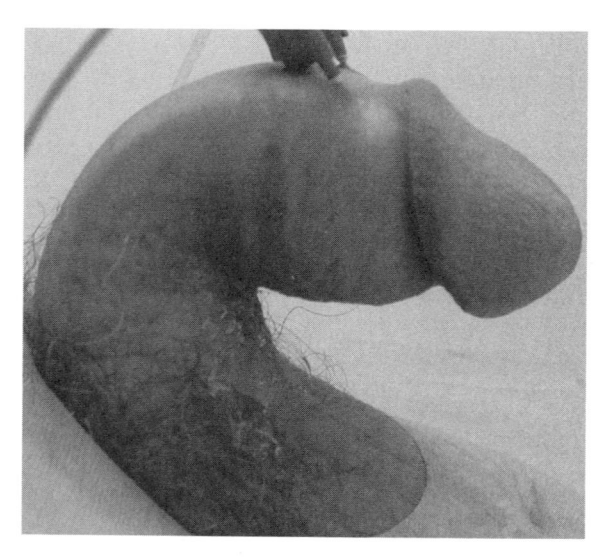

Figure 2 • Photograph of severe downward curvature. The average degree of curvature at presentation is 45 degrees but often 90–degree curvatures are seen.

population, given the very new link between prostatectomy and Peyronie's disease, it is not clear whether this is the case or not.

The major problem with Peyronie's disease, other than the fact that it is a disfiguring condition, is that it results in difficulty having sexual intercourse. It may also be associated with penile pain and with erectile dysfunction. The good news is that the penile pain associated with Peyronie's disease invariably goes away within 12 months of the condition starting. Most often the pain is associated with erection and is generally mild and does not preclude a man being interested in sexual relations. About a third to one-half of men with Peyronie's disease have erection problems, although approximately half of them have erection problems that predated the onset of their Peyronie's disease. Because Peyronie's disease is a scarring condition and scars by their inherent nature contract, most men with Peyronie's disease complain of penile shortening at least in the erect state.

As in most medical conditions where we don't quite understand the cause, treatment can be challenging. There are many medical treatments that have been used over the course of the last century for the treatment of Peyronie's disease, including pills, gels, injections, and shockwaves (Table 3). More than 30 pills have been used over the course of the last 100 years for the treatment of Peyronie's disease and, of course, this typically means that no one pill is a perfect solution. There is little evidence to show that any pill used is better than a placebo for reversing the curvature. However, there is a suspicion that the use of pills may, in fact, stall the progression, that is, the worsening of this condition. Indeed, it is my opinion and the opinion of other experts that medical treatment (pills, gels, injections, etc.) has, as its primary goal, the prevention of progression of the curvature

The pills that have been most commonly used include vitamin E, paraminobenozoate (Potaba), tamoxifen (which is used predominantly in Europe), colchicines, and a drug called pentoxifylline (Trental). I typically reserve the use of pills for men who have plaques that are not amenable to intralesional injection therapy (see a little later in this section) or who refuse to do these injections. There is tremendous interest in the use of gels for treatment of Peyronie's disease, but there is no credible evidence to show that the application of a gel to the penis is of any benefit to men with Peyronie's disease. There is a technology called iontophoresis (also known as electromotive drug administration, or EMDA) where a tiny electrical current is used to drive the agent in the gel across the skin into the plaque. While there is evidence to show that we can in fact measure drug in the plaque by the use of

EMDA, there is as of yet no convincing evidence to show that transdermal gels, whether it be verapamil, dexamethasone, or lidocaine, with or without the use of electrical stimulation, is of any significant benefit.

The primary means of treatment in my practice for the prevention and progression of Peyronie's disease is the use of intralesional injections. Intralesional injections have been used since 1994, when they were introduced by Dr. Laurence Levine in Chicago for Peyronie's disease. There are three drugs that have been explored. Firstly, the one that we use is verapamil. Then there is an interferon, and there is a drug which is not currently available but will be in trials sometime in 2008, known as collagenase.

Intralesional injection therapy involves a series of 6 to 12 injections into the plaque under local anesthetic. It is a procedure that is very well tolerated by patients. Local anesthetic administered at the base of the penis. The penis goes entirely numb and 15 minutes later the medication is injected into the plaque. The plaque is peppered with the needle so that at least 20 to 30 plaque punctures are achieved. After this, a bandage is applied to the penis for approximately one hour and the patient is discharged to return approximately two weeks later for his next injection. I have already told you that 50% of men worsen, 40% stay the same and 10% actually get better when pursuing no treatment. The figures with intralesional verapamil injections in my practice are that approximately 20% worsen, 60% stay the same and 20% get better. So, I tell patients that they have half the chances of penile curvature worsening and we double the chances of it getting better, although the main purpose of the treatment is to prevent worsening of the curvature. The men who come to the office early in the condition (within six months of it starting) are the ones we believe are most likely to benefit.

Shockwaves have been explored in many centers, mainly in Europe. These shockwaves have been used for many years in the treatment of kidney stones and the theory was that the shockwaves might, in fact, cause a breakup of the penile plaque. While some research has suggested improvement in curvature, many have not, and indeed, the most recent study, which was a randomized, controlled trial from Germany, demonstrated no significant improvement in the shockwave therapy group compared to the group that went untreated. Therefore, it is not likely that shockwave therapy in its current form is beneficial to men with Peyronie's disease.

Once a man gets past 12 months after its start and the curvature has been stable, that is, it has not worsened or improved over the previous three months, he then becomes a candidate for surgical reconstruction. Surgery is only indicated in men who have difficulty penetrating, who find it impossible to penetrate, who hurt themselves or hurt their partners during penetration, or who are psychologically distressed by the penile deformity. Most men with Peyronie's disease have curvatures that are in an upward direction. However, there are men who have curvatures in a downward direction or to the right- or the left-hand side. The degree of curvature varies tremendously and we have men who have 10 degrees of curvature and others who have 110 degrees of curvature. When a man has curvature that is more than 45(in an upward direction, it becomes very difficult for him to penetrate, and when more than 30 degrees in a downward or lateral direction, it also becomes very difficult for him to penetrate on. The curvature may be associated with other problems, such as indentations, one or both sides, hourglass deformity, and instability which results in a hinge effect with good rigidity behind and in front of the curvature, but with a grossly unstable penis.

The surgical management of Peyronie's disease is beyond the scope of this book; however, there are generally three types of surgical procedures. First is plication procedure (also known as tucks), which has as its main advantage preservation of erectile function, but as its main disadvantage loss of penile length. The second type of operation is plaque incision and grafting, where the plaque is cut, the penis is stretched, and the defect left behind is filled with a graft. This has a very low incidence of penile shortening, but has a significant incidence of erection problems, that is, reduction of erection hardness. The third procedure is penile implant surgery, which is reserved for special populations, the largest one of which is men with Peyronie's disease who also have erection problems. For further information on surgical reconstruction I urge you to go to the Association of Peyronie's Disease Advocates website at www.peyroniesassociation.org.

V. Fertility Options

It is surprising to me how many men come in to see me after radical prostatectomy who are not aware that they will not ejaculate again. While some physicians may not tell their patients about this, there are patients who are so stressed before surgery that they simply forget what was told to them. Remember that semen is produced by the seminal vesicles predominantly, yet also by the prostate, while the minority of semen is actually sperm from the vas deferens. The prostate and seminal vesicles are removed at the time of radical prostatectomy, and therefore, these men can never ejaculate again.

They are, in fact, completely sterile. After radiation therapy, there is a chronic scarring of the prostate and ejaculation ducts, such that most men three to five years after radiation do not ejaculate semen at all. So, for a man who remains interested in future fertility, it is important that he banks sperm prior to the procedure. Banking sperm is a process by which a man masturbates into a cup and the semen is then examined and frozen (cryo-preserved) for future thawing and use down the road. We don't know a time limit on how long sperm can be frozen, although about 50% of the sperm will die during the freezing process. But the average man, particularly if he has proven paternity (that is, he has children already), will have plenty of sperm if he gives two to three specimens prior to surgery. It is worthwhile knowing that prior to giving a semen specimen, a man should not ejaculate for two to four days prior to giving the specimen so that he can build up an adequate semen volume. However, having periods of absence much longer than this may result in sperm not functioning well as old sperm tend to swim very poorly. Even men who have had radical prostatectomy or those who have had radiation therapy cannot ejaculate, still produce sperm in their testicles. In fact, a man who has a normal testicle examination and is interested in having sperm extraction, will usually have sperm found inside his testicle that can be used for in-vitro fertilization (test-tube baby). It is also important to remember that any sperm that is frozen can only be used with in-vitro fertilization and is not good enough for intrauterine insemination (artificial insemination) or natural conception.

Sperm extraction for most men after prostatectomy, especially those who have had children, is a very simple process whereby local anesthetic is placed into the structure upon which the testicle hangs, known as the spermatic cord. This is a relatively painless injection. The testicle and scrotum go numb and, using a little needle, tissue is extracted from each testicle, placed in special fluid, and transported to the sperm bank where it is analyzed. Any sperm found can be placed into vials that are frozen for future use. This is a very well tolerated procedure, which can be done as an outpatient in an office setting, and most men will return to work the day after the procedure with no significant problems.

CHAPTER 9

PILLS

> I. Viagra and the Like!
> II. Differences and Similarities in the PDE5 Inhibitors
> III. Safety of PDE5 Inhibitors
> IV. Pills for Premature Ejaculation
> V. Summary

I. Viagra and the Like!

The introduction of the little blue pill in the spring of 1998 has revolutionized not just how we treat erectile problems, but also how we perceive sexual health. This medication experienced the most successful launch of any drug in the history of the pharmaceutical industry and has permeated our society on a scientific and secular level. It essentially has become the Coca-Cola or the Kleenex of the drug market. Its discovery is an interesting one. It was originally designed as a drug for angina, that is, for the treatment of chest pain. It was minimally effective for this problem, but during drug trials it was noted that the men were experiencing better erectile function; thus, the start of the Viagra revolution.

Viagra belongs to a class of drugs known as PDE5 inhibitors (phosphodiesterase type 5 inhibitors) or PDE5i for short. PDE5i are medications that

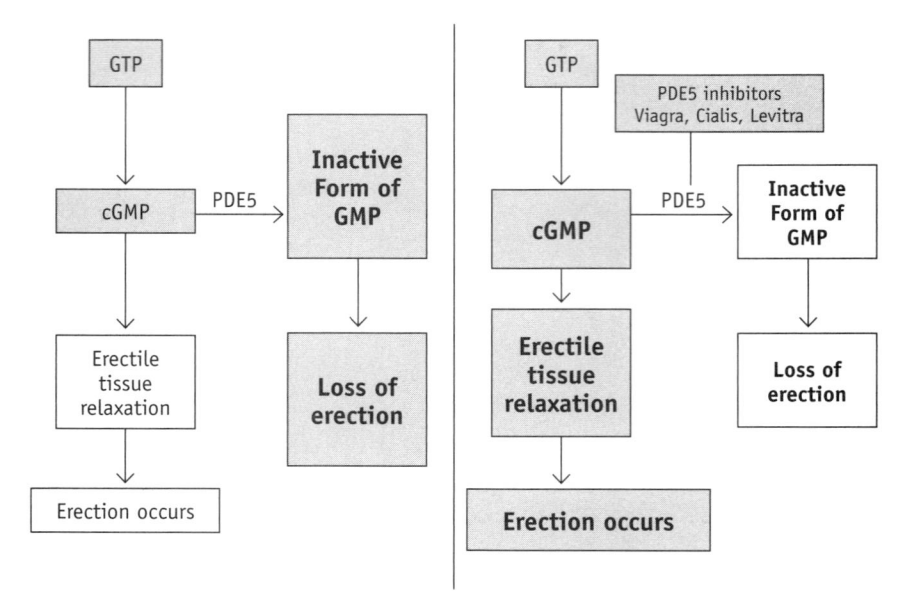

Figure 1 • How PDE5 inhibitors work. The left side of the diagram represents the flaccid state. The right hand side of the diagram represents the effect of PDE5 inhibitors.

increase blood flow into the penis under certain conditions. To understand exactly how they work, you will have to return to Chapter 1 and refresh your memory on the physiology of erection. The cavernous nerves, which travel close to the prostate and end in the erectile tissue, supplying both the smooth muscle and the endothelium, secrete a chemical known as nitric oxide. Nitric oxide is one of the simplest chemicals that exist in our bodies. This chemical sets off a cascade of events that are essential to erectile function. You will remember from Chapter 1 that nitric oxide stimulates an enzyme inside the smooth muscle cell which allows the buildup of an erection-producing chemical known as cyclic GMP (cGMP) (Figure 1). cGMP forces calcium out of the cell, thus resulting in relaxation of the smooth muscle and erection. Cyclic GMP, if allowed to build up in an uncontrolled fashion, would result in a prolonged erection. The body has a mechanism to prevent this and that is an enzyme known as PDE5. Thus the way Viagra-like drugs work is to inhibit this PDE5 and allow the rapid and more complete accumulation of cyclic GMP in the erectile tissue. As you can imagine, if you have problems generating nitric oxide production, then you will have problems responding to PDE5 inhibitors.

The two patient populations most likely to have a problem with their erectile nerves, and thus the ability to generate nitric oxide, are diabetics with nerve injury and radical prostatectomy patients. Thus, in all the drug trials, the groups of people least likely to respond to PDE5 inhibitors are men who have had radical prostatectomy surgery and who have diabetes.

Now before you get too depressed, there is excellent evidence to show that a man who has good function before surgery, who has nerve sparing surgery, and who protects his erectile tissue through penile rehabilitation, has an excellent chance of being a PDE5i responder in the second half of the second year after surgery (18 to 24 months). It is essential for you to understand that the overwhelming majority of men (85%) do not respond to PDE5 inhibitors in the first six months after surgery irrespective of the nerve sparing status. This is because, as we outlined before, even excellent nerve sparing results in temporary cavernous nerve trauma which leads to the inability to secrete nitric oxide and therefore the inability to respond to Viagra-like drugs.

If you have had a radical prostatectomy, by now you should know whether your nerves were saved (spared) or not. As described in an earlier chapter, the nerves are, in fact, not a single nerve, but a bundle of nerves running right alongside the prostate. The number of nerve fibers that are preserved is directly linked not only to the recovery of natural erections, but also to the ability to get a good erection with PDE5 inhibitors. It is well documented that men with both nerves spared are more likely to respond to PDE5 inhibitors than patients who have only one nerve preserved and these men, in turn, are significantly more likely to have good erections with PDE5 inhibitors compared to those patients who have had no nerves spared. Interestingly, patients who have been told they have no nerves spared whatsoever, in some centers will actually have a chance of responding to a PDE5 inhibitor, suggesting that even the surgeon who believes that all the nerves were removed, may have not, in fact, removed every single fiber.

However, as the nerves recuperate over the first two years after surgery, they then become capable of producing nitric oxide, which results in the ability to respond to PDE5 inhibitors. In my experience, the time to peak response to PDE5 inhibitors is approximately two years after surgery. Therefore—and this is a key take-home message for the man post-prostatectomy—if you fail to respond to a PDE5i within the first six months after surgery, even if you fail during the second six months after surgery, this does not mean that you will fail to respond to PDE5 inhibitors in the long term, as the time to best response after radical prostatectomy is about two years.

For those patients who have received radiation, as previously mentioned the average time to onset of erection problems is approximately 12 months after completion of radiation, and for the first year, most men have no significant problem with erection. If they do, they are usually good responders to PDE5i, especially if their function was good prior to radiation. However, in the second, third and fourth years after the completion of radiation there is a reduction in the proportion of patients who get erections with PDE5i. This is related to the slow, progressive damaging effect that radiation has on erection arteries and erection tissue.

Finally, we know as urologists that men who have been prescribed a PDE5i by their family doctors and who "fail" the medication, in some cases are likely not to have failed. Thirty to fifty percent of those men, when re-educated and re-challenged with medication, actually respond because previously, they were on a less than optimal dose or were not using the medication in a correct fashion.

II. Differences and Similarities in the PDE5 Inhibitors

Currently there are three PDE5 inhibitors available throughout the world, although there is a fourth which is available only in Asia (Figure 2). The three available worldwide are sildenafil (Viagra, Pfizer Inc.), vardenafil (Levitra, GSK Schering) and tadalafil (Cialis, Eli Lilly). They all function in a very similar fashion, by blocking PDE5 inhibitor and allowing the accumulation of cyclic GMP. However, there are some differences between the three medications.

The two drugs that are most alike are Viagra and Levitra (Table 1). They are drugs that have a peak blood level at about one hour (this time generally indicates the peak time of action of a medication) and have a duration of effect of about eight to 12 hours. Now, this is important to understand because the package insert (that little piece of paper that comes with your prescription, which nobody reads) for each of these drugs suggests that they last about four hours. However, there is excellent recent evidence to suggest

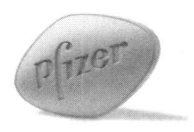

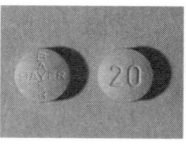

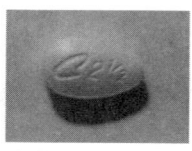

Figure 2 • Photographs of Viagra (diamond-shaped), Levitra (round) and Cialis (tear-drop)

Viagra   Levitra   Cialis

Table 1 • **Comparing PDE5 Inhibitors**

	Sildenafil (Viagra)	**Vardenafil (Levitra)**	**Tadalafil (Cialis)**
Time to onset	1 hour	1 hour	2–4 hours
Duration of action	8–12 hours	8–12 hours	24–36 hours
Food interaction	Yes	Yes	No
Nitrates forbidden	Yes	Yes	Yes
Visual disturbances	+	+	-
Muscle aches	+	+	++
Headache	++	++	++
Nasal stuffiness	++	++	++
Heartburn	++	++	++

+++ common
++ occasional
+ rare
- none

that they last longer. This is no surprise to most urologists as we have been faced with men over the course of the last nine years who not only get a great erection on the night of pill ingestion, but also the following morning.

Cialis is different in that it is a slower-onset drug, but lasts much longer. Cialis is, in fact, a drug that can produce erection for up to 36 hours after a single dose. I tell my patients that Viagra and Levitra are a one-to-12–hour drug, whereas Cialis is a four- to 24–hour drug. Another key difference is that both Viagra and Levitra are significantly affected by the presence of fatty food in the stomach. Fatty food has been shown to reduce the dose from anywhere from 20 to 50 percent, thus limiting the effectiveness of medication when taken with or shortly after fatty food. Furthermore, it doubles the time for which the medication takes to be absorbed from one hour to two hours peak blood level, thus slowing down the onset of action. Thus, I tell all of my patients that during the trial phase (the first four attempts), they should be taking Viagra and Levitra before meals. Given the fact that they are eight- to 12–hour drugs, I tell patients, if they are planning on having sex in the evening and are having dinner at 7 o'clock, to take the medication at 5 o'clock and expect to be ready for sexual relations until after midnight.

Another advantage of this approach is that it distances taking the medication from the actual sexual encounter so that the process is far less mechanical. If you have to take the medication after a meal, then you should wait at least two hours after the completion of the meal. If you are diabetic, then it is inadvisable to use these medications after a meal because of the notoriously poor emptying ability of the stomach in diabetic men. For Cialis, there is no negative impact of food. Therefore, it can be taken with the meal, immediately afterwards or beforehand. However, it is a slow-onset drug, and while there are patients who get a positive response within one hour (as there are patients who get a positive response to Viagra and Levitra in 20 minutes), in the majority of patients, in my experience, it takes quite a bit longer to see a maximum effect. Therefore, I tell patients to take the medication at least four hours before anticipated sexual relations during the trial phase, and that it is fully functional for up to 24 hours after the administration.

I start my patients on the maximum dose of each pill, that is, 100 mg of Viagra, 20 mg of Levitra, or 20 mg of Cialis, and they can decrease the dose if they have an excellent response or if they experience troublesome side effects. Of course, as with most physicians, I encourage my patients to split the pills if they are using less than the maximum dose. For example, we routinely use 25 mg Viagra nightly for penile rehabilitation after prostatectomy or radiation, but we have the patient split the 100–mg pill in four using a pill splitter. This costs a few dollars at your local pharmacy. It is my experience that in the first year following surgery and more than two years after the completion of radiation, most men who require PDE5 inhibitors will, in fact, need to use maximum dose to get a positive response.

The three drugs have very similar side effects, which is what you would expect given the very similar mechanisms of action. They are all associated with headache, facial flushing, nasal congestion, and heartburn. The side effects typically come on within 30 to 60 minutes of taking the pill and last approximately 30 to 60 minutes, and are very mild in nature. Indeed, less than two percent of my patients stop using these medications because of side effects. Both Viagra and Levitra cross-react with an enzyme in the retina known as PDE6, and thus can cause blurred vision, double vision, or loss of color vision (also known as the "blue halo"). These visual side effects are in no way related to the "blindness issue" that was raised by the press in 2006. The visual side effects I have just mentioned are temporary and not dangerous by any means (see the next section of this chapter).

Cialis causes very little inhibition of PDE6 and therefore visual disturbances are rare. It does, however, because of its long duration of action cause pooling of blood in the large muscles in the body, particularly in the back, buttocks and legs, and because of this can cause significant muscle aches. These muscle aches are caused by a different mechanism than the muscle aches experienced by those of you who are using statins (lipitor, crestor, vytorin, simvastatin, pravachol, etc.). The muscle ache that can occur with Cialis is not dangerous (it is related to pooling of blood in the blood vessels of these muscles and not muscle injury), although it are troublesome for some men, (approximately 10%), and for some of these men will require stopping the medication.

III. Safety of PDE5 Inhibitors

In the first year after the introduction of Viagra, more than 100 men died sometime after taking Viagra for the purpose of sexual relations. It highlighted two very important issues. Firstly, men who are using nitroglycerin-containing medications, also known as nitrates (see list at end of chapter), under no circumstances should receive prescriptions for a PDE5 inhibitor. Indeed, in my practice, patients who are even in possession of nitroglycerin, containing medications, even though they may not have used them for more than a year, are not given prescriptions for PDE5 inhibitors. We write a letter to the nitroglycerin-prescribing physician asking him or her if the patient can cease carrying the medication. Approximately 40 percent of the letters we send out return with a response stating that the patient can stop the nitroglycerin medication.

The second issue is that patients are required to have some degree of exercise reserve before initiating a physically exerting activity such as sexual intercourse. I ask all of my patients, "Can you walk up two flights of stairs briskly without the development of chest pain?" If the answer to this question is "yes," and they are not using or in possession of nitroglycerin, containing medications, then they are excellent candidates for PDE5 inhibitors. There is generally tremendous anxiety for some partners about the link between this medication and heart attack. There are more than 100 papers in the cardiology literature demonstrating the safety of Viagra, and there are several on Levitra and Cialis also. Indeed, there is evidence from the drug trials for all three drugs, that the incidence of heart attack is actually lower in those patients who are given the medication compared to the placebo (sugar pill). It is widely believed in the field of sexual medicine that the future use of PDE5 inhibitors will not be mainly in the field of erectile dysfunction, but rather in the field of vascular health (blood vessel protection). The three drugs have been shown to be potent endothelial (endothelium being the inner lining of blood vessels) protectants, have been shown to increase exercise reserve in patients with cardiac condition such as congestive heart failure, and also prolong survival in patients with pulmonary hypertension. Thus, it is plausible that in the future all men and women over, let's say, 40 years of age will be using PDE5 inhibitors regularly to protect their blood vessels and heart, much in the same way that aspirin is used nowadays.

The previously mentioned blindness, also known as NAION (Non-Arteritic Ischemic Optic Neuropathy) is a permanent problem and occurs most commonly in middle-aged men. NAION typically occurs in men and women in their 50s upon waking from sleep. The instance of NAION in the general population is somewhere between 2.5 and 11 per 100,000 persons. Data from Pfizer's very large database (over 13,000 patients have been studied in drug trials for this medication) and from two studies show there is no sign that the instance of NAION is higher among PDE5 inhibitor users. Indeed, there is a sign that it may even be lower than in the general population. The risk factors for the development of NAION are hypertension, high blood pressure, lipid problems, and diabetes. These are the men who are most likely also to have erectile dysfunction, and therefore most likely to be using a PDE5 inhibitor. The FDA agrees with this statement that it is likely that the PDE5 inhibitors are associated with NAION through the sharing of common conditions (diabetes, hypertension, lipid problems), but that there is no clear indication that PDE5i cause blindness. I ask all of my patients if they have any eye problems, including retinitis pigmentosa, macular degeneration, or sudden blindness, and if they answer "yes" to that question, then we refer them to an ophthalmologist for clearance for use of PDE5 inhibitors.

IV. Pills for Premature Ejaculation

As mentioned previously, premature ejaculation is common in men who have erectile dysfunction, particularly in those men who have problems with sustaining capability, who frequently train themselves to have an orgasm more quickly. Of course, the radical prostatectomy patient and many patients

> ## CASE HISTORY 4
> ### PDE5 Inhibitors after Radical Prostatectomy
>
> Leonard is a 60-year-old stockbroker who has been married for the past 12 years to Gladys, who is currently 42 years of age. This is his second marriage. He sees me prior to his radical prostatectomy and is instructed to use a quarter Viagra pill (25 mg) each night for the two weeks prior to surgery, with his catheter in place. He is told to change, once his urinary catheter is removed, to a quarter pill six nights a week and on the seventh night to use maximum-dose Viagra with sexual stimulation. He sees me six weeks after surgery and is obtaining only a 2/10 erection with maximum-dose Viagra. He is encouraged to consider penile injection therapy and opts to do so. He uses a quarter Viagra pill five nights a week and injects twice a week to obtain an erection. He obtains an 80% erection for approximately 60 minutes and is happy. At four months his response to Viagra 100 mg is 2/10, at eight months 3/10, at 12 months 4/10, but by 18 months he is obtaining a penetration hardness erection at 6/10 and by 24 months he has a 8/10 hardness erection with 100 mg. His natural erection response at this stage is 6/10.
>
> This case history illustrates a very important point. That is, that the ability to respond to Viagra, Levitra or Cialis is very dependent on the time after radical prostatectomy. The time to optimal response to these medications is somewhere between 12 and 24 months and for most men, 18 and 24 months after surgery. Therefore, just because a man fails to respond to Viagra at eight or 12 months after surgery does not mean he will not be a responder at two years. This phenomenon is due to the fact that the ability of these pills to work depends on a chemical that comes from the nerves (known as nitric oxide, or NO). If the nerves are "asleep," then there is little NO available, and so the oils don't work. This is why the peak response with pills is around two years after surgery, the point of maximum nerve recovery.

after radiation therapy for prostate cancer have no ejaculation. However, the majority of these patients have the ability to achieve an orgasm, so what we are really talking about is premature orgasm.

Why is this of concern? Because the vast majority of men, once they have orgasms will lose their erections. There are currently no FDA-approved medications for the treatment of premature ejaculation. However, we have, for more than a decade, been using certain drugs off-label (this means when drugs are used for conditions that they don't have an FDA indication for) for the treatment of premature ejaculation. The drug class that is used most commonly for this problem is known as SSRIs (selective serotonin reuptake inhibitors). Belonging to this class are drugs such as Prozac, Zoloft, Paxil, Luvox, Celexa, and Lexapro. The three drugs that have been most studied are Prozac, Zoloft, and Paxil. There is some evidence to suggest that Paxil is probably the most effective medication. However, it is also the medication that appears to be associated with the highest incidence of side effects. Now there are two basic problems with using these medications. Firstly, they need to be used on a daily basis and, once they are stopped, a man will return to his premature ejaculation. Secondly, they have the label of being antidepressants, and for many men this is a turn-off from using them given the stigma that is associated with such medications. Of note, airline pilots are prohibited from using these medications. These medications are effective in something in the range of 70 percent of patients; that is, they increase the time to ejaculation, and the average man gets anywhere from a 100% to 600% improvement in his ejaculation time. It can take three to four weeks to see any significant benefit, as the effect is based on a change in chemicals in the brain, very much like the treatment of depression. The side effects of these medications include sweating, nausea, dizziness, drowsiness, sleepiness, and appetite suppression.

As previously described, premature ejaculation can be broken down into two groups: lifelong, also known as primary, and acquired, also known as secondary. The most common cause of secondary premature ejaculation, whereby the man has had normal ejaculation time for much of his life and suddenly it changes, is the presence of erectile dysfunction. Interestingly, the treatment of men with premature ejaculation that results from chronic erection problems is to firstly treat the erection problem. When treatment of the erectile dysfunction is successful, the majority of these patients will actually return to having a normal ejaculation time.

V. Summary

In summary, PDE5 inhibitors are a safe treatment for men with erection problems. Men after radical prostatectomy may not respond in the first year after surgery and they are more likely to respond as they get toward the end

> ### CASE HISTORY 5
> ### PDE5 Inhibitors after Radiation Therapy
>
> Joseph is a 50-year-old man who is currently single. He has no sexual partner at this time. He underwent radiation seed implantation three years ago. His erectile function prior to his procedure was excellent. However, he started noticing decreasing erectile hardness approximately 12 months after he had his radiation. He used Viagra 50 mg at that point in time with an excellent response. However, over the course of the last two years, he has noticed that his response to the pills has significantly decreased. He is now at a point where he is unable to have penetration using a pill. A duplex Doppler ultrasound of his penis demonstrates decreased blood flow into his penis and venous leak. He starts on penile injection therapy and responds very well.
>
> This case history illustrates three points. Firstly, it can take up to a year after radiation therapy to start noticing any significant deterioration in erectile function. Radiation has a slow-onset, delayed effect on erection arteries and erectile tissue. Secondly, while most men respond to a PDE5 inhibitor in the early stages after radiation, this response may wane over the course of the first three years after radiation. The low point in erectile function after radiation therapy is around three years, at which time the erection function plateaus, and it is not uncommon for a man's response to a PDE5 inhibitor to worsen (sometimes a little, sometimes a lot) over these three years. Finally, even in the presence of venous leak (where the valve in erection chamber is defective), penile injection therapy is very successful. Indeed, even in the presence of venous leak, more than 50% of men will respond to penile injections with good erections.

of the second year after surgery. The effectiveness of these medications in prostatectomy and radiation patients is dependent on a number of factors: in particular, a man's preoperative erectile function, his age, the nerve sparing status of the prostatectomy, the amount of time passed after surgery or radiation therapy, the use of hormone therapy before and after radiation, and the appropriate use of the medication.

APPENDIX
Nitrate-Containing Medications

Nitroglycerin (Deponit, Minitran, Nitrek, Nitrodisc, Nitro-Dur, Nitroglyn, Nitrolingual Spray, Nitrostat).

Isosorbide mononitrate (Imdur, ISMO, Monoket).

Isosorbide dinitrate (Dilatrate-SR, Isordil, Sorbitrate).

Pentaerythritol tetranitrate (Duotrate, Peritrate, Tetraneed).

Sodium nitroprusside (Nipride, Nitropress).

Amyl nitrite (sometimes called "poppers").

CHAPTER 10

INTRAURETHRAL SUPPOSITORIES

> I. How They Work
> II. Advantages
> III. Disadvantages

I. How They Work

In 1997, the intraurethral Alprostadil (a form of prostaglandin E1) suppository manufactured by the VIVUS company from California was approved by the FDA as a MUSE™ (Figure 1). This acronym stands for "Medicated Urethral System for Erection" and, upon its introduction, it was thought that it would revolutionize the treatment of erectile dysfunction. Much of this promise has not been lived up to because of relatively low levels of effectiveness and low levels of consistency when used. Nevertheless, it has a definite role in the management of erectile dysfunction, particularly in patients who do not respond well to pills and are who are fearful of penile injection therapy or find it unpalatable.

It involves the use of a suppository, approximately the size of a grain of rice, which is placed by the patient himself approximately one inch into the urethra (the urine channel) using a special applicator. The patient should urinate prior to administration of the suppository. This urination is aimed at lubricating the urethra for ease of applicator use. The patient should then

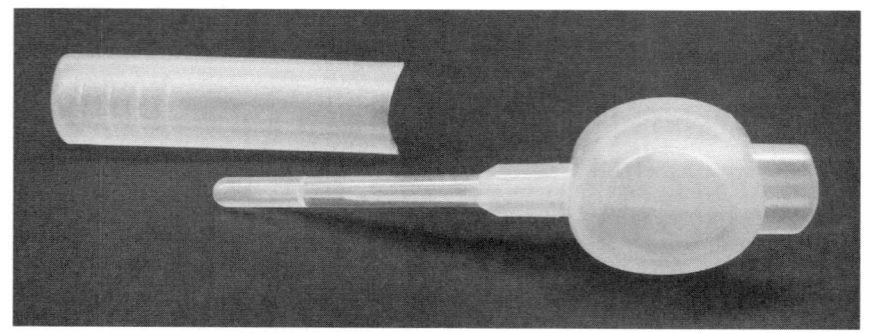

Figure 1 • Photograph of MUSE applicator

stay standing following the administration of the suppository and massage his penis (or have his partner do so) until an erection occurs. This takes anywhere from five to 20 minutes usually, and once the erection has occurred, sexual relations can occur.

The mechanism by which intraurethral suppositories work is that there are blood vessels which pass between the corpus spongiosum (which houses the urethra) and the corpora caverosa (which are the erectile bodies). Upon standing, these blood vessels are swollen (dilated) and on administration of the suppository, the medication is absorbed into these blood vessels and transferred into the erection chamber. There is little doubt that a varying amount of the medication is absorbed into the general circulation and this may cause dizziness or a drop in blood pressure in rare but well documented cases.

Depending on the erectile dysfunction population studied, this medication works in anywhere from 30% to 50% of men. Of note, of men with psychogenic dysfunction, it works in greater than 75%. There are very few studies assessing the use of intraurethral prostaglandin in men after radical prostatectomy or radiation therapy. However, it is believed to be as effective in this population as it is in the general erectile dysfunction population. One of the great problems in the radical prostatectomy population with the use of prostaglandin E1 monotherapy, as we alluded to in the penile injection chapter, is that when the nerves are traumatized, even temporarily, they are hypersensitive to the prostaglandin. This results in aching or burning penile pain in some men. This is true for intracavernosal prostaglandin E1, such as in Caverject or Edex, and is just as true for MUSE.

The intraurethral suppository comes in four doses, 125 mcg, 250 mcg, 500 mcg and 1000 mcg. I have stopped using anything other than 1000 mcg for inducing erection because of the lack of effectiveness of the other doses.

If a patient responds with a robust erection to 1000 mcg, then we consider dropping his dose down to 500 if he wishes.

There is great interest in the use of intraurethral prostaglandin as a penile rehabilitation strategy. There are a couple of small studies using regular very low-dose MUSE (125 mcg either daily or on several occasions per week) as a means of rehabilitating the penis or preventing erectile tissue damage in the early stages after radical prostatectomy. The very preliminary results are encouraging, although it is likely too early to say based on the small studies done to date, whether MUSE has a definite role in rehabilitation. What is interesting is that it is well known that prostaglandin E is capable of turning off the scar-producing chemicals that are produced after nerve injury, and there is a distinct possibility that the use of prostaglandin, whether through penile injections or intraurethral suppositories, may, in fact, have some intrinsic protective effect. This is as of yet unproven, although there is ongoing research assessing this at this time.

MUSE has been used in another group of patients and this is when patients fail Viagra-like drugs alone. Two studies have shown that men who fail Viagra can get an excellent erection when combining Viagra and MUSE. There are two points worth remembering when considering this approach. Firstly, the combination of these drugs is listed as being contraindicated in the package inserts for both drugs. The main reason for this is a concern about priapism (prolonged erection) when two erection-inducing medications are combined. The second concern is that both drugs alone can cause a drop in blood pressure which, when used alone, may not be significant enough to cause any dizziness or fainting, but when used together, may result in a greater blood pressure drop associated with passing out. So, all patients interested in using such a combination approach should have the trial of the combination conducted in the office setting, just in case a serious blood pressure drop occurs.

II. Advantages

The single greatest advantage of MUSE is its simplicity of use. It is foolproof and has a very low incidence of side effects. When it works, it gives an erection similar in quality to that with penile injection therapy, but it is nowhere nearly as consistent as penile injection therapy. Another potential advantage is that it gives a very cosmetic erection, in contrast to vacuum devices. The erection that occurs with MUSE is very normal appearing. It

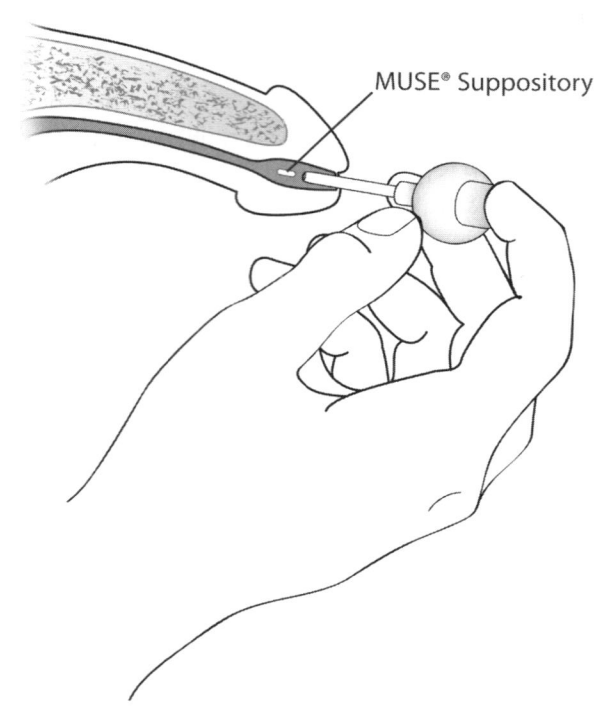

Figure 2 • Illustration of placement of applicator into urethra

is probably even more normal appearing than an erection that occurs with penile injection therapy. With penile injections, the shaft is generally rigid or fully rigid. However the head of the penis tends not to swell. This is not the case with MUSE, where both the shaft and the head swell, and therefore probably gives the most normal-looking erection over pills like Viagra, Levitra, and Cialis.

III. Disadvantages

There are a number of distinct disadvantages, the first being its relative lack of efficacy. Somewhere between 50 to 75% of patients will not respond well to MUSE. The second disadvantage is its lack of consistency, where probably no more than 50 to 60% of the occasions that it is used in men who have previously responded does it give a good erection. The lack of consistency is likely to be related to some degree to the variability in dilation of the previously mentioned blood vessels that pass between the corpus spongiosum and

INTRAURETHRAL SUPPOSITORIES

the corpora cavernosa. One of the great problems under these circumstances is that men often have difficulty gaining confidence in intraurethral suppositories because on one out of every two or three occasions the medication fails to work.

I previously alluded to the problem of pain occurring in men with erection nerve injury, such as a patient with diabetes and patients after radical prostatectomy and after radiation therapy. For many patients, this pain is very mild and well tolerated, but for some it is crippling and prevents them from using MUSE as a treatment. Another disadvantage is its cost. If not covered by insurance, it currently costs about $25 per suppository, which, for many patients is a major obstacle to using MUSE. When you compare this to approximately $12 per pill for Viagra, Levitra, or Cialis, or $1 to 5 for penile injection medication, it is the most expensive of the drug treatment strategies.

There are a number of well documented but not very common side effects, including bleeding from the urethra. This is usually related to poor technique, and when a man has mastered the technique, this is not a concern. Overall, it occurs in less than 5% of all men using MUSE. Approximately 2% of men using 1000 mcg of MUSE will have dizziness upon first administration, and so I recommend that all patients using MUSE have their first doses given under supervision of a health care practitioner in the medical office setting. Should a patient have a significant drop in blood pressure or dizziness, then we would not start that man on 1000 mcg in the at-home setting but rather urge him to use a lower dose.

CHAPTER 11

PENILE INJECTIONS

> I. Historical Perspective
> II. How They Work
> III. Injection Technique
> IV. Medications
> V. Side Effects
> VI. Tricks of the Trade

I. Historical Perspective

Penile injection therapy, or more accurately, intracavernosal injection therapy (as the needle is injected directly into the erectile body, the corpus cavernosum), has been around since 1983. The story of its introduction is interesting as its discovery was pretty much an accident. In 1982, a French surgeon by the name of Ronald Virag, while doing lower limb vascular surgery, injected vasodilators (blood vessel dilators) into the pelvic arteries and the patient obtained an erection. Shortly, thereafter, a British physician by the name of Giles Brindley explored another drug injected directly into the penis; almost simultaneously both of these pioneers in sexual medical research demonstrated that intracavernosal injections may be of benefit to men with erection problems. In 1983, at the National Meeting of the American Urologic Association, Giles Brindley presented his discovery of the erection-produc-

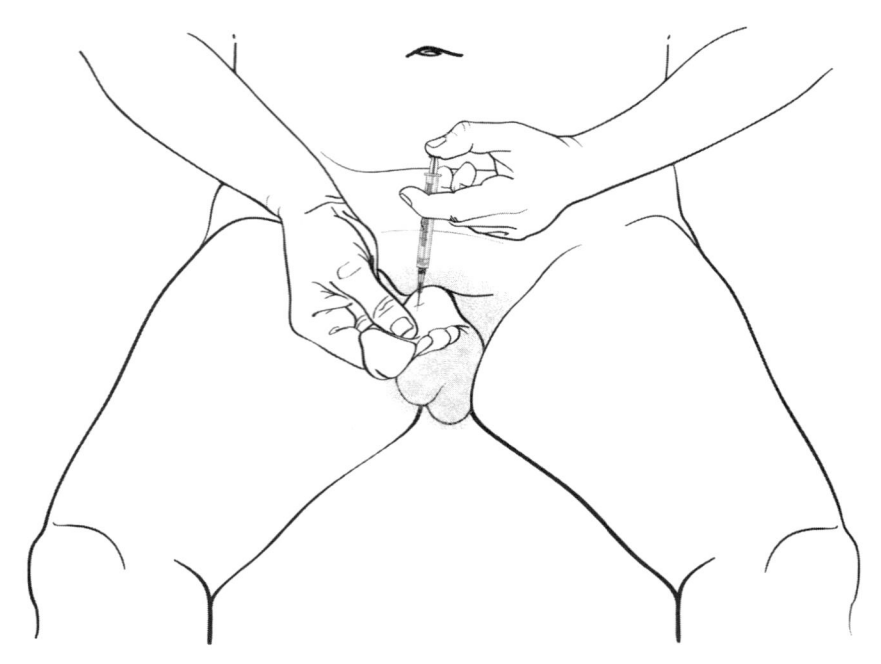

Figure 1 • Illustration of a penile injection being performed

ing potential of a drug called phenoxybenzamine. This drug is no longer used for penile injection. As he presented his data, however, unbeknownst to the audience, he had injected his own penis with phenoxybenzamine prior to his presentation. At the end of his presentation he stood away from the podium, dropped his pants and demonstrated his erect penis for all the audience to see!

Since that time, numerous drugs have been explored for this use, many of which are still in use today. In 1995, Pharmacia (now owned by Pfizer) applied for and received FDA (Food and Drug Administration) approval for their drug, alprostadil, whose trade name is Caverject. Then in Europe, Schwarz Pharma applied for the use of a variant of alprostadil called Edex, and received approval in Europe and subsequently in the United States. These two drugs were the first FDA-approved intracavernosal injection agents. All of the agents that were used prior to that (please see later section for description of the drugs) were not FDA approved. Currently, there is a drug available in Europe (known as Invicorp), but not here yet, that is in trials. One of its touted advantages is the absence of penile pain, which is of importance to those men who have undergone radical prostatectomy (see below).

II. How They Work

Intracavernosal injection therapy delivers vasodilator medication directly into the corpus cavernosum. It is very safe and highly effective. Essentially, this technique applies medication to the erectile tissue and in some respects fools the erectile tissue into believing the erection nerves are fully functional. The chemicals injected work in a variety of ways, all resulting in increased blood flow into the penis. In contrast to oral medications (Viagra and the like), the injection medication requires very little stimulation to achieve full erection. Indeed, it is a true initiator as opposed to the facilitator that pills are.

In the first chapter of this book, I discussed the chemicals required for erection to occur, the most important of which is nitric oxide, which leads to the accumulation of a compound called cyclic GMP (cGMP). A cousin of this agent is cyclic AMP (cAMP). Activation of cAMP also causes erections and that is exactly how alprostadil works. It increases cAMP levels and this leads to smooth muscle relaxation in the penis, which results in erection.

III. Injection Technique

Most side effects and problems that are associated with penile injections can be avoided by thorough education and strict monitoring of the patient. At Memorial Sloan-Kettering Cancer Center, I require two office visits to ensure adequate training of the patient. In a large practice, as I have, the injection training and monitoring is done by a nurse practitioner or nurse who specializes in this form of treatment. The training is provided in two sessions. Firstly, the patient is taught the technical aspects of injection therapy (Figures 1 and 2). While this is not rocket science, our goal is to make sure that he has a good result and does not injure himself. More importantly, however, is that over the course of those two visits, we are trying to determine what dose is safe for the patient to for his first injection at home. I say "safe" because the only real medical problem associated with penile injection therapy is priapism (prolonged erection). If you've been watching TV over the last four years, you may be familiar with the warning during the TV advertisements for erection-inducing pills ("If your erection lasts longer than four hours, you should contact your doctor . . ."). This is priapism (named after the Greek god of lust and fertility, Priapus).

At the first visit, the patient is introduced to the concept of injections by receiving a brief tutorial, with risks, benefits and side effects reviewed, and having a penile injection administered by a sexual medicine clinician. We use a standard starting dose of medication, and the erection hardness and duration of this hardness is monitored and recorded. On the second visit, the patient injects himself under our supervision and the dose he receives depends on what his response was on the first visit. For example, if he had an excellent response of reasonable duration, then he will receive the same dose. If he had an excellent response that is too long in duration, generally more than 60 minutes, then he will receive a smaller dose. In a case where there was an inadequate response, he will receive a larger dose. He is then sent home, a prescription for the medication is organized for him (the medication cannot be purchased at a local pharmacy but is compounded by special pharmacies and shipped to the patient), and over the course of the next two to six injections at home he works very closely with the sexual medicine team to adjust (titrate) the dose to maximize his erectile response.

It is important to understand that close monitoring and dose titration are essential for the safe and effective use of this medication. It is not uncommon for us to see patients trained elsewhere who have never actually been shown how to do injections other than on a model and have been sent home with no instructions regarding duration of erection. I talk in great detail about priapism later in this chapter, but suffice it to say that any penetration-hardness erection lasting longer than two hours is a concern as men experiencing penetration hardness erections of greater than two hours are more likely to eventually experience a full-blown priapism event. Two-hour erections indicate that the patient is on too high a dose of injection medication.

The actual injection process itself is quite simple, easy to learn, and easy to master. The greatest problem for men when they hear about penile injections for the first time is that they imagine this huge needle being used to inject the head of the penis. Penis injections are nothing like a man imagines. Most men experience high anxiety when first introduced to this concept. Interestingly, more than 85% of the patients with whom we discuss penile injection therapy actually choose penile injections, and therefore, you can imagine that it cannot be that bad. Indeed, diabetics who use insulin tell us that injecting their abdomens or thighs with their insulin syringes is identical to the sensation that they experience when they inject their penes. Most men describe it as a "mosquito bite" or like "pulling a hair out of the back of your hand." The syringe that is used is actually an insulin syringe, which is what diabetics use for their insulin injections. There is a 29–gauge needle which is half an inch in length. There is no need to use a larger needle. For example,

PENILE INJECTIONS 145

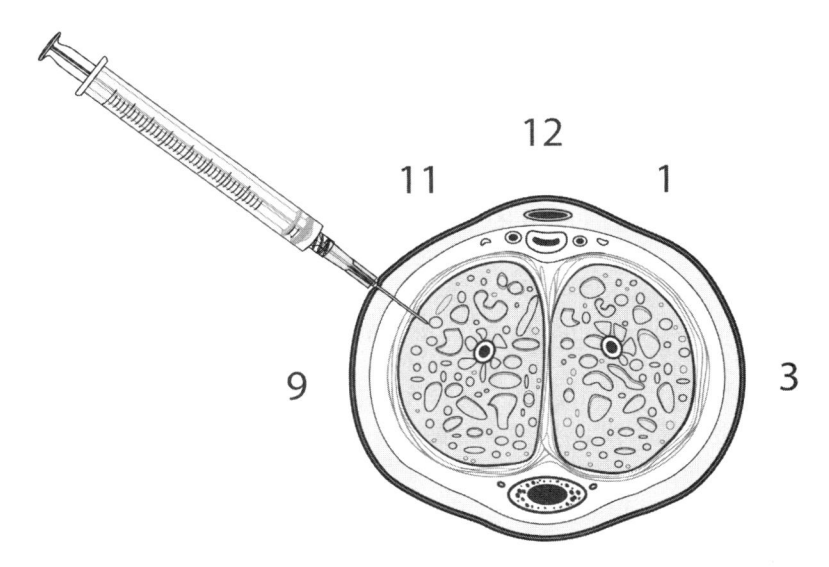

Figure 2 • Diagram illustrating the position and angle of needle placement during penile injection

when you are having blood drawn, it is usually a 20– or 22–gauge needle (the smaller the number, the larger the needle). Likewise, using needles that are smaller than a 29–gauge, for example a 30– or 31–gauge, is associated with potential problems because these needles are very malleable (bendable) and, in fact, can fracture and break off inside the penis. It is interesting to patients that you need to inject only one side of the penis to obtain an erection of the entire penis, and this is because there is communication between the right and left erection chambers (corpora cavernosa). The tissue is termed a syncytium, which essentially means that the electrical impulses pass from one end of the penis on one side to the other end of the penis on the other side in microseconds.

The correct penile injection technique involves a number of key steps. Firstly, the medication needs to be drawn up into the syringe. It is very important that when you are drawing the medication into the syringe that you make sure you are drawing up liquid and not air. The medications I use most frequently are Trimix and Bimix (see later in this chapter), which come in a vial that needs to be stored in the refrigerator. I favor Trimix and Bimix for reasons that I will discuss later.

When you are drawing up medication from a vial, the vial should be held upside-down (Figure 3). A small amount of air is injected into the vial and then, with the tip of the needle below the "water-line," the appropriate dose of medication is drawn up into the syringe. Many physicians use alprostadil either in the form of Caverject or Edex and these syringes come prefilled. The newest version of Caverject, known as Caverject Impulse, allows you to set the dose to be injected by rotating a dial on the syringe. Unfortunately, it is a single-use syringe, and so if you have 20 micrograms in the syringe and you only need 5, then you are wasting 15 micrograms, because the syringe may not be used again.

I recommend to all of our patients that once they are on a stable dose of medication, they make up two or three syringes and leave those ready for use in the refrigerator so that there is not a lot of fumbling around with the medication vial while in the "heat of passion." Once the medication is ready to be used, the cap of the needle is removed and the syringe should be placed on a surface in such a way that the needle does not get dirty before injection. The medication dose is drawn up. For men with impaired vision, a small magnifying reading glass is helpful in making sure the correct dose is drawn up. The penis is then grabbed at its head (the glans) and is stretched with the non-dominant hand. The dominant hand is used to wipe the portion of the penile shaft that is to be injected with an alcohol swab. You do not need to rub this for a prolonged period of time; two or three gentle wipes on the penis will sterilize the area. With the penis in full stretch, the needle is injected in a short, firm stroke directly into the corpus cavernosum so that the entire needle is buried in the skin. Then, and only then, should the plunger be pressed all of the way down. Then the needle should be removed. Using the alcohol swab once again, pressure is applied to the injection site with the thumb of the non-dominant hand and counter pressure is applied to the opposite side of the shaft with the index finger. Pressure should be held for three minutes.

The exception to this is if somebody is on blood thinners, particularly Plavix or Coumadin, I advise patients to hold the pressure for five minutes. Be careful about recapping the needle as you can very easily jab yourself. It is our recommendation that you do not do this, and rather you place the syringe and needle into a household detergent bottle, which cannot be penetrated by a 29–gauge needle. It is worthwhile to check your local city or state regulations with regard to disposal of used needles.

Most men will obtain an erection within five to fifteen minutes. If a man is relaxed, this will happen more rapidly, and if he is nervous it will take a while longer as the adrenaline is fighting against the injection medication.

If men are injecting more than once per week, I recommend that they alternate sides, and when injecting the non-dominant side of their penile shaft, use their non-dominant hand. For example, if you are right-handed and are injecting on the left side using your right hand, there is a higher chance of administering the medication improperly because of poor technique. When practicing using your dominant or non-dominant hand, I recommend a very simple way to perfect your technique: get an orange or a banana, fill your syringe with tap water, and practice injecting with both hands.

For those men who are uncircumcised, it is very important when stretching the penis before injection, that the head of the penis is grabbed and not the foreskin, so you will need to retract the foreskin behind the head, and once you have the penis stretched with your non-dominant hand, then you push the foreskin forward again so that it is not bunched up on the shaft and interfering with identifying the best place for the injection.

Patients are often very concerned about where on the penis the needle is to be injected. The injection is done on one of the least sensitive portions of the penis, the top surface of the middle of the shaft, and this is one reason why this treatment is so well tolerated. I recommend my patients inject in the mid-portion of the penis on the right- or left-hand side. If the penis is thought of as a clock, with 12 o'clock being the top surface as you look down on your penis and 6 o'clock being where the urethra (urine channel) is on the undersurface and 3 and 9 o'clock on the right and left side, respectively, as you look at it, I advise patients to inject at the 2 o'clock or the 10 o'clock position. Once again, you only need to inject one side and should not be injecting both sides in any given session. The needle should be placed at about a 45–degree angle, and, as previously mentioned, the needle should be completely buried before the medication is discharged into the penis. There is some degree of flexibility in where the medication can be injected, but generally speaking, I advise patients to use the mid-portion of the shaft, and should problems arise, other places on the penis can be used for injections.

IV. Medications

I have previously alluded to the fact that there are a number of medications currently available. The most widely used injection agent, in the United States at least, is intracavernosal alprostadil, predominantly in the form of Caverject. The reason that this is used most commonly is that it is readily available, has some insurance coverage, is pre-filled and requires less organization on the physician's behalf. Saying that, it is a medication that works in approximately 60 percent of all men with erectile dysfunction, including prostatectomy and radiation patients. As with any injection medication, this will work better in men who have milder erection problems than those who have severe erection problems.

The standard Caverject doses range from 5 to 20 micrograms and what dose you should be using depends on the rigidity and the duration that you are looking for. I am comfortable with a rigid erection that stays at penetration hardness (6/10 on the hardness scale or harder) for no more than 90 minutes. Most men who are using penile injection therapy are happy with an 80 percent rigid erection that lasts about 30 minutes. The only problem with prostaglandin-containing medications is that a patient who has a cavernous nerve injury, for example, a man after radical prostatectomy or with diabetes, the penis is hypersensitive to prostaglandin. Some of these men complain of penile pain (unrelated to the needle), most of which is mild, but in some circumstances can be severe.

On the other hand, 92 percent of patients in our practice respond to Trimix therapy, so it is easily the most effective medication. It does, however, involve drawing up medication from a vial as opposed to a pre-filled syringe. Trimix contains three drugs: papaverine, phentolamine, and prostaglandin (PGE1). However, the amount of PGE1 (of which alprostadil is a variant) is much lower than that in Caverject, so pain is uncommon. For these two reasons, increased effectiveness and minimal incidence of penile pain, I prefer to use Trimix.

During training with Trimix (or Caverject), if the patient is complaining of any ache or burning sensation in the penis, then he will be switched to Bimix, which is a two-drug mixture containing only papaverine and phentolamine, without the PGE1. There are numerous other medications used outside of the United States, one of which is Invicorp, which is not associated with penile pain after injection. This drug may be useful for the post-prostatectomy patient.

Caverject is covered by some insurance companies, whereas Trimix is rarely covered by insurance. The cost of Trimix, at the time of writing, at the pharmacy Memorial Sloan-Kettering (Bryce Laboratories, Stamford, Connecticut) utilizes is approximately $85 for the vial of medication and shipping. A vial of medication is typically 500 units (5 ml), and this lasts patients anywhere from two to six months depending on the dose they are using and the frequency with which they are using it. Caverject on the other hand, if it is not covered by insurance, is very expensive. Each injection is typically more than $20. The bottom line is that whatever medication works for you and is giving you a satisfactory response is the one you should be using.

V. Side Effects

As I previously stated, if the patient is well trained and closely monitored, then the risk of running into any side effects is incredibly low. I typically see patients approximately three months after they have started injecting and then annually after that. The exceptions to this are men who are enrolled in a penile rehabilitation program post-prostatectomy where they will be seen and on a four-month basis for the first 24 months after surgery, or those enrolled in a penile preservation program after prostate radiation where they are followed every six months for the first three years after radiation is completed. For more details on this, please see Chapter 7.

It is not uncommon to get some bruising on the penis, although if this is more than dime-sized in diameter, then the patient has either not placed enough pressure on the injection site for a long enough period of time (two to five minutes as I mentioned before). It is common for men in the heat of getting ready to make love, to forget to compress, as they are anxious to proceed with sexual relations.

There is much discussion about scarring associated with penile injection, either erection tissue scarring or tunical scarring (remember, the tunica is the outer lining of the erection chamber). Tunical scarring is known as Peyronie's disease (for more details on this problem, please see Chapter 8). I feel comfortable saying that there is no strong evidence to show that penile injections cause any scarring phenomenon in the penis when the injections are used properly. The FDA recommends that penile injections be used no more than three times per week, which is usually more than adequate for the average patient.

Patients ask all the time about the chance of getting infection. In over 12 years of medical practice specializing in sexual medicine, I have never seen a single infection associated with intracavernosal injections. This is likely due to the use of alcohol sterilization of the skin, as well as the tiny size of the needle used. I have mentioned penile pain before, and this is usually related to the PGE1 sensitivity I previously discussed, but it might be due to

> ### CASE HISTORY SIX
> ### Penile Injection Therapy
>
> Klaus is a 65-year-old man with a history of high blood pressure, high cholesterol and coronary artery disease. He had poor erectile function prior to his radical prostatectomy. He commits to penile rehabilitation after his surgery and is using a quarter Viagra pill every night. He fails to obtain a good erection with Viagra 100 mg and because of his prior erectile dysfunction he opts to proceed with penile injection therapy. Within four weeks of starting his penile injections, he is obtaining a 90% erection for 30 minutes with low-dose Trimix. While he has no response to Viagra 100 mg at six months after surgery, by 18 months he is obtaining a penetration-hardness erection with the pill. At 18 months his response is 7/10 and he is using half the initial dose of Tri mix. He is told that he may stop injection therapy now because of his good pill response. However, he opts to continue using penile injections because of its speed, duration and its reliability. He continues to use pills on certain occasions and injections on other occasions over the course of the ensuing two years.
>
> This case history illustrates the acceptability of penile injection therapy to most men. While most men are distressed upon the first mention of penile injections, over the course of time, many of them accommodate and find injection therapy to be an excellent form of treatment. This is because the average erection occurs within five minutes of injection and lasts 30 to 60 minutes. It is also induces an erection with great reliability and therefore gives men a great level of sexual confidence. I have many patients in my practice who are excellent pill responders who still choose to use penile injection therapy, at least intermittently.

Peyronie's disease (especially if the man also complains of penile curvature). If the penile pain is medication-related, the solution is to avoid PGE1–containing medications.

Priapism, an erection lasting longer than four hours, is a true urologic emergency. As interesting as it sounds to patients who have erection problems, it is a lethal and devastating complication, which essentially kills the erectile tissue very much in the same way that a heart attack kills heart muscle. When men have significant bouts of priapism, they are likely to no longer respond to pills or even to injection therapy. Most men who get a significant bout of priapism will require penile implants at some point in their lives. As I mentioned before, priapism can be prevented by excellent education, training, and monitoring of the patient. We have had 11 cases of priapism in the past six years, and nine of these cases happened as a result of poor rule following by patients. The two key situations that can result in priapism are, firstly, when a man injects his penis and does not get an adequate response, then gives himself a second shot; secondly, when a man increases the dose of his injection medication because he wants a more rigid, longer lasting ejection, without clearing this with the sexual medicine staff. Our patients are told that no matter where they are in the country or the world, they are only a phone call away from speaking to one of our sexual medicine experts who can safely tweak the dose to allow them to get the maximum response that is both satisfactory and safe.

Priapism deprives the penis of oxygen and that is, in fact, what kills the erectile tissue. I have previously talked about the importance of oxygen to erectile tissue. Thus, in the properly trained and monitored patient, the chances of experiencing priapism is extremely low. In fact, in our practice it occurs in less than 0.1% of patients. Nevertheless, during injection training, patients are counseled regarding priapism. I tell my patients that if they have a penetration-hardness erection that lasts longer than two hours that they should take Sudafed. They are told to take plain Sudafed and not Sudafed Cold & Sinus or Sudafed Allergy, as the latter medications will cause significant drowsiness. I recommend patients to take 120 milligrams, that is, four 30mg pills at one time. I do not want patients using the 12–hour extended-release Sudafed, as this will not be absorbed rapidly enough. If the Sudafed fails to cause reduction of the erection, I insist that the patient call us at the third hour, no matter where they are in the country or the world and by the fourth hour he should be in an emergency room. If the patient calls us, I will call ahead to the emergency room no matter where that is, and I will talk to the emergency room physician to make sure that the patient is seen promptly, as the longer the priapism lasts the more erection tissue damage occurs.

I actually give our patients a wallet card (see appendix), which describes for the emergency room physician what the patient is using and why he is using it. It also encourages the physician to allow the patient to inject the reversal drug himself. I suggest to the emergency physician that they prepare the reversal drug in the emergency room and then have the patient give himself this injection as its likely the emergency physician has never given a penis injection. The big concern is that the emergency room physician will call the on-call urologist at home. As most priapism typically occurs at 2 o'clock in the morning and it may take the urologist another hour or two to get into the emergency room, this, of course, leads to worsening erectile tissue damage. If the patient experiences priapism, he is not permitted to use another erection-inducing injection until he calls us. If a patient has had to take a dose of Sudafed, this tells us that the dose of medication he is using is too high and needs to be adjusted by us. Thus, I tell our patients "take Sudafed at two hours, call us by three hours and be in the emergency room by four hours." Following these guidelines, it is unlikely patients will ever experience erection damage. Finally, it is important to understand that priapism is only a concern if the erection is at penetration hardness (6/10 or harder), as a 3/10 hardness erection can last many hours without damaging erectile tissue. Only when the penile valve mechanism is closed (this leads to a hard erection) is the penis deprived of oxygen.

VI. Tricks of the Trade

Priapism can be prevented by excellent education and follow-up of the patient. Likewise, the patient has certain responsibilities that we enforce strictly in our program. I do not permit patients to give themselves a second shot within a 24-hour period. We do not permit patients to adjust the medication dose themselves, and insist on them being in contact with the sexual medicine staff to define the best dose. I have patients follow up in the early stages by phone with the one of the members of the sexual medicine team to find the optimal dose, and then in the long term, if patients continue to inject, they need to be seen annually for a penis examination to make sure that there are no side effects from the injections.

Patients are often concerned about traveling with their medication, particularly by air. Caverject can be transported without refrigeration, but Bimix and Trimix I recommend be kept cool. The advice that I give to patients regarding traveling with their syringes and/or their vials of medication has changed with the TSA guidelines for transportation of liquids. Travelling with the vial may result in more rapid deactivation of the drug, so patients are advised to either travel with pre-filled syringes or a smaller (1ml) travel vial of their medication. If travelling with syringes, I recommend that the syringes are placed inside a cigar tube, eyeglass case, or toothbrush holder so that the plunger is not compressed during travel. These containers should

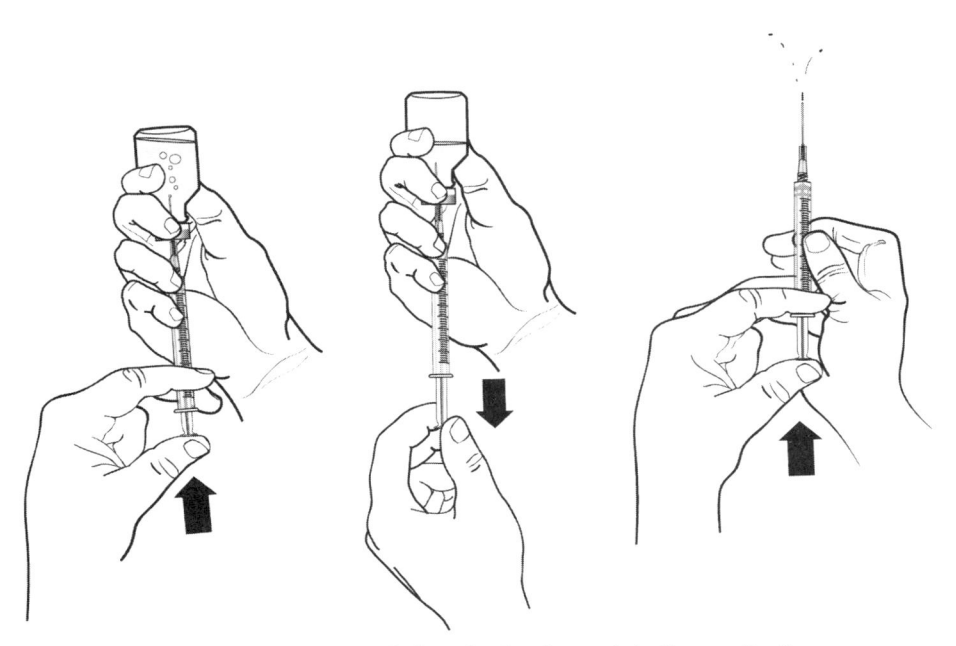

Figure 3 • Diagram illustrating technique for drawing up injection medication (see text)

be placed inside a Ziploc bag, and that Ziploc bag should be placed inside a second Ziploc bag which has refreezable ice packs in it. This can then be placed in a toiletries bag, and with the current security concerns, we recommend that the patient pack that in their checked luggage and not carry it on. It is unclear what the TSA regulations may be in the future, so for further information go to www.tsa.dhs.gov/311.

While penile injections are true initiators of erection, the response can be diminished by high levels of adrenaline. Men have high levels of adrenaline under stress or when anxious or nervous. Sex alone for men with erection problems can become an anxiety-inducing event. Patients are also often anxious in the initial stages thinking about the needle, and some patients are concerned about getting erections that they cannot get rid of (priapism). Thus, minimizing the adrenaline load at the time of the injection is of benefit as it will help maximize the erection response. The effect of adrenaline is to lower the rigidity that occurs with a given dose, and typically speaking, what ends up happening in these men is that once the anxiety-inducing event (the needle) is over with, then the adrenaline level drops and the medication continues to act for a long period of time. The average man, as

I said before, gets an 80 percent rigid erection for about 30 minutes, but for someone with high levels of adrenaline, it is very common to get only a 60 percent rigid erection and this can last for an hour or an hour and a half. So besides paying attention to technique, paying attention to the level of anxiety is also important.

It is important for those of you who have had radical prostatectomy to understand that penile injections are very effective and are used routinely by us in our penile rehabilitation program, but it is likely over the course of the first 18 months that you will need to drop the dose of the injection medication. More than 70 percent of our patients decrease the dose of their injection medication over the course of the first year and a half after surgery. The reason for this is very simple. This is the time frame over which the nerves start recuperating, and as the nerves recuperate, you need less medication to get the same response. Patients typically get a sense that the dose should be decreased, as the duration of the erection increases. A man who is getting an 80 percent rigid erection for 30 minutes will notice, predictably in the second year if he is still using injections, that he will get a 45- and then a 60-minute erection in response to the same dose. Patients are instructed that they may decrease the dose of the medication without checking with us, but they may never increase without talking to us by phone.

In summary, penile injection therapy is effective, is safe when the patient is properly trained and monitored, and is a very useful weapon in our arsenal for the treatment of men with erection problems who are not responding to pills. It is likely that we will have new injection agents in the future (please see Chapter 14), but their arrival is at least 5 to 10 years down the road.

APPENDIX 1
Penile Injection Training: What to Expect

These are the steps that we use in our injection-training program, which is one of the largest in the world. These are excellent guidelines for all physicians who conduct penile injection training, but your local physician may do this slightly differently.

Session #1:
1. You will be escorted to a room.
2. The procedure will be explained to you.
3. Written consent will be obtained from you.
4. You will be asked if you would like to empty your bladder prior to undressing.
5. You will have your blood pressure measured.
6. You will be instructed to undress from the waist down and provided with a hospital gown.
7. You will be asked to sit on the exam table.
8. You will be instructed how to swab the top of the medication vial with alcohol prior to each use.
9. You will learn how to carefully remove the cap from the needle end of the syringe and to take care not to contaminate the needle.
10. You will be shown how to inject a small amount of air into the vial of medication and then invert the vial and withdraw the prescribed amount of medication into the syringe.
11. You will be instructed to gently grasp the head of the penis with the index finger and thumb and pull it straight out.
12. The nurse practitioner will select an injection site at the 10 o'clock or 2 o'clock position in the middle portion of the shaft (avoiding visible veins) and will swab the area with the alcohol wipe.
13. The nurse practitioner will insert the needle as far as it will go and will then inject the medication.
14. The needle will be quickly removed and pressure will be applied to the injection site for two to three minutes.
15. You will be given 10 to 15 minutes of privacy.

continued on the next page

continued from the previous page

16. You may be provided with some adult literature or a DVD to increase arousal.
17. Self-stimulation is encouraged.
18. The peak hardness and the duration at or greater than penetration hardness will be recorded by the nurse practitioner.
19. You will instructed to remain in the physician's office until your erection has subsided below penetration hardness.
20. You may not leave the physician's office with a penetration-hardness erection.
21. You will be provided written instructions regarding what steps to take in the event that priapism (prolonged erection) should occur.

Session #2:

1. The key points from session #1 will be reviewed.
2. The dose of medication used in this session will depend directly on how well you responded during the first session.
3. Under guidance, this time, you will administer the medication as was performed in session #1.
4. You will again be given 10 to 15 minutes of privacy, may be given literature/DVD and self-stimulation is encouraged.
5. Steps 18 to 21 from session #1 will be repeated.
6. If you have demonstrated good aseptic technique in preparing and administering the injection, you will have a prescription organized for medication. The dose you will be started on will depend on how your responded during the second session.
7. The patient is reminded again regarding what steps need to be taken in the event of the occurrence of priapism.
8. You will be instructed to call the physician's office within 24 hours of your injection to report on the hardness and duration of the erection.

APPENDIX 2
Wallet Card for Patients Using Penile Injections

Please show this to your physician or emergency department staff
- The person carrying this card is under the care of _____ for erectile problems.
- The patient is using intracavernosal (penile) injections for his erectile dysfunction.
- The patient has been instructed to be in the emergency department if his erection stays at penetration hardness for 4 hours.
- The patient has been instructed to call _____ staff prior to arriving in the emergency department.
- Erections lasting longer than 4 hours (priapism) are associated with permanent erection tissue damage and this condition constitutes a medical emergency.
- This condition should be treated with the same urgency that you would treat a testicular torsion or a myocardial infarction.
- Failure to deliver appropriate timely care may result in permanent untreatable erectile dysfunction for the patient.
- Most men with priapism lasting less than 6 hours require only the intracavernosal (intrapenile) administration of phenylephrine (Neosynephrine) to achieve detumescence. This agent is not available outside of the United States, so another alpha-adrenergic agonist should be used if not in the United States.
- Upon arrival in the emergency department, the patient should be assessed immediately by the emergency physician and a call placed to the on-call urologist.

continued on the next page

continued from the previous page

- Intracavernosal neosynephrine may be administered by the emergency physician if he/she is familiar with this technique. Alternatively, if the emergency physician is not familiar with the technique of intracavernosal injection and the on-call urologist is not immediately available, the patient himself is capable of administering the injection, provided the physician/nursing staff provide him with the syringe (27- to 29-gauge needle) and medication. We advise that the patient be placed on a cardiac monitor and a continuous blood pressure monitor during neosynephrine administration.
- Neosynephrine usually comes as 10,000 mcg/ml solution. This solution should be mixed with 9 ml of injectable saline to make a 1,000 mcg/ml solution. An initial dose of 500 mcg should be administered. 10 minutes later, if detumescence has not occurred, another 500 mcg should be administered.
- The inability to use this medication or failure of the medication will result in the patient requiring corporal aspiration of blood to achieve detumescence. This should be performed by a urologist.
- The most concerning side effect of this medication is hypertension with reflex bradycardia. This agent is contraindicated in men with a history of profound (malignant) hypertension or who are using (or have used in the recent past) monoamine oxidase inhibitors.
- Rarely, a patient may need to be brought to the operating room for performance of a "shunt" to achieve detumescence. Timely treatment generally prevents the need for this.
- We ask that a call be placed to the prescribing doctor's answering service when the patient has been seen by the emergency physician.

CHAPTER 12

VACUUM DEVICES

> I. How Do They Work?
> II. Advantages
> III. Disadvantages

I. How Do They Work?

Vacuum erection devices, also known as vacuum constriction devices, have been used for improving erectile function for more than a century. From a historical perspective, vacuum devices were first described in 1874 by Dr. John King. He stated, "When there is impotency with diminution of the size of the male organ, the glass exhauster should be applied to the part." In 1917, Dr. Otto Lederer developed a surgical device to produce erections with a vacuum and first applied constriction rings for maintenance of the erection. In the 1960s, Geddings Osborn developed his version of the vacuum device, which he called the "youth equivalent device" and became commercially available in 1974. Of note, sales of this device were banned by the United States Postal Service and the FDA withdrew its approval in 1976. It was reapproved in 1982 and has since then gone on to be a routine form of treatment in the management of erectile dysfunction. However, the introduction of oral agents for ED has significantly decreased the use of these devices for ED.

There are a number of medical equipment companies that have specially designed and FDA-approved devices (Figure 1). These approved devices are carefully constructed so that a limited amount of pressure is allowed to develop. The principle involves the use of negative pressure applied to the penis, specifically the erectile bodies (corpora cavernosa), which results in inflow of blood into the erection chambers and erection ensues. The constriction band is applied to the base of the penile shaft to reduce blood flow draining out of the penis to promote maintenance of erection. The system involves a cylinder, a vacuum pump, and a constriction ring. The cylinder and constriction rings vary greatly between the various companies; however, they all function very similarly. I favor the battery-operated versions, which can be used in a one-handed fashion, as opposed to the manual pump, which requires two hands: one for stabilizing the cylinder on the penis and the other for pumping the device.

FDA-approved devices have pressure pop-off valves to reduce the likelihood of pressure induced penile injury. The pressure that is permitted is approximately 200 to 250 mmHg. In contrast, there are devices, available over the internet, through mail order, or in sex shops, known as "penis developers," which have not been tested and can expose the penis to pressures well in excess of the above figure. It is important for physicians and patients to be aware that these instruments are potentially dangerous and have no FDA approval, much in the same way that nutriceuticals (over-the-counter sexual health supplements) have no FDA approval.

I give the patient a prescription for the device, which he can pick up at his local pharmacy or order directly from one of the companies that manufacture FDA-approved devices. If the patient has difficulty or fails to obtain a usable erection, he returns to the office for a training session where my nurse practitioner goes over the key points in getting the best out of the vacuum device. It takes anywhere from two to 10 minutes to obtain a functional erection, and our experience indicates that it takes approximately four attempts at using the vacuum device before patients become proficient with the technique (see Appendix).

Prior to using the device, it is important to understand that the penis after vacuum device use is hard beyond the point of the constriction band but soft behind it; therefore, it is important to place the constriction band as close to the base of the penis as possible. Behind the constriction band, the penis is soft and somewhat unstable, and therefore, if the constriction band is placed on the shaft of the penis, this will result in a hinge effect and the penis

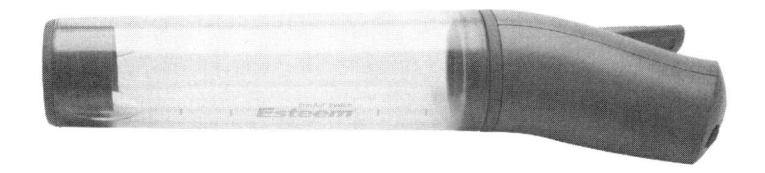

Figure 1 • Photograph of one type of vacuum device. The cylinder displayed is a one-hand operated version.

will buckle during attempts at penetration. It is estimated that 75% of men achieve adequate rigidity, allowing them to obtain vaginal penetration. To the best of my knowledge, there is no literature on the use of vacuum devices in gay men, so what proportion of those men who use vacuum devices are able to obtain a penetration-hardness erection is not well known, although I have gay patients who have used them successfully. Another point of importance is that to achieve a negative pressure using a vacuum device, a tight seal must be achieved at the base of the penis (at the open end of the device). To accomplish this, gel needs to be applied around the open end and some men will need to trim the pubic hair to maximize this seal.

The vacuum device is indicated for men with erectile dysfunction. There are no specific conditions that would interfere with the use of these devices. However, there are certain groups of men who should probably avoid the use of vacuum devices: 1) men using blood thinners (Coumadin, Plavix) or have a history of bleeding disorders, 2) men with diminished penile sensation, 3) men who have significant penile curvature, 4) men with a history of priapism (prolonged erection) or who are at risk for its development, and 5) men with spinal cord injury.

Blood thinning medications may cause the patient to develop bruising and swelling of the penis due to rupture of the superficial veins in the shaft of the penis, which is in turn, due to pressure from the constriction ring. In the patient who is not on blood thinners, this trauma is uncommon, and if it occurs, usually resolves on its own. In an anticoagulated man, this bleeding can result in a blood collection under the skin (hematoma), which is not only unsightly, but will cause significant discomfort. Given this, we avoid the use of vacuum devices for patients who are on anticoagulants. We have never experienced any such problems in men using aspirin alone. Likewise, patients with a history of bleeding disorders should be directed toward other treatments. Patients who have reduced sensation in the penis, especially a man with spinal cord injury, are at risk for skin injury with repeated use of the constriction band. The band may cause ulcers on the skin because these patients cannot sense the trauma. In general, constriction bands should be used with extreme caution in all patients and should be applied for only a very short period of time (usually no longer than 30 minutes).

There is controversy as to whether men with Peyronie's disease (acquired penile curvature) or penile curvature that is congenital (from birth) in nature should be allowed to use a vacuum device as the straight cylinder may exert significant stress on the curved penis, potentially resulting in trauma to the already bent shaft of the penis. We discuss this with the individual with Peyronie's disease and if the patient is motivated to use this device, we permit it, but monitor the patient very closely. Other than these groups of men, there is no restriction to the use of the vacuum device in men post-prostatectomy or who have had radiation therapy for prostate cancer or are on hormone therapy.

II. Advantages

It is estimated that somewhere between 80 to 90% of men can obtain a successful erection with the vacuum device. In fact, studies have shown that it is possible to obtain 80% rigidity with the use of such devices. The overall patient satisfaction rate cited in the medical literature is somewhere between 60 to 80%. However, it is my experience that for young to middle-aged men with a reasonable frequency of sexual relations, there is very poor compliance, that is, long-term usage of the device. There is no doubt, however, for those patients who take to this technique, that significant improvement in erection quality, frequency of intercourse, frequency of orgasm, and sexual satisfaction can be achieved. As previously mentioned, for a man with ED, improvement in his erectile function will likely translate into improvement in sexual satisfaction, not for just him but also for his partner. The biggest advantage of the vacuum device is that it is a simple and safe form of treatment. It also typically receives good insurance coverage, and, most importantly, it is totally reversible. If the patient does not wish to continue with this therapy, it is easily stopped and if it was used in a proper fashion, no long-term negative effects will have occurred.

There is great interest in the use of vacuum devices currently for penile rehabilitation post radical prostatectomy. At this point, however, there is no animal evidence and little human evidence that there is any real advantage

VACUUM DEVICES

from a penile rehabilitation standpoint. It is worth remembering that we believe that delivery of increased levels of oxygen to the penis (cavernosal oxygenation) is required for rehabilitation. What is interesting is that the vacuum device typically increases the oxygen content within the penis only minimally, as approximately 50% of the blood that is brought into the penis with the use of the vacuum device is arterial (high level of oxygen) and 50% is venous (low oxygen level) in nature. Furthermore, when the constriction ring is applied to the penis, the oxygen level drops further. Thus, if you believe that penile rehabilitation revolves around cavernosal oxygenation, the vacuum device is not likely to play any significant role based on the evidence available at this point in time.

However, might there be some intrinsic value to stretching of the penis? This is possible, and this is why we need large studies looking at the use of the device in the radical prostatectomy population. A couple of reports in the medical literature, which are heavily flawed, suggest that the vacuum device after radical prostatectomy translates into improved erectile function. It is difficult to decipher from these studies whether there is a significant effect or not. In my practice, as previously mentioned, penile rehabilitation revolves around two strategies: the regular use of PDE5 inhibitors (Viagra, Levitra, Cialis) alternating with the generation of erections, which for most men in the early stages after surgery requires penile injections. We discourage patients from using vacuum devices as monotherapy (single therapy), but if somebody is enthusiastic to use these devices, he is permitted to use them as the third arm in a multimodal strategy (pills, shots, and vacuum device). If a man is going to use it, we suggest he use it for 15 minutes at least once a day without the use of the constriction band. Remember that our patients use Viagra, for example, nightly at bedtime, and then two to three times a week, they are instructed to use injections for the purpose of erections. So adding the use of the vacuum device on top of these is somewhat burdensome for patients.

III. Disadvantages

Probably the most significant disadvantage of the device is that it generates a non-cosmetic erection. By this I mean that the penis, particularly in a Caucasian male, does not appear pink or red; in fact, it tends to be blue or grey. This is because the blood that is passing into the penis is largely venous and therefore carries very low levels of oxygen. This is cosmetically a turn-off for some men and for some partners. Furthermore, because the blood is not arterial, it has a lower temperature (it is about 1 to 2 degrees lower than the rest of the body), so one of the most common complaints of partners is that the penis feels cool to touch and upon penetration. The use of the vacuum device results in swelling of the veins underneath the skin, and so there is what appear to be varicose veins on the penis when the device is applied.

The second potential problem is many men will require a very tight constriction band to maintain blood within the corporal bodies and this translates into discomfort and in some men causes significant penile pain. In the very rare case, the constriction band is so tight that it can cause an injury to the penile sensation nerves and temporary penile numbness may occur while the band is in place.

Thirdly, when traveling, the device (bands and gel) need to be transported with you. So it is not exactly discreet. For the single man, concealing this from his partner may be a challenge. Finally, the continued use of any treatment for ED (pills, shots, or devices) revolves around the integratability of the treatment. Essentially, this means how easy the treatment is to integrate into a couple's sex life. This is a complex issue with many factors impacting it, such as how good an erection is achieved, how quickly the erection occurs, how long it lasts, and how natural the erection is, among others. The erection with a vacuum device is not fully rigid, looks different in Caucasians, and takes 10 to 20 minutes to generate. So, many users find it somewhat difficult to integrate into their sexual relations and it is my experience that, in other than elderly patients, the long-term use is poor.

VACUUM DEVICES

APPENDIX
How to Use Your Vacuum Device

1. Urinate.
2. Stand.
3. Ensure there is not too much hair around the base of your penis.
4. Apply enough gel around the base of your penis to ensure a seal.
5. Place the constriction band that you will be using over the cylinder about 2 inches from the open end.
6. Place the cylinder over the penis.
7. Push the cylinder firmly against the pubic bone.
8. Activate the device (with the button if it is battery-operated or the separate hand-pump if it is a manual device) until you are about 50% hard, and release some of the pressure by pressing on the valve. Then re-activate and pump some more. Deflate a little. Perform this "double-pumping" for a few minutes until you get a rigid erection.
9. Slide the constriction band down the cylinder over the base of the penis as close to the body as possible.
10. Remove the cylinder.
11. Now you should have an erection sufficient for intercourse.
12. Remove the constriction band within 30 minutes.

CHAPTER 13

PENILE IMPLANTS

> I. Historical Perspective
> II. Who Are Candidates for Penile Implant Surgery?
> III. Device Types
> IV. Device Selection
> V. Surgical Technique
> VI. Complications
> VII. Summary

I. Historical Perspective

Up until the late 1960s/early 1970s, it was felt that most of the causes of erectile problems were psychological. This was related in large part to a lack of understanding of the physiology and pathophysiology of erectile dysfunction. Since that time, an explosion in our understanding of these factors has led us to a better sense of appropriate treatment of individual patients. Penile implants (also known in the medical field as penile prostheses) have been around since the 1950s, when very primitive implants were used. Plastic rods were placed under the skin of the penis outside of the erection chambers, and one can imagine how poor the function of these devices was as well as the artificial appearance of the erection. It was not until the early 1970s when pioneers such as F. Brantley Scott and William Furlow introduced the concept of the inflatable penile prosthesis. Since that time, these devices have undergone significant change and modifications. Currently, penile implant surgery is recognized as a third-line treatment (first-line treatment being pills, reversal of medical conditions associated with erectile dysfunction, and psychological counseling, and second-line treatment being intracavernosal injections, transurethral suppositories and vacuum erection devices). Penile implants have some distinct advantages and some definite disadvantages.

On the advantage side, it generates a 100% rigid erection. All of the inflatable (pump up/pump down) implants give a fully rigid erection. It also takes somewhere between five to 15 seconds to generate the erection. Furthermore, based on medical literature, penile implants have the highest satisfaction of any treatment that we use for men with erection problems, for both the man and his partner. This is almost certainly related to the speed and rigidity that one can get with an implant.

On the disadvantage side, it involves an operation; therefore, it is more invasive than pills or injections. We will describe the surgical technique and pre- and postoperative care later. However, the average man will experience anywhere from one to three weeks of pain, bruising and swelling after the surgery. Most men tolerate the procedure very well, and I tell my patients that the most important predictor of postoperative pain control is the patient's personality. Usually the patient's partner will know best whether the man has a "high" or "not so high" pain tolerance.

It is associated with complications, the two most significant of which are infection, which occurs in about 2 to 3% of patients, and mechanical breakdown, which occurs in about 15% of patients over the course of the first ten years or so after the original operation. I tell patients that 10 years after surgery, one has about an 85% chance of having the same implant as day one and a 97% chance of not having had an implant infection.

A number of modifications have occurred over the course of the three decades since implants have been available commercially. There have been tremendous advances in biomaterial sciences, such that the material that is used today is both supple and has incredible strength. There are a number of devices, but the majority of devices use either silicone or polymers such as Bioflex (which is a polyurethane polymer). These materials allow rapid and repeated expansion and deflation of the cylinders without significant injury to the device wall. Modification to the tubing has also occurred, which again increases the reliability and survival of the implant.

Currently, there are two major companies involved in manufacturing penile implants (Figures 1 to 3): Coloplast, which has a series of three-piece implants (I will explain this in greater detail later), and AMS (which stands for American Medical Systems), which has both a two-piece device and a series of three-piece devices. The AMS cylinders are made of silicone, while the Coloplast cylinders are made of Bioflex. One of the problems with silicone is, over the course of time, with inflation and deflation of the cylinder, the silicone may crack, causing device breakdown. Another potential problem with the older silicone devices was that after repeated inflation, the cylinders were known to undergo a ballooning (like a bubble on a bicycle tire). To this end, a couple of modifications have occurred in the AMS devices to prevent both of these problems, primarily the introduction of a three-layered device, with the middle layer being a synthetic material which prevents over-inflation of the cylinder. Thus, the AMS three-piece devices are considered "controlled expansion" devices. Cylinders are also now lined by a special coating called Parylene, which adds further strength and mechanical reliability to the device.

Another modification is the introduction of a lock-out valve. I will explain later in this chapter what auto-inflation is. In short, it is when the device inflates of its own accord without it being activated by the patient. This is usually due to excess pressure being placed on the reservoir and saline being forced into the cylinders. The way to prevent this is to have a lock-out valve. Coloplast have devices with the lock-out valve on the reservoir and the three-piece AMS devices have a lock-out valve on the pump. These innovations have reduced significantly the incidence of troublesome auto-inflation.

The next modification in chronological order has been the introduction of antibacterial coating. The AMS three-piece devices are coated with a combination of two antibiotics (rifampin and minocycline) which, over the course of the first few days after implant surgery, leak into the tissue around the cylinder. The Coloplast device has an anti-adherence coating, which, when the device is soaked in antibiotic solution at the time of surgery, absorbs the antibiotic solution, and again leaks this over the course of the first few days after surgery. I will discuss penile implant infection in far greater detail later in this chapter; however, there is some evidence to suggest

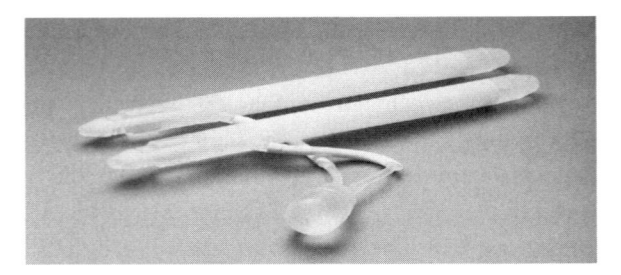

Figure 1 • Ambicor™ two piece penile implant

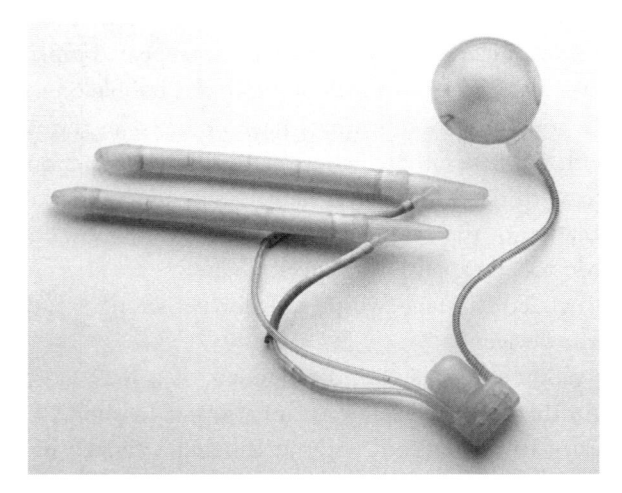

Figure 2 • Antibiotic coated AMS 700 CX three piece penile implant (Inhibizone)

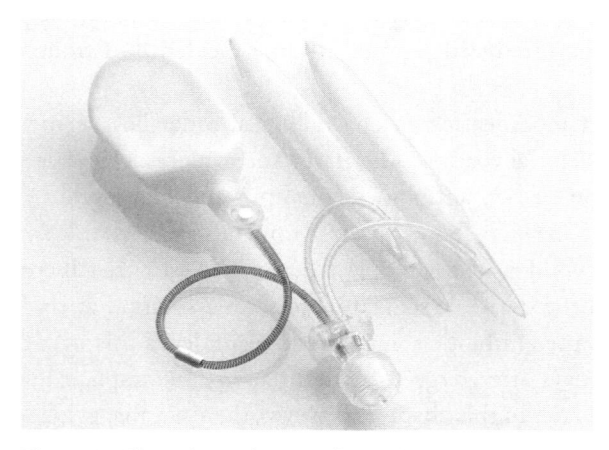

Figure 3 • Titan three piece penile implant

that both of these innovations have led to a slight reduction in the incidence of implant infection.

The final innovation still being developed by both companies is ongoing and involves changes in the pump mechanism. The pump on the three-piece device is a complex one in that it acts as both the inflation and deflation mechanism, and this is sometimes a source of concern for the patients in terms of learning. The pumps today are far easier to use than they were two decades ago, and further refinements are expected in the near future.

II. Who Are Candidates for Penile Implant Surgery?

As I mentioned previously, penile implant surgery is a third-line treatment, and therefore, in my practice, patients undergoing penile implant surgery have failed pills (Viagra, Lavitra, Cialis) or have responded but have experienced significant side effects that have caused the patient to stop using the pills. The most common side effects that cause drop-out and discontinuation of Viagra and Levitra are headache, nasal congestion, heartburn, and facial flushing. In my practice of Cialis users, drop-out for side effects occurs most commonly because of headache or muscle aches (mylagia).

All implant patients have previously been counseled about intracavernosal penile injection therapy, and the vast majority of our patients who undergo implant surgery have failed to respond to penile injection therapy. I encourage all of my patients to at least try one penile injection before making a decision regarding moving from pills directly to penile implant surgery. I dislike my patients basing their decisions about injection therapy on mental imagery (the needle and penis concept), which of course is a negative mental image. I would much prefer the patient to experience what the injection feels like, and the vast majority of patients, when they try penile injections, tolerate it very well. However, in my practice, something in the range of 10% of our patients will fail to respond to injection therapy and these are the patients who are the ideal candidates for implant surgery. The overwhelming majority of patients who fail injection therapy have a condition called venous leak. We have described venous leak in great detail in previous chapters. As I mentioned previously, the penis gets erect through a simple hydraulic mechanism. Just like a bicycle tire, there is a hose (actually there are two hoses) and a valve. The two hoses are the erection arteries (cavernosal arteries) and these carry blood into the right and left erectile bodies (corpus cavernosam). The valve mechanism allows the blood to be trapped in the penis so that good rigidity can be generated as well as maintained for a sufficient period of time for intercourse to happen. The valve mechanism is dependent on the health of the erectile tissue, the smooth muscle that I talked about previously. When the smooth muscle undergoes scarring (fibrosis), the valve becomes leaky and this is venous leak. The most common causes of venous leak include diabetes, radical prostatectomy surgery, and prostate radiation. Thus, the majority of patients who undergo penile implant surgery in my practice either have diabetes with subsequent erectile dysfunction, or have had radical prostatectomy or prostate radiation for prostate cancer management.

There is much discussion about the ideal timing of penile implant surgery after radical prostatectomy surgery. To the patient who had good erectile function before surgery, had reasonable nerve sparing, commits to penile rehabilitation, and has a significant chance of recovery either of his natural erections or at least a pill response, we would wait at least 12, if not 18 months, after surgery to see if he is going to recover natural erections. There are patients who develop venous leak within the first 12 months after surgery. Although this is not common, these patients would move directly to a penile implant discussion.

There are surgeons, sadly, who try to convince patients to have penile implant surgery in the first six months after surgery, essentially preventing them from ever gaining natural erections or becoming a pill responder. The argument that many of these surgeons use to encourage patients to proceed with implant surgery at such an early time is the prevention of penile length loss. I previously talked about penis length loss in Chapter 12 and I mentioned that this was related to erection tissue damage. So the patients who are most likely to have penile length loss are the patients who have venous leak and those most likely to be undergoing penile implant surgery. However, if a patient commits to penile rehabilitation and has had reasonable nerve sparing surgery, the chance of penile length loss may be lower, which goes against the argument for early implant surgery. Those patients in my practice who end up getting early (in the first 12 months) penile implant surgery have typically had very poor erectile function before their radical prostatectomy and have failed at least pills if not injection therapy before surgery.

While not commonly performed, there are some men who have such poor erectile function before surgery and have failed all medical treatments, who are candidates for simultaneous radical prostatectomy and penile implant insertion. While there is very little medical literature on the advisability of this, there is a small amount of evidence that would suggest that there is no higher incidence of penile implant infection or excessive bleeding for this simultaneous approach, and therefore, is believed to be a safe option. In my practice, when such a patient sees me and has been educated how to use pills and has clearly failed them and has failed injection therapy, we will insert the reservoir of a three-piece device in the pelvis at the time of the radical prostatectomy, but we will not place any cylinders or scrotal pump at that time. If the patient wishes to have a two-piece device, then this will be postponed until at least three months after his radical prostatectomy. This is because the most challenging part of the implant operation after radical prostatectomy surgery is placement of the reservoir. Once the reservoir is placed at the time of the radical prostatectomy, cylinder placement is easily accomplished a few months later. There is only a single medical paper addressing simultaneous placement of the penile implant and prostatectomy. While there appeared to be no higher incidence of implant infection, infection is of such concern that, in my opinion, leaving the cylinder placement until after the patient has recovered from his radical prostatectomy is a good idea. Furthermore, most men are not going to be interested in sexual intercourse in the first couple of months after radical prostatectomy.

One of the other causes of erection tissue damage that results in venous leak is the use of long-term hormone therapy (Lupron or Zoladex), the medications used for high-risk prostate cancer or metastatic prostate cancer. These drugs, when used for longer than six months, are notoriously associated with erection tissue damage, and thus, many of these patients will be required to consider penile implant surgery. Go back to Chapter 8 for a refresher on hormone therapy for prostate cancer.

Given that the profile of erectile dysfunction development after radiation therapy is different; that is, it is slow in onset (it may take up to five years for the patient to get to the low point in his erection function), penile implant surgery is used as it would be for any other patient, such as a diabetic who has not had radical prostatectomy. Firstly, the patient is treated with pills, and if pills are giving a less than satisfactory response or associated with significant side effects, the patient is moved to penile injection therapy or urethral suppositories, and if he fails these or finds these unpalatable, then penile implant surgery is discussed.

III. Device Types

Penile prostheses are generally of two types, malleable (also known as semi-rigid, or non-inflatable) and inflatable devices. The malleable devices have an outer coating with a central core of metal or plastic. These implants are paired solid devices implanted in the erectile bodies, and produce constant penile rigidity. The primary advantage of these devices is the ease of implantation, while the disadvantages include a constantly rigid penis that does not look normal in the flaccid or erect state. There is some difficulty with concealment and an increased risk for device erosion because of constant pressure. These devices have fallen out of favor as the modern inflatable devices are so reliable and better cosmetically. The surgeons most likely to use malleable devices are those that do only a few implants a year.

There are three malleable devices made by three different companies: American Medical Systems (the AMS 650), Coloplast (Acu-Form device) and TIMM Medical Technologies (Dura-II device). I have limited contemporary experience with these malleable devices as the vast majority of our patients undergoing implant surgery receive an inflatable device.

Inflatable devices are of two varieties: a two-piece and a three-piece. As previously mentioned, the only two-piece available is made by AMS (the Ambicor) and this company has a series of three-piece devices. Coloplast has a series of three-piece devices. Each company has a standard implant cylinder as well as a narrow base cylinder which is used for men with short and/or narrow penises, and particularly in patients who have tremendous amounts of erection tissue scarring so a narrower device is required. AMS has a third device which is known as the Ultrex device, which expands in length (all other devices do NOT expand in length), although this device is not widely used, and it is not clear from the medical literature how much length increase men actually gain from using this device.

The Ambicor two-piece device consists of paired cylinders which are pre-connected to a pump (Figure 1). Each cylinder is placed into each corporal body (corpus cavernosum) and the pump is placed into the scrotum between the two testicles. When a man is ready to attain an erection, he squeezes on this pump and this inflates the device. Because there is no reservoir of saline, the device is prefilled with saline and most of the saline is maintained inside the back portion of the cylinders, that is, the portion that is not actually inside the external penis. When the pump is activated, the fluid is transferred from the back portion into the front portion of the device and gives a rigid erection. Because the device does not have a reservoir, not all of the fluid can be stored in the back portion of the cylinder and, therefore, some fluid will always be left in the front portion. For this reason I tell my patients that using a 10–point hardness scale, where 10 is fully rigid, 6 just about good enough for penetration, and 0 completely soft, most patients will have a 3/10 with the Ambicor device in the deflated state, and that it will be, as with a three-piece, 10/10 when inflated. The big advantage of the two-piece device for some men is its ease of use. It is inflated by squeezing on the pump, but is deflated by simply bending the device at the junction of the penis and the scrotum. This activates the valve and fluid rushes from the front portion to the back portion of the cylinder. Thus, for men with poor manual dexterity, this is an excellent device.

Three-piece inflatable implants have paired cylinders, a small scrotal pump, and a large-volume fluid reservoir (Figures 2 and 3). The pump is placed in an identical position to the two-piece, that is, inside the scrotum between the testicles. Patients are often concerned that they will not be able to identify the pump between the testicles, but this, in my experience, is never the case. The pump is usually firmer than the testicles and usually quite a bit smaller and easily felt inside the scrotum. The three-piece devices have two cylinders, just as the two-piece does, although because there is a reservoir, these cylinders, when deflated, can empty completely, and therefore, a man may have a completely flaccid penis in the deactivated state. The difference between the two- and three-piece is that the three-piece device has a reservoir. This reservoir is usually placed behind the pubic bone through the hernia ring on either the right- or left-hand side. Approximately 90% of all penile implants that I perform use a three-piece device, while 10% are two-piece, and I will explain later in this chapter which patient gets which device.

IV. Device Selection

The ideal penile prosthesis will enable a man to control when he has an erection and will allow penile flaccidity and an erection that approximates as closely as possible a natural erection. To achieve these goals, fluid must be transferred into the expandable cylinders for erection and back out of the cylinders for flaccidity. I routinely use the Coloplast three-piece inflatable prosthesis, but that is not to say that surgeons who use the AMS device are wrong.

Indeed, there is likely no significant difference between these two in infection, mechanical reliability, ease of use, cosmetics, or patient satisfaction.

There are a number of populations in which we consider using a two-piece device. By the way, all of my patients before implant surgery do three things. Firstly, they get our reading material which does not just have product brochures, but also has a run down of potential complications (see Appendix) as well as medical literature on penile implant surgery. Secondly, they see watch the two- and three-piece implant videos so that they can make an informed decisions regarding which device they feel is most appropriate for themselves. Thirdly, I encourage all of my patients to speak to one of my patients who has previously undergone penile implant surgery so they can get a clear idea what to expect before and after the operation.

There are six populations in whom we consider two-piece implants: (1) Patients who have had radical cystectomy surgery (bladder removal for bladder cancer), and this is due to the fact that the space behind the pubic bone is disrupted at the time of surgery and, therefore, the reservoir may come in contact with bowel. It is probably a theoretical concern that this reservoir can erode into bowel and there are many centers in the country that routinely use three-piece devices for such a patient population. (2) Patients who have had kidney transplant surgery or may receive a kidney transplant in the future. Because the kidney transplant is placed down in the pelvis, we are concerned about placing a reservoir too close to the site where the transplant is or will be in the future. (3) Certain patients who have had radical prostatectomy. In our experience, approximately 10% of radical prostatectomy patients present great difficulty in permitting the placement of a reservoir in a proper location, because of scarring of the usual reservoir space after radical prostatectomy. When this occurs, there are two options. One is to place a two-piece device, and the other is to make an incision on the abdomen and place the reservoir inside the belly, not in its usual position. It is important to understand that failure to make an adequate space for the reservoir will result in auto-inflation. (4) Likewise, patients who have had bilateral inguinal hernia surgery, especially where mesh has been used. This will make it very difficult, if not impossible, to place a reservoir in the usual fashion and, just like the radical prostatectomy patients who have an obliterated space behind the pubic bone, these patients can either have a two-piece or have the reservoir placed inside the belly. (5) Spinal cord injury patients who desire penile implant surgery, not just because of erection problems, but also to allow the application of a condom catheter (a condom attached to a catheter for urine drainage) because the solid nature of the end of the two-piece device aids in supporting the condom catheter for such patients. (6) As mentioned previously, patients with poor manual dexterity, particularly aged patients, who may benefit from having a two-piece device.

I make certain that the advantages of the two- versus three-piece device are explained to the patient so that he can make a more informed choice. Assuring that a patient has realistic expectations prior to proceeding with implant surgery is essential to ensuring high postoperative satisfaction, specifically discussing infection rates, rates of re-operation, and the lack of penile length increase with penile prosthesis surgery. It is very common for a patient to think that a penile implant will lengthen his penis, and this is not the case. At the time of surgery, the penis is actually measured in its length and this includes not just the external penis that you see from the outside, but includes the entire penis from the tip (glans) all the way to the very back portion of the penis, which is attached to the bone we sit on when we are on a bicycle seat. Thus, probably something between 50 to 66% of the penis is external, but the remainder is inside the body. The penis length is what the penis length is, and we cannot increase that. It is important for patients to understand that this is the case. I tell patients to stand in front of a mirror and pull their flaccid penis to stretch it and that the length they see in the mirror will approximate that of the erect penis after implant surgery.

While malleable devices have some perceived advantages—specifically ease of placement and lower cost—we utilize inflatable devices in almost all patients because of the rigidity and flaccidity profile of these devices as well as their more natural appearance and function. In the modern era, the breakdown rates for malleable and inflatable devices are approximately the same. If a patient is given a choice between a two- and a three-piece device and opts for a two-piece device, it has been my experience, and the medical literature supports this, that these men are extremely happy. The unhappy two-piece implant patients that I have seen have come from other surgeons where they were not counseled regarding the availability of a three-piece device.

V. Surgical Technique

Preparing for Surgery

Once I have determined that a patient is a candidate for implant surgery, we have at least one lengthy discussion regarding this, and as mentioned previously, the patient reads our literature, watches the videos, and also speaks to one of our prior implant surgery patients. The patient is counseled about two- and three-piece devices and signs an informed consent form prior to surgery. The patient is brought back to the office seven to 10 days before surgery for pre-surgery testing. For the implant patient, this is very important as it includes not just blood work, and potentially a chest x-ray and EKG depending on the patient's age and health status, but also includes a urine culture to ensure that the urine is sterile. The reason this is very important is that the presence of infected urine is a significant risk factor for the development of penile implant infection. At this preoperative visit, the patient is also instructed to scrub his penis and scrotum with Chlorhexidine soap once per day while showering on each of the seven days prior to surgery. We also use preoperative oral antibiotics.

It is worth noting that there is tremendous debate and controversy about the role of antibiotics in patients who are having implant surgery. There are some high profile centers that use no preoperative or postoperative oral antibiotics, but most centers do. We use Ciprofloxacin 500 mg twice a day for the two days prior to the operation. On the morning of surgery, the patient is admitted to the preoperative holding area, having been NPO (nothing by mouth) after midnight. He has an intravenous line started and has the administration of two antibiotics, Gentamicin and Vancomycin. These antibiotics are chosen because they act against the two most common types of bacteria that cause implant infection. Vancomycin is a very good drug for a bacterium called *Staphylococcus epidermidis* and the other bacteria are called gram-negative rods (including such bacteria as *E. coli*, *Pseudomonas*, *Proteus*, and *Klebsiella*). The patient receives a single dose of Gentamicin and a single dose of Vancomycin. Of note, some patients are allergic to these drugs, in which case we will use Aztreonam for the Gentamicin allergic patient and Ampicillin for the Vancomycin-allergic patient.

It is worth mentioning here that Vancomycin is associated with an uncommon side effect called the "red man" syndrome, which is really the result of a massive histamine release after infusion of the Vancomycin antibiotic. This results in a red tinge to skin which is usually very short lived and is in fact usually of no concern, but clearly indicates to the patient that he should not be using Vancomycin at any point in the future. We try to ensure that the antibiotics are being instilled somewhere between 30 to 90 minutes prior to the start of the operation so that the blood and erection tissue levels are highest to minimize risk of infection.

PENILE IMPLANTS

Operation

The patient is brought into the operating room and is laid on the operating table. Patients ask me all the time which is the best form of anesthesia. It really makes no difference to me whether the patient has general or spinal anesthesia. This is a decision that is left up to a discussion between the anesthesiologist and the patient himself. As long as the patient has no sensation in the penile area, then I am happy and this is readily obtained with both general and spinal anesthetic.

The patient then has his genitalia shaved. Patients are instructed not to shave themselves the night before or the morning of surgery as this is associated with higher rates of implant infection. He is scrubbed and painted with antimicrobial solution, either Chlorhexidine or Betadine, and then has the surgical drapes placed on him with only his penis and scrotum being exposed. A Foley catheter is placed into his bladder. For those of you who have already undergone radical prostatectomy, you will be only too familiar with the Foley catheter! Throughout the procedure, large amounts of antibiotic irrigation solution are typically used to wash the operative area, once again in an effort to try to minimize infection rates.

Operative Technique

There are two types of incisions that are used: one in the scrotum, known as transverse scrotal or penoscrotal, and the other at the very base of the penis as it joins the abdominal skin, known as an infrapubic incision. The majority of high-volume implant surgeons use a transverse scrotal incision, as a small incision can be made and it is cosmetically more acceptable. The only advantage of an infrapubic incision is that it is closer to the hernia ring so that the reservoir can be placed under direct vision, but reservoirs are placed routinely with ease through a transverse scrotal incision.

Once the incision has been made and the penis has been exposed from underneath with a transverse scrotal incision, the erectile bodies are cut. An incision is made approximating one to two inches, depending on the surgeon, on either side of the urethra. The erectile bodies are then dilated. That is, the natural erection tissue is crushed to make space for the implant cylinders. Making space for the cylinder within the erection chamber can be accomplished in a number of ways. There are special surgical instruments designed to do this and each individual surgeon has his/her own method. Once the corpus cavernosum has been dilated, it is measured with a special instrument as previously mentioned, from the very tip all the way down to the most back portion of the penis.

The two most notorious complications in the operating room are crural and urethral perforations. Crural perforation, which is placing a hole in the very back portion of the penis through over aggressive or misdirected dilation. This makes the operation somewhat more difficult, but should not present too much of a problem for the surgeon who has expertise in penile implant surgery. Urethral perforation (perforation occurring in the urine channel) may lead the surgeon to consider abandoning the case entirely because of the concern for future implant infection (the urethra is an inherently bacteria-laden structure).

Once the corporal bodies have been dilated and measured, then a cylinder length is chosen that best fits the individual patient. Implant devices range anywhere from 12 to 27 cm in length, and each individual patient is given the length that is measured for him. If a patient has a corporal body that measures 18 cm (and this is measured on stretch), then it is completely inappropriate to put in a larger device to try to increase his penis length. This will only result in buckling of the device upon inflation, which is routinely associated with penile pain and poor function.

If the patient is having a two-piece device, that is, a device without a reservoir, then at this time, the cut in the erection chamber is sewn up. If the patient is having a three-piece device, then a reservoir is placed through the hernia ring on the right or left side, into the space behind the pubic bone. The proper place for the pump is in a midline position within the scrotum so that it is separate and easily differentiated from the testicles. It is usually fixed in place with a stitch so that it does not move out of position. There are no connections that need to be made with a two-piece device. With a three-piece device, there may be connection that needs to be made between the pump and the reservoir, and this is easily done with special connectors that are included with the device.

Prior to closing the incision, the device is inflated and deflated to insure that the patient has a rigid, straight erection with the tips of the device present within the head of the penis. The incision is then closed. I routinely use absorbable (dissolvable) stitches for the skin, which typically fall out between three and six weeks after surgery. The implant device is routinely left deflated at the end of the operation. Because we use a transverse scrotal incision, we put an athletic supporter on the patient, inside of which are gauze pads which act as a compression dressing, and as soon as the patient gets to the recovery room an ice pack is placed to minimize swelling.

What to Expect after the Operation

It is not unusual that patients have significant pain for the first 48 hours. All of our patients get sent home with a prescription for a narcotic (typically something like Tylenol with codeine, Vicodin, or Percocet). Most patients tolerate the pain very well, although they waddle around the house for the first several days! Swelling of the scrotum and bruising of the base of the penis, scrotum, and sometimes the inner thigh are not uncommon in the early stages after surgery. However, every effort is made during the operation to try to limit the amount of bleeding, and the compression dressing and ice packs are aimed at trying to reduce the swelling and amount of bleeding. The concern about a scrotal hematoma (a collection of blood, not just bruising) is that this hematoma may, in fact, get infected and lead to implant infection.

It is not uncommon for men to experience some nausea within the first few hours after surgery. This occurs in some men after anesthesia and is usually related to the use of the narcotics that the anesthesiologist gives the patient during and at the end of the operation. We make sure before surgery that all patients have in hand a prescription for pain killers as well as antibiotics. My patients are told to use Ciprofloxacin for seven days after surgery beginning on the evening of surgery.

Once again, as previously stated, there is controversy about the role of antibiotic use in patients having implant surgery. I use it and have a very low infection rate and so continue to use these medications. I have my patients come back within 10 to 14 days after surgery to make sure the wound is healing well, that the swelling is reducing, and that the pain control is good.

I instruct my patients to keep the compression dressing on until the fourth day after surgery. If the dressing becomes soiled, I insist they replace it with a similarly sized clean compression dressing. The swelling support stays on until the patient sees me for the first time after surgery, again, usually 10 to 14 days later. I encourage the patient to position the penis upwards on the abdomen as much as possible. I believe this contributes to the reduction of swelling of the penis. I advise patients to use an ice pack inside the scrotal support for the first two to three days after surgery, but never directly in contact with skin as an ice burn can occur. I also encourage patients in the early stages to drink plenty of fluids.

CASE HISTORY SEVEN
Penile Implant Surgery

Jerome is a 70-year-old man six years after radiation therapy. He has a 70-year-old wife with whom he has an excellent sexual relationship. Erectile function prior to radiation therapy was good. He was routinely obtaining a 7/10 hardness erection with Viagra 50 mg. However, over the course of three years after radiation, his erections diminished and he required penile injection therapy for sexual intercourse. He comes to me now using high-dose, high-strength Tri mix with a 5/10 hardness erection which is short-lived and generally better while standing than lying down. He is diagnosed with venous leak. He is counseled regarding penile implant surgery. We discuss the pros and cons, risks and benefits. He reads the literature, views the videos, and speaks with two patients who have had the procedure. He opts to proceed with a three-piece inflatable penile prosthesis. He had it performed, stays one night in hospital, and goes home the next day. Four weeks later, his pain and swelling are minimal and he is taught how to use his device. He is instructed to inflate his device every day for the next three months. At six months after surgery, he has had an excellent technical outcome, with his device easy to inflate and deflate. He now routinely has successful and satisfactory sexual intercourse.

This case history illustrates the role of penile implant surgery in my practice. Penile implant surgery is generally reserved for patients who have tried penile injection therapy and in whom it has either failed, or who no longer find the therapy acceptable. It also illustrates the excellent outcome for the majority of men who have this procedure. Only 1 to 3% of implants get infected and only 15 to 20% will break down mechanically over the course of the first 10 years after surgery. Therefore, 85% of men at 10 years have the same implant they had originally received and 97% will never have had an infection of the device.

The patient has a Foley catheter in during surgery, and if the patient is going home the day of surgery as most of our patients do (unless they are older, less healthy or admission is insisted on by their insurance company), then the catheter is removed at the end of the operation. If the patient is staying in hospital overnight, then the catheter will stay in overnight and will be removed at 5 o'clock on the morning after surgery. It is common for men who have had a catheter in place, once it is removed, to have some burning sensation for a few hours to a few days afterwards. This is due to irritation of the lining of the urethra. If this is a real problem, Pyridium or Urised, which are mild anesthetics for the urethra, can be prescribed.

My patients eat within a couple of hours of surgery and usually tolerate a full meal later on that day. It is worth noting that the narcotics that are used for any operation are incredibly constipating, and if you have any tendency towards constipation, then it is worthwhile starting the day of surgery using a stool softener, such as Colace. If you have a strong history of constipation, you may need to use Milk of Magnesia or even suppositories to make sure the bowels move well.

I ask my patients not to shower until the fourth day after surgery so that the incision does not get wet and can seal before being exposed to water, and we discourage our patients from using baths or swimming pool or swimming in the ocean for a full two weeks after surgery. Most of our patients walk around the day of surgery, particularly if they are operated on in the first half of the day, and they may go up and down stairs with care. I encourage my patients to raise their legs when sitting, and we tell them they should not drive for the first seven days after surgery. We discourage the patient who has had a three-piece implant from lifting any heavy objects (greater than 10 pounds) for at least two weeks after surgery so that the reservoir which has been placed has a chance to get sealed in its position and does not slip out of position. Finally, the narcotic pain killers are very constipating, so if they are being used for more than a couple of days, stool softeners are worth taking to keep the bowels moving.

VI. Complications

The concept of the patient making an informed decision essentially mandates that a discussion of postoperative complications are included in the preoperative discussion. There is always discussion as to how common a complication needs to be before it should be discussed. For example, if a complication occurs in 1/1,000,000 patients, is this something that should be discussed with a patient prior to surgery? This is left to each individual surgeon's discretion, but usually surgeons confine their complication discussion to either life-threatening complications or those that occur in more than 1% of patients.

It is worth mentioning at this time that there has been much controversy over the last 15 years regarding the use of silicone implants, although this has been more of an issue for breast implants than for penile implants. A decision was made by the FDA in 1993 to prohibit the use of silicone for breast implants based on some very weak medical evidence. Indeed, I feel comfortable telling you that there is no clear evidence that the use of silicone is associated with any auto-immune disease or medical problem. Once again, the Coloplast three-piece cylinders are made of polyurethane polymer called Bioflex and it is only the AMS cylinders that are made of silicone. However, the tubing that goes from the cylinders to the pump and the reservoir tubing on all devices is also made of silicone. The Ambicor device, that is, the two-piece device, is made entirely of silicone.

Implant Infection

The complication of most concern is implant infection, and this occurs in anywhere from 1 to 3% of men. It is due to bacteria getting onto the device at the time of surgery and it is likely that infection risk is reduced by the use of antibiotics in and around the time of surgery, as well as irrigation during surgery, whether with saline alone or an antibiotic solution. The introduction of the antibiotic coating and anti-adherence coating in the AMS and Coloplast implants, respectively, has likely contributed to a further reduction, although the magnitude of this infection rate reduction is fairly small given that the overall rate of infection itself is low. The great problem with penile implant infection is that this is not an infection that can be treated with the use of oral or intravenous antibiotics. When a penile implant is infected, it needs to be removed. The signs of implant infection are very clear. There is usually drainage of pus from the incision, worsening of the swelling, pain that is increasing, redness of the incision or scrotum, hardness of the incision or scrotum, fixation of the pump to the skin (that is, the pump being stuck to the skin on examination), and fevers and chills. I tell all of my patients that if any of these symptoms occur, they need to call us immediately, regardless of where they are in the world and what time of day or night it is. Of note, the vast majority of penile implant infections occur within the first eight weeks after surgery, although uncommonly, it can occur up to 12 months after surgery. Thus, if I can get my patients to the eighth week after surgery without an infection, we feel confident telling them that the chance of getting an infection in the future is very low.

The historical approach to dealing with penile implant infection is to remove the penile implant, irrigate the penis and scrotum with antibiotic solution, and then close it with the intention putting an implant back in somewhere between two and six months after the removal procedure. The problem with this approach is that, once the implant cylinders are removed, there is no erection tissue left behind and the space is filled with collagen (scar). As scars contract, these men have a 100% chance of experiencing penile length loss, and many of these patients lose significant length, some losing up to 50% of their penile length. Because of this, pioneers like Dr. John Mulcahy and Dr. Steven Wilson introduced the concept of salvage implant surgery. This more modern approach, which has gained widespread accessibility and use, involves removing the infected implant and irrigating the penis and scrotum as usual, but in this case using a very prolonged antibiotic and antibacterial irrigation, and replacing the device immediately. Obviously, the great concern about this is a repeat infection. However, literature would suggest that only between 20 to 25% of patients who have this approach actually end up getting another implant infection. I have had many patients who have had penile implant infections with very aggressive bacteria who underwent salvage procedure with excellent results. Those patients in whom salvage implant surgery should probably not be considered are those who have dead tissue within the penis or scrotum (due to severe infection) or who are immunocompromised (for example, those patients who are on immune suppressants for a prior transplant procedure).

The final thing I would like to mention about implant infections is that there is recent evidence to suggest that patients who have had penile implants, who undergo surgical or dental procedures in the future may be at higher risk for developing a delayed implant infection. I recommend that all patients who have previously undergone penile implant surgery, who are about to undergo another surgical or dental procedure, take a Ciprofloxacin pill the night before the procedure and then the night of the procedure to try to minimize the risk of delayed implant infection. This is something that should be discussed with the surgeon who did the penile implant.

Mechanical Breakdown

The next complication to be discussed is mechanical breakdown (or malfunction in "medicalese"). I tell patients that they have approximately a 15% chance of requiring reoperation for mechanical breakdown over the course of the first 10 years after surgery. It is my experience that the younger and more sexually active men are the ones most likely to develop a problem with mechanical malfunction. Essentially what happens is that a tear occurs in the cylinder or a blow-out in the tube going from the pump to the reservoir in a three-piece device, and the saline leaks out and the device can no longer be inflated. The saline that leaks out is not dangerous as it is sterile. One of the problems with implant surgery is that once you have a penile implant, the only way to obtain an erection at any point of time in the future is to have another implant procedure performed. So, if the device breaks down, another implant will be required if sexual intercourse remains important for the patient.

Other causes of mechanical malfunction, such as reservoir rupture and scrotal pump malfunction, are generally very uncommon. When a implant malfunctions, as the patient squeezes on the scrotal pump, it remains flat and does not re-inflate and fluid does not re-accumulate in the pump, so the cylinders remain deflated. The device can be removed and a new device placed, although this does require a second operation, very similar in nature to the first implant operation. The infection rate with this operation, goes from 1 to 3%, to 3 to 6%. There is much medical literature on the reliability of these implants with mechanical failure rates ranging anywhere from 1.5% to 20% over the first decade after implantation (Appendix 3). The bottom line is that the design of these devices has come a long way, and they are very reliable and result in very high levels of patient and partner satisfaction.

Auto-Inflation

Auto-inflation is a condition where the device inflates itself, slightly or significantly during physical exertion. Great care is taken during the procedure to prevent this by creating an adequately sized space for the reservoir. Auto-inflation is rare with a two-piece device. In men who are obese, or in men in whom an inadequately sized reservoir space is created, straining and increased abdominal pressure will put pressure on the reservoir and fluid may leak out into the cylinders with inflation of the device. The use of the newly developed lock-out valves on the reservoir or the pump has significantly gone some way toward reducing the likelihood of auto-inflation. It is my experience that most patients who report auto-inflation are getting very mild filling of their penes. However, every so often, I will see a patient who has auto-inflation to the point of developing a fully rigid erection. If auto-inflation is bothersome, and it is probably bothersome in less than 5% of patients, then the reservoir needs to be repositioned either in the same location or on the opposite side by a small surgical procedure.

Erosion

Erosion is where the cylinders or the scrotal pump burrow their way through the skin. This is generally a sign of penile implant infection, in which case the device will need to be removed. However, under certain circumstances, this can occur without infection being present. This is most commonly seen with malleable implants, which are consistently rigid and the pressure can cause burrowing of the implant out of the head of the penis. Erosion is very uncommon in patients having a three-piece implant, because these are low-pressure devices when the device is inflated and they spend most of the time in the deflated state.

Device Migration

Device migration refers to the problem where the device slips back out of the head of the penis and is due to one of three scenarios. The first scenario is migration due to crural perforation, typically the case when migration occurs with only one cylinder. As previously mentioned, this is where a hole is made in the back portion of the erection chamber during overly vigorous dilation or misdirected dilation. If this happens and goes unrecognized during the operation, later on after surgery, the device may slip back. This will require a second operation to correct. If crural perforation is identified during the operation, it is not a concern as it can be fixed right then and there.

The second scenario is where the device is incorrectly sized, for example, in a man who has a 20–cm corporal body and has only an 18–cm device implanted in the penis. This is very uncommon in the hands of a surgeon familiar with implant surgery.

Finally, there is a group of men who each have a hypermobile glans (which is difficult to define in the flaccid state) and, despite the fact that they have insertion of properly sized implants, because of the hypermobility of the glans, the head of the penis off the end of the implant, resulting in what is known as the "supersonic transporter deformity" (or in Europe is known as the "Concorde deformity"). If this is the case, then the glans can be repositioned using a simple surgical procedure called glanulopexy. If the cylinders are undersized, then the only way to ensure filling of the head of the penis is to replace the cylinders.

Reservoir Herniation

Reservoir herniation is an uncommon event occurring in less than 1% of patients, and involves the reservoir of a three-piece device popping out through the hernia ring and is due to one of two reasons. Firstly, it can occur in men who overexert themselves in the early stages after surgery, and before the reservoir has been sealed in place, it gets forced outwards during abdominal straining. Secondly, in patients who have a hernia and have a wide hernia ring, the device may fall out if it is not adequately fixed in place. This leads to a bulge present in the groin when the device is deflated, but when the device is inflated, this bulge goes away. For most patients, this is not particularly bothersome, but when it is bothersome, the reservoir can be repositioned and fixed in place by a small surgical procedure so that this will not happen again.

Penile Length Changes

Finally, there is a lot of debate about penile implants causing penile length loss. There is very little to suggest that implants actually shorten the penis. In fact, there is very new literature to suggest that penis length at the beginning of the operation is the same as that at the end of the operation and six months after surgery.

It is likely that men who are complaining about penile length are experiencing one of four problems. Firstly, men who have implant surgery for Peyronie's disease will, by definition, have had penile shortening even before their implants are put in place. The scar that occurs during Peyronie's disease contracts and this results routinely in penile length loss even before an implant is placed.

Secondly, men who have had radical prostatectomy have a significant chance of having some shortening of the penis, albeit not very great, but there is strong medical evidence, as mentioned in a previous chapter, to suggest that there is an association between radical prostatectomy and penile length and volume loss.

Thirdly, it is often the case that a man after implant surgery is comparing his penis length to what it was when he last had a good erection. For most men undergoing implant surgery, this duration is anywhere from one to five years. So during the one to five years that the erection tissue is not being exercised properly, it undergoes atrophy and there is a shortening of the penis. This is not related directly to the penile implant surgery itself.

Finally, while penile implants do not lengthen the penis, they do, in fact, increase the girth of the penis, and this altered penile aspect ratio (length-to-width ratio) may, in fact, make the penis look shorter than it actually is. Think of two columns that are equally tall, yet one is narrower and the other much wider. It will appear that the wider column is shorter than the one is thinner.

VII. Summary

In summary, therefore, penile implants are an excellent option with very high levels of patient and partner satisfaction in the properly selected patient. In my practice, this means that the patient has failed pills or has had significant side effects with pills and have explored the concept of penile injections, preferably even trying penile injections before making a decision about implant surgery. Good preoperative counseling, good preoperative and postoperative care, and excellent operative technique lead to the highest rate of good function, good cosmetic appearance, and long-term mechanical reliability of the device. I would encourage all patients considering penile implant surgery to discuss the surgery with someone who has undergone implant surgery previously so that they have realistic expectations prior to proceeding.

APPENDIX 1
Penile Implant Information Sheet

Advantages of an inflatable penile implant
1. It allows full rigidity (hardness) of the penis.
2. Erection usually occurs within half a minute after starting to pump the device.
3. It does not require taking pills or preparing injection medicine.

Disadvantages of an inflatable penile implant
1. It requires an operation. Typically, patients have their operations in the same-day surgery center and leave a few hours later.
2. The surgery is irreversible. This means that if the implant needs to be removed or the patient changes his mind, no other treatment will work well for him.
3. Implant surgery is associated with some complications, which, while not common, need to be discussed. These complications are listed below.

Potential complications of penile implant surgery
- Infection: This occurs in 2% of men with a first-time implant. This figure increases significantly for repeat surgery. If the device gets infected, it may need to be removed. Infections usually occur in the first eight weeks after surgery but may occur up to one year after the operation.
- Early mechanical breakdown: This occurs in about 2% of cases and involves the malfunction of the pump or cylinders in the early months following surgery. In this case, the device will need to be replaced.
- Re-operation: There is approximately a 15 to 20% re-operation rate within the first 10 years after the original surgery because of wear and tear. However, almost six out of seven men will not experience this problem and will have their implants for life.
- Autoinflation: Under certain circumstances, the device may inflate itself slightly during physical exertion. Great care is taken during the procedure to prevent this. However, in certain cases (heavy men, men following radical prostate surgery), this may occur despite good surgical technique.

continued on the next page

PENILE IMPLANTS

continued from the previous page

- Scrotal hematoma: Swelling and bruising of the scrotum, lower abdomen, and inner thighs may occur after this operation. Sometimes this bruising collects and causes significant swelling. This is prevented by the application of a good compression (scrotal support) after the operation and adhering to the doctor's instructions postoperatively.
- Other complications include device erosion (generally associated with implant infection) and device migration; however, these problems are much less common than those listed above.

What to expect

- There will be pain/swelling for about two weeks after the operation.
- You will be required to take at least 10 days off work.
- No sexual activity is allowed for four to six weeks following the operation.
- It may take more than six months for the penis to feel normal again.
- There should be no change in the quality of ejaculation or orgasm.
- There will be NO change in penile length.

APPENDIX 2
Post Penile Implant Surgery Instructions

You are to expect

- Small amounts of drainage on your dressings.
- Pain, tenderness, swelling, and bruising for several days after your surgery.
- Nausea on the day of your operation after you return home.
- That you should leave with prescriptions for pain medicine and antibiotics.
- That you should also leave the hospital with an appointment for a post-operative visit with your doctor within the first two weeks after your surgery.

continued on the next page

continued from the previous page

Instructions

- Keep the compression dressing on until the fourth day after your surgery.
- If the dressing becomes soiled, replace it with a similarly sized clean compression dressing.
- Keep the scrotal support on until your first postoperative visit with your doctor.
- Position your penis upwards on your abdomen as much as possible.
- For two to three days, place an ice pack inside the scrotal support (not directly in contact with skin).
- Drink plenty of fluids.
- Eat lightly the remainder of the day of surgery, then return to normal diet as tolerated.
- Make sure your bowels function normally, as pain medications are constipating. You may need to use stool softeners to help your bowels function normally.
- Finish your antibiotics completely.
- You may shower on the fourth day after surgery, but avoid tub baths for two full weeks.
- You may walk around the home and up stairs immediately, but carefully.
- When sitting, raise your legs.
- Do not drive until at least one week after surgery.
- Do not lift any heavy objects (greater than 10 lbs) for at least two weeks after surgery.

Call for the following reasons

- Fevers over 101 degrees.
- Excessive drainage from your wound, especially blood or pus.
- Pain or scrotal swelling that is not improving after the first week following surgery.
- Redness around the wound.
- If you need to have any further surgical or dental procedures, because you will need antibiotic coverage to start the night prior to treatment and for 24 hours after treatment. Please call to have a prescription called into your pharmacy.

CHAPTER 14

FUTURE THERAPIES FOR SEXUAL PROBLEMS

> I. Drugs for Nerve Protection
> II. Drugs for Erectile Dysfunction
> III. Gene and Growth Factor Therapy
> IV. Stem Cell Therapy
> V. Multimodal Therapy

This chapter attempts to predict the future to help you understand what therapies we may be using in the coming years to treat sexual problems that occur in patients with a diagnosis of prostate cancer, whether they have been treated by surgery, radiation, or hormone therapy. The main potential developments in the near future include drugs that protect nerves from injury or help them regenerate (neuromodulators), new drugs for the treatment of erectile dysfunction and other male sexual problems, as well growth factor, gene therapy, and stem cell therapy for the treatment and potentially the prevention of sexual disorders.

I. Drugs for Nerve Protection

Since the introduction of nerve sparing prostatectomy by Dr. Patrick Walsh in 1983, it has been well recognized that the degree of erection nerve preservation is directly related to the recovery of erectile function. Irrespective of the technical expertise of the surgeon, even perfect nerve sparing on both sides results in trauma to the nerves. This occurs because the nerves are pushed out of the way or traction is applied to the nerves during the procedure. This results in temporary nerve injury, somewhat like a concussion injury, where the nerves are stunned. These nerves may spend many months dormant before waking up and it may take up to two years before the nerves are fully recovered. Wouldn't it be exciting if we could use a medication that would prevent the nerves from injury or help those nerves regenerate after injury? This concept is called neuromodulation and is being explored, not just in the radical prostatectomy patient, but also in patients with neurologic diseases and diabetics with nerve injury.

There is a vast amount of experimental evidence from studies looking at these types of drugs in animals with experimental nerve injury and even cavernous nerve (erection nerve) injury. We know that even temporary nerve trauma results in damage to the smooth muscle and the endothelium components of erectile tissue. It appears that nerve transection leads to greater erectile tissue damage than a blunt injury to the nerve and that bilateral nerve injury has greater effects than unilateral injury. I previously outlined the changes that occur in erectile tissue after radical prostatectomy, including erection nerve injury, collagen deposition (scarring), increased production of scar-inducing chemicals, and actual death of smooth muscle cells.

The most widely studied group of neuromodulatory compounds are known as immunophilin ligands. Immunophilins are proteins that are found in immune tissue and are found in far greater concentrations in nerve tissues, both in the spinal cord and in the peripheral nerves. As previously mentioned, the erection nerves are combined sympathetic and parasympathetic, the former turning off erection and the latter turning on erection. Immunophilins are proteins that act as binding ports (receptors) for a family of medications which are predominantly immunosuppressant (drugs that are used to suppress the immune system in patients who have undergone transplant to lower the risk of rejection of the transplanted organ). Drugs in this class include cyclosporine, tacrolimus (also known as FK506 and marketed as Prograf), and rapamycin.

The major concern about these agents, of course, is that they suppress the immune system. However, the doses of tacrolimus, for example, that are being studied for nerve protection are the same doses that have been used in large trials of this drug in patients with rheumatoid arthritis. The dose that is used for nerve protection purposes is approximately half of that which is used in transplant patients, and in the large rheumatoid arthritis studies to date, there have been no cases of immunosuppression. This is likely due to the low doses of tacrolimus used in these studies. Nevertheless, great interest has existed in the development of compounds that protect nerves but DO NOT suppress the immune system. Guildford Pharmaceuticals has developed a series of GPI compounds, which, while they are immunophilin ligands, have no immune suppression effects.

Dr. Bud Burnett from Johns Hopkins was the first person to show that rats that had their erection nerves injured had greater recovery of erections after the trauma if treated with tacrolimus compared to a placebo treatment. My laboratory has shown that the use of tacrilimus in rats who have undergone bilateral crush injury to their erection nerves results in significant improvement in erectile function, significant preservation of erectile tissue, and significant regeneration of the erection nerves after injury.

So far in the USA, there have been two large trials conducted looking at immunophilin ligands in the radical prostatectomy population. In the tacrilimus study, patients were randomly chosen (flip of a coin) to either receive the drug or a placebo (sugar pill). They received the medication for seven days prior to surgery and for a total of six months after surgery. It is too early to determine whether this treatment is of benefit, but hopefully by mid-2009, we will have results from this study.

The side effects in this trial that were most frequently encountered were gastrointestinal upset, elevation of potassium levels in the blood, and reduction of magnesium levels in the blood, all of which have been well documented in the transplant and rheumatoid arthritis literature. No patients had the medication stopped because of side effects. This was a large study involving multiple centers lead by Memorial Sloan-Kettering but also including Baylor College of Medicine, UCLA Medical Center, The Cleveland Clinic, New York University Medical Center, and University of Michigan Medical Center. The results of these studies are eagerly awaited. It is likely that, should there be significant improvement in erection function recovery with tacrolimus, urologists will start using it in the radical prostatectomy population.

GPI-1485 has also been studied in a randomized, controlled study. This trial has been completed and six months data have been presented at the American Urological Association Meeting in 2007, but not yet published. At the six-month time point, there appeared to be no significant difference in erection function recovery between those patients who were treated with placebo compared to either a low or a high dose of GPI-1485. Long-term data is awaited.

The nightly sildenafil post-prostatectomy study that I previously discussed, which demonstrated that there was a seven-fold increase in the likelihood of a man returning to his preoperative erection hardness raised some interesting questions. When this data was originally presented, it was thought that the beneficial effects were related to that fact that men using Viagra in the early stages after surgery were getting nighttime erections and therefore bringing oxygen into the penis, which we now believe is critical to the health of erection tissue. However, we know that most men in the early stages after prostatectomy are not having a significant response to PDE5 inhibitors. At Memorial Sloan-Kettering, 86% of patients do not respond to these drugs within the first few months. So this study has forced us to look at other mechanisms by which PDE5 inhibitors may protect erectile tissue. I previously alluded to the fact that the endothelium is essential for the health of erection tissue and the development of erections, and there is excellent evidence to show that PDE5 inhibitors are potent endothelial protectants.

One of the other mechanisms by which PDE5 inhibitors might have a benefit is through neuromodulation. Indeed, there are now two studies, one with sildenafil (Viagra) and the other with tadalafil (Cialis), which demonstrate a beneficial effect of the use of these medications in animals who have had a stroke induced. In both of these studies, the animals treated with the drug compared to placebo have significant improvement in their ability to walk properly after stroke and ongoing research is being conducted to look at the role of PDE5 inhibitors in neuromodulation.

It is my personal opinion that we will have a neuromodulatory drug in the future, whether it be an immunophilin ligand or some other kind of compound. Other groups of drugs that have been looked at include minocycline (which is an acne antibiotic), PARP inhibitors, and a compound known as erythropoietin. It is interesting that the latter medication is used routinely in patients with chronic anemia, as it generates production of red blood cells from the bone marrow. Dr. Bud Burnett's group at Johns Hopkins has shown in animal studies that there is a benefit to the use of erythropoietin in the erection nerve–injured rat. No large-scale human studies have been conducted with erythropoetin at this point in time.

II. Drugs for Erectile Dysfunction

Currently in the United States of America, there are three drugs approved for the treatment of erectile dysfunction: Viagra, Levitra, and Cialis. In Europe and the rest of the world, there is another drug called Uprima, which is apomorphine administered sublingually (under the tongue). In Asia, there is a fourth PDE5 inhibitor, Udenafil, which has been used with significant benefit.

There are, however, several pharmaceutical companies that have drugs in development for the treatment of erectile dysfunction, including new PDE5 inhibitors being studied. The question needs to be raised, however, as to how many PDE5 inhibitors the erectile dysfunction drug market can sustain. It is likely that any new PDE5 inhibitor is going to be no more effective than the ones that are available at the moment. However, they may be quicker in their onset of action, longer lasting in their duration of effect, and may be associated with fewer side effects. The two drugs that are furthest along in development are being studied by Vivus (the makers of MUSE) and Surface Logix. Early human data has been presented and it is expected that both products will move forward to FDA submission in the not too distant future.

For some time, there has been significant interest in the use of gels that are applied to the penis to help erection. Obviously, this has tremendous palatability to the patient because no pill needs to be taken, no injection needs to be used, and no suppository needs to be applied. Two companies have been in this field for quite some time, NexMed and MacroChem. MacroChem had an agent that contained prostaglandin E1, which was applied to the head of the penis; however, preliminary studies have failed to show any significant benefit in men who have physically based erection problems. It is not clear at this point in time where this MacroChem product is headed. NexMed has a gel called Alprox-TD which is applied to the urethral meatus (opening of the urine channel). This product is also being looked at for women for clitoral application for which it is known as Femprox-TD. Preliminary data are encouraging, although it is not clear to me whether the patients studied have significant erectile dysfunction or not. The side effects with these treatments tend to be skin irritation at the site of application. These drugs are of mild-to-moderate effectiveness.

There is also great interest in the delivery of centrally acting drugs. By this I mean drugs which have their primary effect in the brain rather than in the penis. Sublingual apomorphine, which is available outside the United States, is one such drug. This agent stimulates dopamine receptors in the brain, particularly in the center that triggers erection. Known as Uprima, this drug is relatively weak, but may play some role in the treatment of men with psychogenic erectile dysfunction or men with mild erectile dysfunction. Unfortunately, as with any of the centrally acting agents, nausea and vomiting are potential side effects. Men may rarely also experience significant drops in blood pressure and pass out (syncope). This drug has been marketed by Abbott Pharmaceuticals outside of the United States. It was rejected by the FDA and is not likely to be approved in this country in its sublingual form.

Another company, Nastech, has been looking at this drug in a nasal spray formulation, delivered very much in the same way that you would use a nasal spray for seasonal allergies. Trans-nasal delivery of apomorphine in very early studies has been shown to be as effective as the sublingual form of the medication.

One of the drugs furthest along in its development and with results that are eye-catching, is the drug known as bremelanotide (previously known as PT-141; Palatin Technologies). This is a centrally acting agent, known as a melanocortin agonist which is currently being studied for trans-nasal delivery. It acts in a very similar fashion to the dopaminergic agonist, apomorphine, in the same area of the brain although it functions through different receptors than apomorphine. In early studies in men with mild to moderate erectile dysfunction, this medication has been shown to be of significant benefit and large phase III studies are awaited before Palatin Technologies submits this drug to the FDA for a final evaluation.

One of the most interesting things about this compound is that, in early studies when the drug was administered subcutaneously (injected under the skin) rather than by a nasal spray, as it is now, there was a significant improvement in some men in their libidos (sex drive). It is my opinion that the newer oral, transdermal and trans-nasal drugs will be no more potent than the drugs that we have available at the moment (Viagra, Levitra and Cialis) and that centrally acting drugs will be used for men with only the mildest forms of erectile problems. Therefore, I think that the role of these drugs as single therapy in patients who have undergone radical prostatectomy or radiation therapy will be limited. However, the future of erectile dysfunction treatment in prostate cancer patients or any man with erectile dysfunction is going to be combination therapy, very much in the same way that we treat high blood pressure and high cholesterol levels with multiple medications. It is likely that we will be using pill/pill, pill/gel, pill/nasal spray combinations in the future. I believe that we will see the number of men, currently 60%, who are responding effectively to PDE5 inhibitors increase in the future with the use of combination therapy. It is impossible for to me to see that there will not be a role for penile injection therapy or penile implant surgery in the future. Men who develop venous leak (erectile tissue damage), which occurs frequently after radical prostatectomy and prostate radiation will always require a drug more potent than oral agents (or penile implants if they fail such drugs).

III. Gene and Growth Factor Therapy

Genes, which are pieces of DNA, are located on the chromosomes inside every cell of our body and are the master controllers of all chemical processes within the human body. There are genes that give us our hair color, our hair type, our eye color, our body shape, and our risk for developing conditions such as autoimmune diseases like rheumatoid arthritis, heart disease, and even cancer. The idea behind gene therapy is to inject a gene into an organ or tissue, which may restore function in that organ. There are a number of ways that are used to get the gene into the tissue (this is known as transfection), the most common one thus far being the use of viruses. This is because viruses are excellent at penetrating cells, so by attaching a gene to them, these genes can be delivered to the area that we are interested in.

Gene therapy has been looked at in animals for the treatment of Parkinson's disease, immune disorders, heart disease, several forms of cancer, and cystic fibrosis. Gene therapy has been explored in the treatment of erectile dysfunction, predominantly in rats so far. The two genes that have been most studied are the nitric oxide synthase (NOS) gene and the hSlo gene. I previously alluded to how important nitric oxide is in the penis.

Nitric oxide is produced by an enzyme, nitric oxide synthase. There are several medical conditions that are associated with reduced nitric oxide synthase presence, particularly conditions where the erection nerves are injured, for example, after radical prostatectomy or prostate radiation. The idea is that we could inject this gene into the penis and that this would restore nitric oxide levels, which would lead to improved erectile function. In aged rats, where erectile function is significantly reduced compared to young animals, several centers have shown that the transfection of the nitric oxide synthase gene has resulted in significant improvement in erectile function, such that the erectile function in the old animals returns to the level seen in young rats.

Another gene that has gone through the animal research phase and has recently gone into human research is the hSlo gene. This gene is involved in the regulation of the calcium in erectile tissue. Calcium is critical to the ability of the smooth muscle in the penis to contract and relax. In a recently conducted pioneering trial, Dr. Arnold Melman at Montefiore Medical Center, along with the esteemed researcher George Christ PhD, has shown in a small number of men with severe ED that significant improvement in erectile function was achieved when they were treated with the hSlo gene.

While not gene therapy, growth factor therapy has also been explored. Growth factors are chemicals produced by cells that nourish other cells or tissues and are essential for normal tissue health and growth. Dr. Craig Donatucci at Duke University has looked at vascular endothelial growth factor, also known as VEGF. This growth factor is very important for the production and protection of blood vessels. You will remember me stating that the penis is essentially one large blood vessel that is similar to a vein in the flaccid state and an artery in the erect state. VEGF is critical to the health of erectile tissue. In the rat model, Dr. Donatucci's group injected VEGF into the penes of old rats, and very similar to the nitric oxide synthase gene transfection experiments, they have shown that significant improvement occurs in the erectile function of these animals. No human studies have occurred to date.

IV. Stem Cell Therapy

Stem cell research has received a huge amount of attention over the course of the last five years. This is a highly controversial issue that raises all kinds of emotions for patients. There are political concerns, religious concerns, and ethical concerns associated with stem cell therapy. Stem cells are precursor cells which, irrespective of where they are obtained from in the body, are capable of dividing and renewing themselves for long periods. They are also unspecialized and can give rise to many different types of specialized cells and tissues, including muscle, nerve, blood cells, and erection tissue. There are two different types of stem cells: embryo-derived stem cells and adult-derived stem cells. Embryo-derived stem cells are derived from embryos and not from human eggs. These embryos have typically been generated during

FUTURE THERAPIES FOR SEXUAL PROBLEMS

in-vitro fertilization and have been donated for research purposes by couples. Adult stem cells, on the other hand, are found in many different types of tissue and can still generate specialized cell types or tissue. These cells are present so that they can help maintain and repair tissue in the organ in which they are found. Far more readily available than embryo-derived stem cells, they are more limited in their ability to produce different types of specialized cells in the body.

The list of medical conditions that have potential applications for stem cell therapy is long, including rheumatoid arthritis, autoimmune diseases, connective tissue diseases, diabetes, neurologic diseases, heart disease, spinal cord injury, and several forms of cancer. Dr. Tom Lue at UCSF Medical Center has demonstrated very recently that fat-derived stem cells can differentiate into smooth muscle and endothelial cells (the components of erectile tissue). The prospects for adult-derived stem cell therapy in erectile dysfunction, I believe, is bright if appropriate funding can be raised for the ongoing research. The hope is that stem cell therapy in the penis will not only prevent injury to erectile tissue after prostate radiation or radical prostatectomy but that it may, in fact, help regenerate tissue. It is believed at this point in time that the presence of venous leak, which results from erectile tissue scarring, is irreversible. However, it is conceivable that stem cell therapy may help regenerate and reverse the scarring process and may, in fact, be a curative therapy for venous leak in the future.

In speaking with Dr. Lue, he has stated that they are very close to being ready to go into human studies with fat-tissue-derived stem cells. Think of how easy it would be to have a pound of fat excised and to have these cells injected for the purposes of regeneration of a variety of tissues in the body.

V. Multimodal Therapy (Figure 1)

Very much in the same way that I am advocating multidrug therapy for erectile dysfunction, I believe the future of treatment of erectile problems for men after prostate surgery, prostate radiation, or hormone therapy will be multimodal. If we consider that there are three factors that are critical to erectile function, that is, erection nerve integrity, smooth muscle integrity, and the integrity of the endothelium, then I believe that in the future we will be using treatments, pharmaceutical or otherwise, that will be used to protect each of these three components. I have already discussed in this

```
                    /\
                   /  \
       Endothelial/    \Neuroprotection
PDE5 inhibitors  Protection           PDE5 Inhibitors?
Statins        /        \             Erythropoetin?
              /          \            Immunophilin ligands
             /_____\
           Smooth muscle protection

         Penile injections   Gene therapy?
         PDE5 inhibitors     Stem cells?
               MUSE?         Vacuum Device?
```

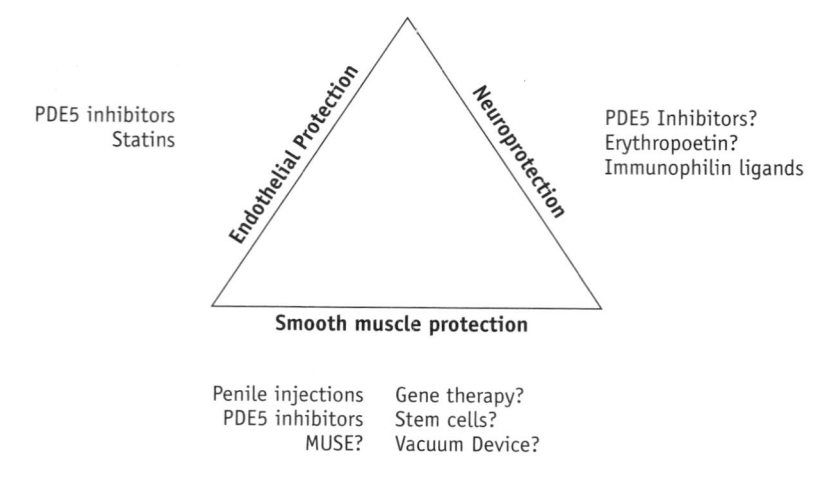

Figure 1 • Diagram illustrating the concept of a multi-modal approach to penile rehabilitation

chapter neuromodulary drugs which may potentially include PDE5 inhibitors, erythropoietin, PARP inhibitors or immunophilin ligands in the future or other drugs that are as of yet not in development.

It is believed that erection itself protects the smooth muscle and endothelium, and we know that PDE5 inhibitors in some men, transurethral prostaglandin suppositories in some men, and intracavernosal injection therapy in most men generate erection. In this chapter, I have also discussed that gene and growth factor therapy and stem cell therapy may be used in the future for protection or regeneration of smooth muscle. And finally, I have discussed the fact that PDE5 inhibitors are potent endothelial protectants and, for men who come to my office to see me before their surgeries or radiation, we use endothelial preconditioning by using PDE5 inhibitors even before the treatment has begun.

There is now excellent evidence to show that the statin drugs, those drugs that reduce blood cholesterol levels, such as Lipitor, Crestor, Zocor, Vytorin, and others, are also excellent protectants of the endothelium. I believe that it is likely that in the future, endothelial preconditioning and penile rehabilitation in the radiation and surgery patient will involve not just neuromodulators and erection-inducing agents, but also the combination of PDE5 inhibitors and statins, for the protection of erection tissue.

There are a couple of small animal experiments and one small human study that have suggested that there is an accumulated beneficial effect for combining PDE5 inhibitors and statins in the radical prostatectomy population. The bottom line is that at no point in time prior to this has there been such an amount of research in this field. I believe the future is bright and that we will be using multimodal therapy in the future. Whether we will ever have a single agent that will accomplish all three tasks of nerve protection, smooth muscle protection, and endothelial protection is not clear, and I think that we will most likely be using several medications or strategies to protect and help regenerate erectile tissue in these patients.

CHAPTER 15

TESTOSTERONE AND THE PROSTATE

> I. Testosterone
> II. Hypogonadism
> III. Symptoms of Low Testosterone
> IV. Evaluation of a Man with Low Testosterone
> V. Risks and Benefits of Testosterone Supplementation
> VI. Testosterone and Prostate Cancer
> VII. How Testosterone is Supplemented
> VIII. Monitoring of the Patient Receiving Testosterone Supplementation

I. Testosterone

Testosterone is the major sex hormone in the adult male. The family of hormones that testosterone belongs is called androgens and includes two other high-profile hormones: DHEA, which is widely used as an over-the-counter sexual health supplement, and androstenedione, which has been used in professional sports as an anabolic steroid (Figure 1). The state of low testosterone levels is termed hypogonadism. Testosterone plays a crucial role in the developing fetus and at puberty, and it is critical for muscle development and preservation, reducing body fat, bone density, sex drive, and erectile tissue health, as well as mood, energy, and motivation.

In men, testosterone is produced predominantly by the testicles. The cells that produce testosterone inside the testicle are called Leydig cells. Testosterone is also produced in very small amounts in the adrenal glands, which sit on top of the kidneys on both sides. The production of testosterone (see Chapter 6, Figure 1) is stimulated by a hormone from the pituitary gland (a small organ sitting directly under the brain and attached to the major bodily function area of the brain known as the hypothalamus). This hormone is called luteinizing hormone, more commonly known as LH. LH travels from the pituitary gland in the blood to the testicles and stimulates the Leydig cells to produce testosterone. The production of LH is stimulated by a luteinizing hormone releasing hormone, more commonly known as LHRH, from an area of the brain known as the hypothalamus. Interestingly, the production of testosterone involves what is called a negative feedback system, which when testosterone levels are normal, suppresses the production of LH and LHRH by the brain. This mechanism keeps testosterone levels in check. Testosterone tends to decrease as we age; it is estimated that there is anywhere from 10 to 25% reduction per decade of life after the thirtieth year of life, and this occurs for a variety of reasons. These include reduced secretion of LHRH by the hypothalamus, decreased receptivity of the pituitary gland to LHRH, decreased ability to produce LH by the pituitary gland, and decreased number of Leydig cells in the testicle, as well as decreased sensitivity of Leydig cells to LH.

Testosterone is broken down into two very important hormones. The first one is dihydrotestosterone, more commonly known as DHT. The conversion of testosterone into DHT occurs by an enzyme called 5–alpha reductase. This enzyme is located in numerous tissues, but in large quantities in the prostate and skin. You will remember from the chapter on benign prostatic enlargement that 5–alpha reductase inhibitors, such as finasteride (Proscar, Propecia) and dutasteride (Avodart), by blocking conversion of T to DHT, may reduce the size of the prostate. This is also the enzyme that causes hair loss, as DHT is the primary androgen responsible for hair loss in men. This is why 5–alpha reductase inhibitors may be useful in men with early onset balding.

The second breakdown product of testosterone is estrogen. It is surprising to many men that we have the female sex hormone estrogen in our blood. The enzyme that breaks testosterone down to estrogen is known as aroma-

TESTOSTERONE AND THE PROSTATE

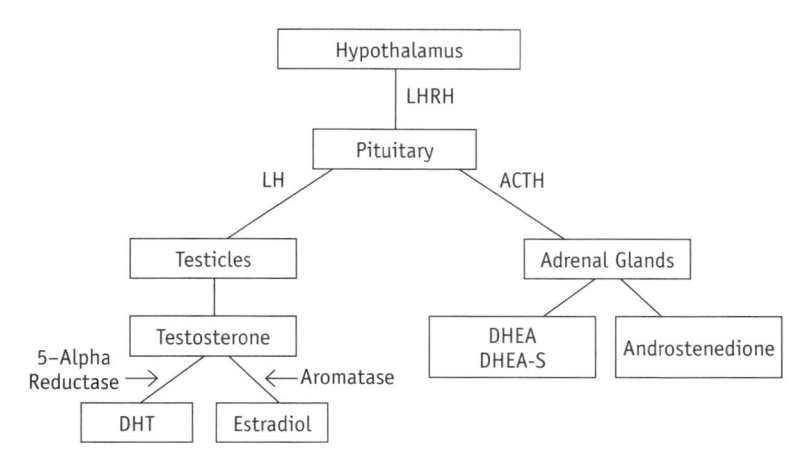

Figure 1 • Diagram showing the mechanism of testosterone production
LHRH: luteinizing hormone releasing hormone - stimulates pituitary gland to make LH
LH: luteinizing hormone - stimulates testicles to make testosterone
ACTH: adrenocorticotrophin - stimulates adrenal glands to make androgens
5 alpha reductase - an enzyme that degrades testosterone to DHT
Aromatase - an enzyme which degrades testosterone to estradiol (the major estrogen)

tase. This typically occurs in the fatty tissues of the body. In fact, men who are obese and have very large amounts of subcutaneous fat have high levels of aromatase and are more likely to break their testosterone down to estrogen. Estrogen, while present in the blood, is supposed to be there in only very small quantities and, when these levels are increased, it results in symptoms very similar to the symptoms that occur in men with very low levels of testosterone. There are a group of drugs known as aromatase inhibitors which are used predominantly in women with breast cancer; however, these may be of benefit to some men who have low levels of testosterone associated with high levels of estrogen. We will discuss this later in this chapter.

Within the blood, 40 to 50% of testosterone is tightly bound to a protein known as sex hormone binding globulin (SHBG) and is not readily available for use. Another significant proportion is bound to a protein known as albumin, and only 2 to 4% of testosterone is actually circulating freely. This is known as free testosterone as opposed to the total testosterone level and this will be important when we talk about evaluating a man with symptoms of low testosterone. Interestingly, DHT also binds to androgen receptors but with a greater affinity than testosterone, causing DHT to be a more potent hormone.

II. Hypogonadism

Hypogonadism is due to one of two causes: firstly, failure of the testicles to produce testosterone, and secondly, failure of the pituitary gland to secrete enough LH to stimulate the Leydig cells in the testicle to make testosterone. It will be no surprise that in a man who has no testicles, there is very little testosterone produced, and likewise, in a man who has had a testicle removed for trauma or testicle cancer, testosterone levels may be low. There are men who have had undescended testicles at birth (where the testicles fail to make their way into the scrotum prior to birth), and these testicles often do not grow to full size and may be deficient in their testosterone production. Anabolic steroids turn off the testicle's production of testosterone, and if used for long enough, may cause irreversible damage such that once the man stops the anabolic Steroids, there is no testosterone production, leading the man to a lifetime dependency on testosterone supplements.

Chemotherapy has a significant negative effect on the testicles, as well as on their sperm-producing function and their testosterone-producing cells. Obviously, at Memorial Sloan-Kettering Cancer Center, we see many men who have had bone marrow transplants and stem cell transplants, who have received total body irradiation and chemotherapy, and a significant percentage of these men have low testosterone after their transplants.

There are certain syndromes and conditions that cause the pituitary gland to fail to produce LH. The most well known is a condition called Kallman's syndrome, where the cells that produce LH (and its cousin, follicle stimulating hormone, also known as FSH, the primary fertility hormone) are unable to produce these hormones. These men may also have problems with the absence of smelling ability (known as anosmia). The good news for a man with Kallman's syndrome is that, when we replenish the LH and FSH by injectable drugs, they, in fact, frequently have significant growth of the testicles and greater production of testosterone, and dramatically increase their fertility potential.

It is estimated that there are 4 to 5 million men in the United States alone who suffer from hypogonadism, and that it is age related (Figure 3). Hypogonadism is relatively uncommon in men under 50 years of age. It is estimated that approximately 5 to 10% of men will suffer from it over the course of their lifetimes, but this may be a gross underestimate. However, at 60 to 70 years of age, this incidence rises to somewhere near 20% and that figure rises closer to 30% in men above 70 years of age.

Hypogonadism is associated with certain medical conditions such as diabetes, steroid use (for example, in patients with asthma, the chronic use of prednisone is often prescribed), COPD (which is a chronic pulmonary condition), AIDS, chronic renal failure, rheumatoid arthritis, alcohol abuse, chronic liver disease, and, as previously mentioned, radiation to the testicle or cancer chemotherapy. For those of you reading this who are diabetic, if your physicians are not checking your testosterone levels with some degree of regularity, then I believe they should be doing so. Likewise, any man with chronic ongoing medical problems is at risk for having low testosterone. Two other conditions are associated with low testosterone: one is depression and the second is chronic stress or fatigue, both of which suppress the production of LH by the brain and result in low levels of testosterone. Both of these are reversible as opposed to the other medical conditions that were previously mentioned.

III. Symptoms of Low Testosterone (Table 1)

There are many symptoms of low testosterone, and unfortunately, the symptoms associated with this condition are also symptoms that occur in men with chronic fatigue, major stress, and depression. The presence of these symptoms should prompt the clinician to order blood work to determine whether the testosterone level is actually low or not, although many conditions can cause the same symptoms.

The classic signs and symptoms of hypogonadism include reduction in general well-being, decreased sexual desire (libido), increased fatiguability, loss of energy, depressed mood, decreased productivity at work, reduction in strength, increase in body fat, anemia (that is, low red blood cell count), erectile problems, and osteoporosis (or a lesser version of this, known as osteopenia).

While testosterone is the major sex hormone in men, my primary concern in men with low testosterone is reduced bone density. Osteopenia and osteoporosis put a man at increased risk for fractures, particularly in the lumbar spine, resulting in compression fractures and loss of height, as well as in his hip, resulting in hip fractures. Hip fractures are very common, but it is important to understand that in people over 50 years of age, the incidence of significant complications with hip fracture is very high and some of these complications are serious.

There is no doubt that low testosterone levels translate into reduced sexual fantasy, reduced sexual activity, and an overall reduced interest in sex.

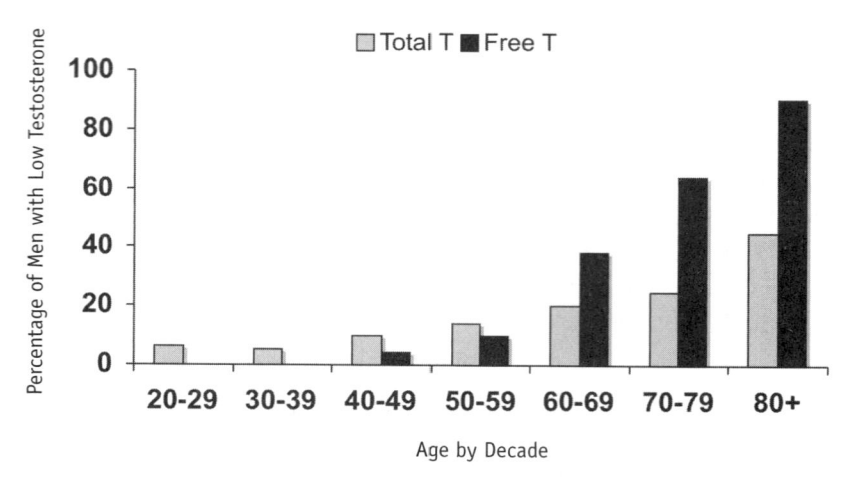

Figure 2 • Incidence of low testosterone (total and free levels) as men age (adapted from the Baltimore Longitudinal Study on Aging).

However, it is not absolutely clear whether it is directly linked to erectile dysfunction or not. Much of the literature linking erectile problems with low testosterone actually study men with practically no testosterone as opposed to men who have a slight or moderate reduction in their normal testosterone levels.

There are a number of questionnaires used for the assessment of a man with symptoms consistent with low testosterone, the most famous of which is known as the ADAM questionnaire designed by Dr. John Morley from St. Louis University. A copy of this questionnaire is appended to the end of this chapter. This is a useful screening test for you, as answering more than three of these questions with a yes is associated with low blood testosterone levels.

With regard to hip fractures, it has been estimated that approximately 70% of men with hip fractures have low testosterone versus about 30% of men who have not had hip fractures. Therefore, you can see the significant impact of low testosterone on bone density. Likewise, in men who have histories of depression and low testosterone levels, when their testosterone levels are supplemented, the incidence and severity of depression decreases dramatically. In diabetics who have hypogonadism, normalization of the testosterone level actually increases metabolic rate, decreases body fat, decreases insulin resistance, and improves sugar control. So, screening men who have diabetes for low testosterone is a critical element in their overall treatment.

Table 1 • **Symptoms of Low Testosterone Levels**

• Erectile dysfunction	• Depression
• Decreased sexual desire (libido)	• Loss of muscle mass
• Fatigue	• Weight gain
• Loss of energy	• Osteoporosis
• Sadness	• Anemia
• Grumpiness	

Finally, within the past two years there have been three studies that have clearly shown that a low level of testosterone is associated with an increase in cardiovascular disease and certain forms of cancers. I believe that men over 40 years of age should be screened regularly by a blood test to determine if the testosterone level is low.

IV. Evaluation of a Man with Low Testosterone

Evaluation is broken down into history, physical examination, and laboratory/radiology testing. I have already discussed the symptoms associated with low testosterone, so when your physician sees you, he or she should be asking you about these symptoms if you complain of low libido, decreased energy, or fatiguability.

Examination should be focused primarily on the size of the testicles. In the average male, the testicles are approximately 18 to 24 ml in size and testicular sizes that are much smaller than this are usually associated with low testosterone levels. Another important part of the examination is to examine the man's chest for the presence of breast tissue, a condition called gynecomastia. The presence of gynecomastia is frequently related to low testosterone or increased estradiol levels.

The main means of evaluating the man who may have low testosterone levels is the use of blood work. If cost is a consideration, then measuring a total testosterone level alone is all that is required. It is important to remember that this testosterone level should be performed early in the morning, probably before 10 o'clock. The reason for this is that the serum testosterone level is highest in the morning and lowest in the afternoon. It is common for me to see patients who have had a blood test showing a low testosterone level where the blood test was done at 4 o'clock in the afternoon, and when this test is repeated in the early morning, the testosterone level is actually normal. This circadian rhythm of testosterone is not as pronounced in older men as the peak and trough levels in any given day are closer together than in young men. However, we still advise that all men having a testosterone level checked should have this done in the morning. We also measure the free testosterone level, sex hormone binding globulin level, and the estradiol level (estradiol is the main estrogen in the male). If this blood test demonstrates that either the total or free testosterone levels are low, then we will repeat it. The evidence suggests that up to a third of men who are reported to have low testosterone levels on initial measurement have normal testosterone levels upon repeat testing. This may be related to variations in testosterone production from day to day or the timing of the blood draws. We never base treatment decisions on a single testosterone level. If the first testosterone level is low, then the second test is done, including the brain hormones FSH, LH, and prolactin. Prolactin is an interesting hormone in the sense that it is relatively redundant in men. However, when it is at high levels, it may indicate a benign tumor in the pituitary gland and, when it is very high, may, in fact, it suppress LH production, resulting in a low testosterone level.

All men who have documented low testosterone levels on both of the blood tests, are advised to have bone density testing. This will define whether the man has osteopenia or osteoporosis. Should the man have bone density loss, then he is an excellent candidate for testosterone, or at least the use of osteoporosis-reversing medications (known as bisphosphonates). This latter class of drugs includes such well known medications as Fosamax, Actonel, Forteo, Zometa, and Boniva.

V. Risks and Benefits of Testosterone Supplementation

The American Association of Clinical Endocrinologists, one of the groups of physicians most commonly managing patients with diabetes and hormone problems, states that men with symptoms of hypogonadism and a total testosterone level of less than 300 are candidates for testosterone replacement therapy. Some authorities suggest that levels below 400 should raise the possibility of testosterone replacement therapy.

It is important for you to understand that one or two levels of testosterone within a month of each other do not give the physician a clear sense of the testosterone profile of the patient over the course of the prior decade.

There are men who live their lives with testosterone levels of 350, and if their levels drop to 300, they may, in fact, have very few symptoms. However, there are men who live their lives with testosterone levels of 700, and if their levels drop to 300, this will translate into significant symptoms of low testosterone. Therefore, the actual amount of testosterone in the blood is not the most important thing, and its likely that the change in testosterone levels over the course of time, probably a decade or more, actually indicates whether that man will develop symptoms or not. What is interesting is that the normal range of testosterone is tremendously variable, and varies significantly from lab to lab. The functional range is probably in the 300 to 800 ng/dl range. However, some laboratories go down to 250 as the lower limit and some labs go up to 1200 as the upper limit. My recommendation to you is, if you are having your blood work done for testosterone levels, that you have the blood test done at the same lab consistently so that the different lab tests can be compared using the same reference range.

In a man with low levels of testosterone, the benefits are obvious. If you remember the symptoms of low testosterone, pretty much all of these symptoms can be improved to some extent by increasing the testosterone level in the blood. It may take two to three months with a normal testosterone level to start seeing some improvement in symptoms, but it is common for men to report increased libido, increased energy level, less fatiguability, better mood, better productivity at work, and on occasion, improvement in erectile function. If a man has osteopenia or osteoporosis, it is not uncommon to see reversal of this over a six- to twelve-month period once the testosterone level is normalized. It is not uncommon for men to lose body fat and weight when their testosterone levels are increased. Men will often claim when they have low testosterone that even though they are working out regularly, they do not see the positive results in their bodies that they used to see when they were younger. However, when we restore testosterone levels to normal, they will claim that they are now starting to see benefits from their work-out schedules.

As switch any medication, there are potential side effects. The first one is increase in red blood cell count (this is measured as a percentage known as hematocrit). Now, while low levels (anemia) are bad for us, very high levels are also bad. The reason for this is that, when red blood counts get to very high levels, they actually increase the viscosity of the blood and the blood tends to get thicker; this may be associated with conditions such as stroke. Generally speaking, if a man's hematocrit level before treatment is over 50, he should see a hematologist for evaluation of this before being given any form of testosterone supplementation. Of note, it is common for cigarette smokers to have very high levels of red blood cells in their blood.

Testosterone therapy–associated elevations in red blood cell count, hematocrit and hemoglobin are reported to be more common and significant in men using injectable testosterone compared to those using patches or gels. Historically, there have been concerns about lipid (cholesterol, triglycerides etc) levels. However, there is excellent accumulating evidence to show that lipid levels may actually be decreased by normalization of testosterone levels and, as stated previously, that a man's cardiovascular risk is actually reduced when having a normal testosterone level versus a low testosterone level.

Rising testosterone levels may be associated with some adverse effects. In men who have sleep apnea, the condition may be worsened by achieving very high levels of testosterone in the blood, and likewise, men with very high testosterone levels can develop gynecomastia. This is due to the fact that the testosterone is being broken down by aromatase to estradiol, and high levels of estradiol will cause gynecomastia. It is my experience, in hundreds of men on testosterone treatment, that if their blood levels remain in the middle of the normal range, then neither sleep apnea or gynecomastia are concerns.

We are trying to place the vast majority of men into the middle of the normal range. If the normal range is 300–800, we are trying to get men into the 550–point (plus or minus 50) range. This is readily achievable for most men using most testosterone supplementation strategies.

Still, there is great concern about the impact of testosterone supplementation on the prostate gland. The development of the prostate is dependent on testosterone during fetal life. As we age, DHT becomes the major androgen in the prostate, resulting in enlargement. In men with low baseline levels of testosterone who are treated to increase their testosterone levels, there is a mild increase in prostate size, but this increase has been shown to be no greater than in healthy age-matched controls, suggesting that the impact of supplementing a man's testosterone into the normal range is insignificant. We also know from using scoring systems to assess a man's urinary function (the International Prostate Symptom Score, for example) that there is no significant increase in the IPSS when men have their testosterone levels normalized.

After testosterone supplementation, PSA (the prostate cancer blood test) levels increase although the amount by which it increases is relatively small. In reports, anywhere between 0.2 to 0.75 unit increases have been seen over a 12–month period. However, these are not believed to be clinically significant. While the precise cause of benign prostate enlargement (BPH) is not well understood, the presence of androgens, in particular testosterone and DHT, although not causative, is required for the development of BPH. Interestingly, despite decreasing levels of testosterone in the blood as we age, levels of DHT within the prostate remain high, and lowering of DHT using 5–alpha reductase inhibitors results in a reduction in prostate symptoms.

VI. Testosterone and Prostate Cancer

In 1941, Huggins and Hodges demonstrated that men with metastatic prostate cancer could be treated by castration. In fact, Charles Huggins went on to win the Nobel Prize for this research. It is this finding that has caused tremendous concern among patients and physicians about the use of testosterone supplementation in men with a diagnosis of prostate cancer, because physicians and patients alike have become accustomed to the concept that "testosterone feeds prostate cancer cells." However, the literature, both animal and human, is murky regarding the role of testosterone in prostate cancer development. The bottom line is that there is no large long-term study that has looked at the use of testosterone supplementation in men with prostate cancer diagnosis, post-prostatectomy, or post–radiation therapy. It is safe to say that most studies to date have not found a significant association between testosterone levels and the development of prostate cancer, although there are rare reports to the contrary on this issue.

What is interesting is that men tend to develop prostate cancer at a time in their lives, when their testosterone levels are at the lowest point, as opposed to 21–year-old men, who have the highest testosterone levels, yet essentially zero incidence of prostate cancer. Another interesting fact is that men with very low levels of testosterone cannot produce normal levels of PSA. PSA is a chemical produced by the prostate cells which needs testosterone for its production, and failure to have testosterone at a level results in a relative absence of PSA. There is some evidence that men with low testosterone who are diagnosed with prostate cancer have higher grade (level of aggressiveness) and higher stage (level of invasion) prostate cancer compared to men with normal testosterone levels. This suggests that men with low testosterone levels, when diagnosed with prostate cancer, may have a delayed diagnosis. Some authorities talk of a "testosterone challenge," which means that men with low testosterone levels should have testosterone supplemented to see if their PSA levels rise significantly. This may allow the early diagnosis of prostate cancer, which otherwise would have gone undiagnosed until it became advanced, perhaps metastatic in nature. I have personally seen men with low testosterone levels and PSA levels of 2.0 (well in the normal range) who, when supplemented with testosterone, have normalization of the testosterone levels into the middle of the normal testosterone range, but their PSA levels now shoots up above 4 (the level above which prostate biopsy is advised).

In a highly informative study by Dr. Abraham Morgentaler in Boston, patients who had the precursor to prostate cancer known as PIN (prostatic intraepithelial neoplasia), who had low testosterone, were supplemented with testosterone. There were only 20 cases. However, after 12 months follow-up, only one patient with PIN was actually diagnosed with prostate cancer after repeat biopsy for an abnormal prostate exam. In this study, there were slight increases in PSA but no significant difference between the men with PIN versus those men who did not have PIN in the study. Thus, this study would suggest that even in men with precancerous changes in their prostates when supplemented with testosterone, experience no significant incidence of prostate cancer development.

There are several small series reporting the use of testosterone in men after radical prostatectomy. These series number anywhere from five to 20 patients, and none of them show any significant concern for PSA recurrence after prostatectomy. At Memorial Sloan-Kettering Cancer Center, patients who have low testosterone after radical prostatectomy, who are symptomatic, are sent to see me by the cancer surgeons. If these men have documented low testosterone levels on two blood tests, if they have symptoms classically associated with low testosterone, if they have two PSA blood tests after surgery that are undetectable, and if they have cancer confined to the prostate and a Gleason score of 7 or less, they are considered candidates for testosterone supplementation. We have a serious, face-to-face, pros-and-cons, risks-and-benefits discussion with the patient and the bottom line, in my opinion, is that testosterone supplementation in any population, but especially in this population (that is, men post-prostatectomy or with a diagnosis of prostate cancer), is a negotiated one. We have had several patients in my clinic who had low testosterone prior to surgery, and then underwent radical prostatectomy. Then, their cancer surgeons would not allow them to receive testosterone supplementation after surgery and the patients came in to see me

CASE HISTORY EIGHT
Testosterone Supplementation after Radical Prostatectomy

Victor is a 48-year-old man. At the time I saw him, he was married to a 38-year-old woman and had three children. He indicated then that they were not planning on having any more children. He had undergone a radical prostatectomy for Gleason 6 organ-confined prostate cancer. He first saw me four months after surgery to start penile rehabilitation. At that time, on examination, his testicles were approximately half the normal size and he had varicose veins (varicoceles) around both his testicles. On closer questioning, he had a low sex drive, low energy, would fall a sleep after meals routinely, and had also noticed a decrease in productivity at work. He had a total testosterone level of 200 upon first testing, and when repeated, it was 250, both levels being well below normal (normal range 300 to 800). He had a bone density scan which demonstrated softening of his bones (osteopenia, the step before osteoporosis occurs). By five months after surgery, he had three PSA levels measured, all of which were undetectable. His chance of having an undetectable PSA at 10 years after surgery using the Memorial Sloan-Kettering nomogram was 95%. We discussed testosterone supplementation, its pros and cons, risks and benefits, including the absence of long-term safety data on testosterone supplementation in men after radical prostatectomy. However, I informed him of several small studies suggesting testosterone supplementation in a radical prostatectomy patient was safe. We discussed the concept of a three-month trial and he started on a testosterone gel at 2.5 g/day. Two weeks later, his total testosterone level was 380 and he experienced a mild improvement in symptoms. His dose was increased to 5 g/day and his repeat testosterone level was 520 with a dramatic improvement in his energy, his libido, and his work productivity. Two years later he has had no change in his PSA level and his symptoms have remained improved. His bone density normalized within 12 months of starting testosterone supplementation.

This case history discusses a very controversial area in sexual medicine. Five years ago, the thought of giving a man after radical prostatectomy, testosterone supplementation would have been considered unacceptable. However, there has been a shift in thinking over the course of the last few

continued on the next page

continued from the previous page

> years, and currently, in highly select individuals, specifically, men who have a very good prognosis, and who have organ-confined cancer and definite symptoms of low testosterone, testosterone supplementation is considered. The supplementation of testosterone in this population is a negotiated decision. The patient needs to be made aware of the pros and cons and the risks and benefits. This man had symptoms that were classic for low testosterone levels including osteopenia, and had significant improvement in testosterone level and symptoms within the first few months after starting testosterone supplementation and, most importantly, at two years after starting testosterone gel, there was no increase in his PSA level.

complaining of suicidal thoughts resulting from such a low level of testosterone. At the time of writing, we have approximately 25 patients who are after radical prostatectomy at Memorial Sloan-Kettering Cancer Center with the features outlined above, who have been placed on testosterone supplementation in some fashion, and no PSA recurrence has occurred.

I am not aware of any literature that addresses the use of testosterone in men who have had radiation therapy for prostate cancer. Conceptually, it is a great concern to me if a man who underwent radiation therapy for prostate cancer, who has his prostate remaining, who may have dormant cancer cells remaining in the prostate, goes on testosterone because of the concern of waking up the dormant prostate cancer cells. As testosterone supplementation is a negotiated decision, I have a small number of patients post-radiation for prostate cancer who, after a serious discussion about risks, opted for testosterone treatment. These men have all been more than 5 years after radiation, have stable PSA levels, had an endorectal MRI which did not raise suspicion for recurrent cancer, and had repeat prostate biopsy which failed to show any remaining cancer. Only under these circumstances would I even consider testosterone supplementation in the prostate radiation patient.

VII. How Testosterone Is Supplemented

Testosterone levels can be supplemented in a number of ways (Table 2), including pills, injections, patches, gels, and non-testosterone-based strategies. Let us start off with the latter. There are two major concerns of testoster-

Table 2 • **Means of Increasing Testosterone Levels**

Testosterone-based supplementation	
Gels	Androgel
	Testim
Patches	Androderm
	Testoderm
Intramuscular injections	Testosterone enanthate (Delatestryl)
	Testosterone cypionate (Depo-testosterone)
	Testosterone propionate (Testrona)
	Testosterone undeanoate (Nebido)*

Subcutaneous pellets**

Non-testosterone-based supplementation
Clomiphene citrate (Clomid, Seraphene)
Intramuscular human chorionic gonadotropin (hCG)

* Available currently only outside of the United States
** Not used commonly

one supplementation. Firstly, testosterone is a relatively good contraceptive. It turns off the brain hormones that produce sperm (FSH), and therefore men for whom fertility is a concern, in my opinion, are poor candidates for testosterone supplementation. When a man receives testosterone supplements in a regular fashion for more than six to twelve months, he runs a significant risk of having irreversible damage to his testicles, such that when the testosterone supplement is stopped, the man's testicles will no longer be able to produce any sperm.

Secondly, when men are given testosterone supplements for a prolonged period of time (the exact duration is unclear), then the testicles will shrink and they will no longer be able to produce testosterone; therefore, the man will be dependent on testosterone supplements for the rest of his life. So, in my practice there is a three-month trial period during which the patient has the testosterone level normalized, and then we review the symptom improvement. If there is significant symptom improvement and the patient is interested in continuing testosterone supplementation, then we will do so. If there is no significant improvement in symptoms, then the patient will have the testosterone supplementation stopped.

There are also two strategies that can be used that do not entail the use of testosterone. The first is the use of a pill by the name of clomiphene citrate (more commonly known as Clomid). This pill is probably better known to women than men as it is used for female fertility problems. What is interesting about clomiphene is that it actually increases LH levels from the pituitary gland and may, in fact, result in significant increases in testosterone levels. Men who are good candidates for this treatment are men with low levels of testosterone who have symptoms and have normal or low levels of LH. Men with high levels of LH typically will not benefit from clomiphene. Clomiphene is a pill that is taken daily or every other day at full dose (50 mg) or half dose (25 mg). It has practically no side effects other than some potential for weight gain (usually seen at higher doses than what we use) as well as some blurred vision. It is very well tolerated and there is no known time limit on its use. There is a concern about tolerance to the medication; in a small percentage of men, repeated usage will result in decreased effect. For this reason, we start patients off at a daily dose of 25 mg and one month later they have their blood tests rechecked to ascertain what level of improvement they have experienced. For young men, for men concerned about fertility, and for men concerned about permanent testicular shrinkage, we routinely use clomiphene citrate.

Another, slightly more invasive strategy for men which does not involve testosterone directly is the use of intramuscular hCG injections. hCG (human chorionic gonadotropin) is another fertility hormone which induces ovulation in women. It is very similar from a structural standpoint to LH, the hormone that causes testosterone to be produced by the Leydig cells in the testicle. It can be given as an injection into muscle (shoulder, buttocks) and can cause the testicles to produce testosterone. Once again, men who have high levels of LH are not likely to respond very well to this strategy. We use between 1,000 and 1,500 international units and inject it three times a week, and once again, blood work is checked approximately one month after commencing this treatment.

In the history of supplementing testosterone, testosterone pills have been used previously but are currently not available in the United States. They come in a variety of forms and the reason they are not available in this country, although they are available in Canada and in Europe, is that some of them are associated with irreversible liver damage. Practically speaking, there is no longer any role for oral agents in the management of low testosterone, at least in the United States.

There are a variety of injectable testosterone agents that can be self-administered by patients under the supervision of a physician. These include testosterone enanthate (Delatestryl), testosterone cypionate (Depo-testosterone), and testosterone propionate (Testosterona). These agents need to be injected regularly (every one to three weeks), and the dose and the frequency of injection depends on blood test results. The ideal way to do blood tests in a man using intramuscular testosterone is to do two blood tests: the first (peak) level is checked one day after the intramuscular testosterone injection and the second (trough) level is checked the day of the next injection prior to the injection being given. The peak and trough levels will give a clear sense for what dose and what frequency should be used. The average man starts with 200 mg given intramuscularly two weeks apart. We do have some men who use it weekly and we have men who require it only once every three weeks.

The downside to injectable testosterone is that it results in very wide variations in testosterone levels. For the first three to five days after injection, patients typically have levels above normal. For the ensuing seven days, the levels are in the normal range, although they drop over the course of the week. For the last three or so days of the cycle, the testosterone levels are below normal. It is likely that these wide variations result in greater side effects, particularly with red blood cell count, sleep apnea, and lipid profile changes.

While not available in the United States at the time of writing this book, there is a drug being tested in trials at the moment called Nebido, which is testosterone undecanoate, an intramuscular injection given once every three months or so. Nebido has shown some significant effectiveness in getting steady normal testosterone levels in European studies (no peaks and troughs in the testosterone levels). It is likely that medication will play a significant role in the treatment of men with low testosterone levels. When I talk to men about this drug, they are interested in the fact that they will need only four injections a year rather than having to take a pill every day, a shot once every two weeks, or rub a gel on daily. This drug is eagerly awaited and may be available in 2010.

Testosterone patches and testosterone gels (known together as trandermal therapy) have played a large role in testosterone supplementation over the course of the last decade. These result in stable testosterone levels without the large peak and trough levels seen with injectable drugs. Testosterone patches have fallen significantly out of favor over the course of the last five years since the introduction of the gels. Patches were applied either to the scrotum (Testoderm) or to a non-hair-bearing part of the body (Androderm). While 85% of our patients were able to achieve normal levels of testosterone with the patches, there was a significant incidence of skin reaction because of an allergic reaction to the vehicle present within the patch. For this reason, the gels have essentially taken over for the patches.

There are two gels available: Androgel and Testim. Androgel comes in a pump as well as in tubes. These are gels that are rubbed on skin and are absorbed directly through the skin. We are interested in the pump delivery because one pump equals 1.25 gm of testosterone. The average man starts at 5 gm, and so we can titrate very accurately and in very small increments, and this is very important to us in a man who is post-prostatectomy or radiation, as we are trying to ensure that he does not get too high a level.

Testim comes only in a tube and has a slightly musky smell. However, the vehicle that is used in Testim is more potent than in Androgel and it absorbs more readily. For patients who fail to absorb testosterone effectively using maximum-dose Androgel, we will switch them to Testim; we have had significant success in converting an Androgel failure to a Testim success. It is worth mentioning that, from a cost effectiveness standpoint, intramuscular testosterone injection is the least expensive. The testosterone gels are relatively expensive at approximately $150 to $200 per month, and for some men testosterone gels are not covered by their health insurance carriers.

The concern about transfer of testosterone gel from the patient to his partner or his children has not been seen in my practice. So, as long as the patient is given clear instructions how to use the medication, this issue is not a concern. The vast majority of the agent is absorbed within ten to fifteen minutes and if the man knows that he is going to come in contact with another person, then he just needs to cover up that area using some clothing. Of note, when applying the gel, avoid the area in front of the elbow where blood is drawn. The reason for this is that when blood is being drawn for measuring the testosterone level, any testosterone gel on the skin at the point where the needle is placed will result in an artificially high testosterone level result.

Finally, there was a testosterone pellet available, which was placed under the lip against the gum, known as Striant. This never really took off and, to the best of my knowledge, is not used very much any more. There are also subcutaneous testosterone pellets that can be injected under the skin of the abdomen, for example, but once again they are not approved in the United States nor are they used with any great degree of frequency.

VIII. Monitoring of the Patient Receiving Testosterone Supplementation

Prior to starting testosterone supplementation in any of the fashions outlined above, a man, of course, will have his testosterone level checked, should have his red blood cell count, hemoglobin, and hematocrit checked, should have his PSA level checked, and should have a prostate exam to make sure there are no abnormalities. Approximately one month later, I will check total testosterone, free testosterone, hematocrit, and PSA and estradiol levels to define the impact of the testosterone supplementation. If these levels are abnormal, then we will switch the dose of the medication or even change the route of administration. At three months, the patient has repeat testosterone levels checked along with hemoglobin, hematocrit, and PSA levels, and a prostate exam performed. We insist all of our patients on testosterone replacement have testosterone levels checked every six months after this, along with a PSA, and if the patient has a history of a radical prostatectomy, he will have his PSA levels checked every three months.

APPENDIX 1
ADAM questionnaire about symptoms of low testosterone (Androgen Deficiency in the Aging Male)

1. Do you have a decrease in libido (sex drive)?	Yes	No
2. Do you have a lack of energy?	Yes	No
3. Do you have a decrease in strength and/or endurance?	Yes	No
4. Have you lost height?	Yes	No
5. Have you noticed a decreased "enjoyment of life"	Yes	No
6. Are you sad and/or grumpy?	Yes	No
7. Are your erections less strong?	Yes	No
8. Have you noticed a recent deterioration in your ability to play sports?	Yes	No
9. Are you falling asleep after dinner?	Yes	No
10. Has there been a recent deterioration in your work performance?	Yes	No

APPENDIX 2
AMS Testosterone Deficiency Questionnaire

Which of the following symptoms apply to you at this time? Please, mark the appropriate box for each symptom. For symptoms that do not apply, please mark "none".

Symptoms	none	mild	moderate	severe	extremely severe
1. Decline in your feeling of general well-being (general state of health, subjective feeling)	☐	☐	☐	☐	☐
2. Joint pain and muscular ache (lower back pain, joint pain, pain in a limb, general back ache)	☐	☐	☐	☐	☐
3. Excessive sweating (sudden episodes of sweating, hot flushes independent of strain)	☐	☐	☐	☐	☐
4. Sleep problems (difficulty falling asleep, waking up early, poor sleep, sleeplessness)	☐	☐	☐	☐	☐
5. Increased need for sleep, often feeling tired	☐	☐	☐	☐	☐
6. Irritability (feeling aggressive, easily upset about little things, moody)	☐	☐	☐	☐	☐
7. Nervousness (inner tension, restlessness, feeling fidgety)	☐	☐	☐	☐	☐
8. Anxiety (feeling panicky)	☐	☐	☐	☐	☐
9. Physical exhaustion/lacking vitality (general decrease in performance, reduced activity, lacking interest in leisure activities, feeling of getting less done)	☐	☐	☐	☐	☐
10. Decrease in muscular strength (feeling of weakness)	☐	☐	☐	☐	☐
11. Depressive mood (feeling down, sad, on the verge of tears, lack of drive, mood swings)	☐	☐	☐	☐	☐
12. Feeling that you have passed your peak	☐	☐	☐	☐	☐
13. Feeling burnt out, having hit rock-bottom	☐	☐	☐	☐	☐
14. Decrease in beard growth	☐	☐	☐	☐	☐
15. Decrease in ability/frequency to perform sexually	☐	☐	☐	☐	☐
16. Decrease in the number of morning erections	☐	☐	☐	☐	☐
17. Decrease in sexual desire/libido (lacking pleasure in sex, lacking desire for sexual relations)	☐	☐	☐	☐	☐

CHAPTER 16

GETTING BACK A SEX LIFE

> I. What Is a Normal Sex Life?
> II. The Effect of Aging on Sexual Function
> III. Seeing a Doctor for Sexual Problems
> IV. Re-establishing a Good Sex Life

I. What Is a Normal Sex Life?

So now that you have read through all the aforementioned evidence, figures, and scientific mumbo-jumbo, what about getting back to actually having sex? Over the course of my 12 years as a sexual medicine physician, I have seen thousands of couples and I can therefore say without hesitation that there is no such thing as a "normal" sex life. I see many 50–year-olds in my practice who rarely have sex and I have many 80–year-olds who have sex on a regular basis. It is, however, safe to say that men and women tend to either be sexual beings or non-sexual beings. One of the predictors of continued sexual activity in old age is a high level of activity at a younger age. Nobody feels comfortable thinking of their parents or even their grandparents being sexually active. It is estimated that 80 to 90% of men in their 40s are having sex weekly versus approximately one-third of men over 60 years of age. The Cologne male survey suggested that 70% of 70–year-olds were having sex and 40% of them were having sex weekly. While it is likely that not all of them are having sexual intercourse but rather other forms of sexual activity, it does indicate that older people are sexually active. Couples ask me all the time how often they should be having sex and there is no right answer to this question. However, in older couples, men are typically interested in sex on a more regular basis than their female partners.

Research conducted in developed countries has shown that 18– to 30–year-olds have sex an average of eight times per month, in 30– to 40–year-olds about seven times a month, and in 40– to 50–year-olds an average of five times per month. About a quarter of unmarried men and women report that they have not had sex in the past year. In married men, 13% report having sex only a few times in the past year, almost half reported having sex a few times in the past month, and a third of them report having sex two to three times a week, with about one in seven reporting having sex four times or more a week. These figures are approximately similar for married women.

So you can see that the majority of even young people are having sex no more than one to two times per week. Just as some people can be described as sexual or non-sexual beings, couples also conduct sex in generally two patterns, that is, planned or spontaneous, and some couples will use either approach depending upon the circumstances. The older a couple gets, it has been my experience, the more planned relations are, and the younger the couple, the more spontaneous relations are. The average 65–year-old man has been married for 35 years may have sex once per week or once every two weeks and typically has a clear idea when that will happen through either verbal or non-verbal communication with his partner.

A very large study sponsored by the Pfizer Corporation called the Global Study of Sexual Attitudes and Behaviors questioned almost 30,000 men and women from many countries throughout the world about the importance of sex in their lives. Eighty-three percent of men and 63% of women said that sex was very, extremely or moderately important to them. When asked about whether they had sexual intercourse over the past 12 months, 83% of men answered yes compared to 66% of women.

It is clear that orgasm is far more important to men than it is to women and the overwhelming majority of men are orgasmic with either self stimulation or with partner sex. Indeed, orgasm is the general focus for most men, particularly young men. Women in general are more likely to be orgasmic without a partner being present. It is estimated that approximately one-third of women have never had an orgasm, approximately a third of women have had an orgasm only on their own, and only one-third of women have had an orgasm in the presence of a partner.

Our understanding of the sexual lives of people, in particular Americans, rests on the shoulders of several key researchers. Kinsey (and now the Kinsey Institute), Masters and Johnson, and Dr. Edward Laumann, an eminent sociologist at the University of Chicago, have all made huge contributions to this field. It is well documented that men think about sex, and have more sexual fantasies and more sexual desires than women, regardless of age or relationship status. The discrepancy in these factors is greatest in young men and lowest in older men.

The sexual script of any couple is dependent upon many different factors, including cultural, relationship, and personal factors. The majority of men initiate sex and men tend to use more direct methods to initiate sex. For women reading this book, it is important that you understand that, generally speaking, men do not like to perform on demand. A classic example of this is a man who is in an infertile relationships who get a phone call in the middle of the day from his partner saying, "Today is the day that I'm ovulating," and that they have to have sex that night. Under these circumstances, somewhere between a third and one-half of men will develop erection problems. This on-demand erection performance is very adrenaline-producing and, as I previously mentioned, adrenaline is very much an anti-erection chemical.

One of the most common reasons in my practice for men failing to initiate sexual encounters is erectile dysfunction. You will read several times in this book that confidence is critical for a man's erection. As men, we often believe we are only as good as our last erection and, if the last erection was poor or less than what we were looking for, we will be worried the next time we walk into the bedroom. This lack of confidence leads to a reduced libido, avoidance behavior, and reduced sexual activity frequency.

II. The Effect of Aging on Sexual Function

Aging affects both male and female sexual health and function. In men, aging is associated with increasing incidence of erectile dysfunction, decreased sex drive, decreased sexual fantasy, and decreased sexual frequency. The Massachusetts Male Aging Study, which was a study conducted originally between 1987 and 1989 in the Boston area, studied almost 1,300 men and assessed their erectile function. The subjects were aged between 40 and 70 years, and over those 30 years 52% of men had some degree of erectile dysfunction and a third had clinically significant erection problems. It was estimated that one in twenty 40–year-old men and one in five 70–year-old men had the complete inability to have sexual intercourse.

While the incidence of erectile dysfunction in international studies varies between 10 to 35%, one thing that is clear that is erectile dysfunction is a common problem and is associated with aging. Whether age itself is the major factor or not is unclear and it may be that erectile dysfunction is associated with other factors, such as the increased likelihood of having high blood pressure, high cholesterol, or diabetes, and the cumulative effect of cigarette smoking. Men with diabetes are four times more likely to develop ED, men with benign prostate enlargement three times more likely, and men with high blood pressure and elevated cholesterol levels two times more likely. Cigarette smoking has also been shown to be a significant risk factor for the development of erection problems. Another message from the Massachusetts Male Aging Study is that changing lifestyle factors, such as weight, activity level, and cigarette smoking in mid-life may be too late to have any real impact on future erectile function and thus, it appears that these changes need to be made as a young adult.

With regard to libido, I have talked about this in great detail in the chapter on testosterone (Chapter 15). Testosterone, which is produced by the testicles predominantly, is the primary libido hormone for both men and women. As men age, there is an approximate 10% reduction per decade of life in the testosterone levels in our blood. For some men, there is a 25% reduction per decade in life. The symptoms associated with low testosterone while including low libido, also include decreased energy levels, fatiguability, decreased motivation, sad mood, decreased productivity at work, falling asleep after meals, as well as some other symptoms. As we age, our testicles tend to become softer and sometimes smaller. Given that this occurs, men's testosterone levels drop. The normal range for testosterone is approximately 300 to 800 ng/dl. However, it is not known what testosterone level is required for a man to have an excellent libido. Low testosterone is not the only cause of low libido. In fact, low libido is associated with conditions such as depression, chronic fatigue, and chronic stress.

As we age, the amount of semen that we ejaculate also reduces. This is partly related to the reduced testosterone levels that occur in older men, as semen production is heavily dependent upon the testosterone level in the blood. It may also be related to the fact that most older men have a slightly enlarged prostate, and the prostate compresses the urethra and may obstruct the flow of semen through the penis. Some men with very large prostates have retrograde ejaculation, where the semen is transported back into the bladder rather than out through the penis, due to the blockage the prostate is causing. For some of these men, the retrograde ejaculation is worsened by prostate medications such as Flomax (tamsulosin) or Uroxatral (alfuzosin).

The time it takes to achieve an orgasm from the start of sexual stimulation increases as we age. This is probably related to multiple factors, including penile sensitivity issues. Interestingly, however, very recent evidence suggests that the incidence of premature ejaculation in older men is very similar to that in younger men. One of the most common causes of premature ejaculation that is primary in nature (that means where the patient has not had the premature ejaculation all of his life) is the presence of erectile dysfunction. A man who has problems with sustaining capability of his erections will sometimes train himself (subconsciously) to ejaculate more quickly so that he does not lose the erection prior to orgasm.

While female sexual dysfunction is beyond the scope of this book, I refer you to several excellent resources for information on female sexual health at the end of the book. Female sexual dysfunction is divided into four categories: low libido (medically termed hypoactive sexual desire disorder), problems with lubrication and clitoral engorgement (medically termed female sexual arousal disorder), orgasmic disorders, and sexual pain disorders. As women pass through menopause, the ovaries fail to function and they lose the majority of their estrogen and up to 60% of their testosterone. Given that testosterone is a primary libido hormone, it is not difficult to see why postmenopausal women may have decreased sexual desire. However, it is not as simple as a straightforward hormonal issue. There are many factors that impact a woman's libido and, when speaking with women in my practice, relationship issues tend to be the most significant factor.

There is tremendous controversy about what defines sexual dysfunction in women versus a state of sexual health. It is true that there are many women who lubricate poorly and who have low sexual desire who are not bothered by these symptoms. It is difficult to conclude that these women have dysfunctions. The hormonal changes that occur around menopause may lead to a condition known as atrophic vaginitis. This condition, which is related to low estrogen levels in the genital area, results in stiffening of the tissues at the opening of the vagina (the introitus). This combined with poor lubrication may cause significant pain upon vaginal penetration.

While erectile dysfunction is a problem effecting men, it has a huge impact on the couple. It has been shown that women who are sexually active tend to have better vaginal health than women who are not sexually active. The vagina is a muscular structure which, if not being used, can contract; if a couple has not had sex for two years, then going straight to having sexual intercourse is inadvisable. The vagina, in effect, needs to undergo a period of dilation so that discomfort is minimized. This can be achieved in a number of ways, including through the use of vaginal dilators. It is important not to underestimate the negative impact that sexual pain has on a partner's interest in having sex. The concept of psychotherapy and hormone treatment for women with sexual dysfunction is well beyond the scope of this book; these are highly controversial issues even in the field of sexual medicine.

III. Seeing a Doctor for Sexual Problems

Patients often struggle with deciding which type of physician they should see for their sexual problems. If you have had prostate surgery, radiation, or hormonal therapy for your prostate cancer, then the first person you should bring this up with is your treating physician, whether it be a surgeon, radiation oncologist, or medical oncologist. The greatest level of expertise lies in urologists (this is not to say that there are not primary care physicians, internists, cardiologists, or endocrinologists who have specific expertise in sexual problems). Among the 9,000 urologists in the United States of America, there is a select number who specialize in sexual medicine. These experts can be found on the website for the Sexual Medicine Society of North America (www.sexhealthmatters.org). Among this group of 300 urologists, there is an even smaller group whose members conduct research and have very busy practices focussing on the prostate cancer patient, as is the case with me.

There are several obstacles to the delivery of good sexual health care to patients. The first is physician discomfort. It is shocking to the public that most medical students during medical school obtain no more than two hours of education in adult sexual health. It is impossible to prepare a young physician for the complexity and sensitivity of a sexual health discussion in two hours. It is common for a patient or couple to tell me that they brought up the subject with their physician, but it was clear to them that their physician was uncomfortable. There is research that suggests that two-thirds of patients who fail to bring up sexual health to their primary care physicians do so because they are afraid that the physician would be embarrassed. Furthermore, it is estimated based on the Global Study of Sexual Attitudes and Behaviors that less than one in seven physicians ever ask their patients about sexual health. It is easy to see why the primary care physician will not do this. In addition to the discomfort level, there are significant time constraints.

In the current health insurance environment, physicians have to see more patients to make a smaller amount of money than they were earning 10 years ago. So when a patient goes to his primary care physician to discuss his high blood pressure, high cholesterol, cigarette smoking, and weight, the physician will focus on the correction of his blood pressure, his cholesterol level, and his weight, and try to encourage the patient to stop smoking. At the bottom of the list of things for the physician to talk to him about is his sexual function.

There is tremendous pressure on family physicians and internists to treat every aspect of your medical health when, in fact, there is significant benefit to seeking expert help when it comes to sexual function. It is estimated that a third to half of men who are prescribed Viagra-like drugs by their primary care physicians are using them improperly. Furthermore, when patients are counseled and re-educated by a urologist, they may, in fact, then respond with good erections to these medications. It is also estimated that one-third of men stop from using Viagra-like drugs within one prescription and half of them by six months, and one of the factors causing this is the failure of physicians to follow-up with patients.

If you had high blood pressure, your physician would give you a medication to treat that and would monitor your blood pressure while on treatment, Right? Due to time constraints and physician discomfort level, it is common for physicians not to schedule follow-up visits with patients regarding their response and satisfaction with erection medications. This lack of follow-up results in patients giving up the medication. Your physician should interview and examine you in a private environment, speak to you at a level that you can understand, not be judgmental, and have a sense of optimism with regard to your treatment. I tell patients that 95% of patients can get back to having sexual intercourse in the future.

During your interview, you will be asked questions about your erections. These questions will address how long you have had problems, how you would grade your erection hardness, your ability to get and keep an erection, whether you have night-time erections, your sexual activity level both on your own and with a partner, whether you have consistent or intermittent problems, and whether the onset of erection problems was sudden or gradual. Of course, for the man who has had a radical prostatectomy, the onset of erectile dysfunction, if he had normal erections before surgery, is very acute. You may be asked about the difference in your erection hardness between a sexual erection and a masturbatory erection. Men who have sudden-onset erection problems or who experience some good erections alternating with poor erections may have psychologically based erection problems.

You should also be asked about your libido, your ejaculation, and your orgasm function. Your physician should also inquire as to whether you have any penile curvature or deformity. With regard to hardness, we use a 10–point scale, where 10/10 is fully rigid, 6/10 is just about good enough for vaginal penetration (7/10 for anal penetration), and 0/10 is completely soft like it is when we walk around during the day. Thinking about answers to these questions before going in to see your physician will speed up the interview process and may help inform the physician as to what questions are important to you. The physician will want to know what your goals and expectations are. For most patients, the goal is to have sexual intercourse again. For some younger patients, the goal is to be off all medication and be cured. Some older patients come in on a fact-finding mission and really have very little interest in sexual activity but are concerned that their erection problems may be the manifestation of an underlying medical condition that might be serious.

Your doctor will then perform a physical examination, with the majority of the time spent examining your genital area. Your penis will be examined and its stretch will be assessed. The penis is a muscle very much like your hamstring and should be very stretchy. Penises that have poor stretch either have erection tissue damage or tunical damage, such as in Peyronie's disease. Your testicles will be examined and their size and consistency will be noted, and any other important features that are linked to testosterone deficiency will also be recorded. If you are over 50 years of age and have not had your prostate checked recently, you likely will also have a prostate exam. As part of your evaluation, you may have some blood work done to check your hormone levels as well as a PSA if you are over 50 years of age.

It is unfortunate, but many patients tell me that when they see their family doctors/internists and sometimes even their urologists, the questioning regarding their sexual health occurs at the very end of the interview, when the physician is trying to move on to the next patient. The physician has a hand on the doorknob and the patient is forced to bring up the subject without the physician ever having mentioned it. Often, this leads to the physician giving the patient a sample of Viagra, Levitra, or Cialis without ever going over instructions as to how to use the medication.

I encourage my patients to bring their partners in for the interview. There are many reasons why this is advantageous for the physician and for the patient. Firstly, most patients have some level of anxiety when they are seeing a physician to talk about their sexual function. Under these circumstances, it is not uncommon for patients to forget some of the information that was given. Having a partner present will increase the amount of information that will be remembered. Secondly, the purpose of a sexual medicine physician is to restore the couple, if the man is in a physical relationship, to satisfactory sexual relations. This needs to take into account not just erection, libido, and ejaculation status for the man, but also partner factors. Having a partner present may allow the physician to discuss some of these factors and determine what is the best course of action for the couple as opposed to just for the man. Even something as simple as assessing a patient's erection hardness when taking a medical history is often impacted by whether the partner is present. It is common for a man to overestimate his erection hardness, and having a partner present to corroborate his erectile rigidity before and after prostate cancer treatment is helpful to the physician. Finally, men are poor at listening to instructions, following instructions, and complying with the instructions that physicians give them. It is my experience that having the partner present helps improve the patient's compliance with treatment.

Most of all, I would encourage you to be proactive about your sexual health. Given the factors that we have discussed above, physician discomfort and time constraints, sexual health is often ignored by the medical profession. I would encourage you to go into this interview with a clear sense what it is you want to discuss and what your goals and expectations are. Most physicians will welcome you walking in with a note pad with questions listed so that you do not forget anything and so that you can take notes during the discussion. Remember that it is not essential that you obtain every piece of information and have a definitive plan after one single discussion. Sometimes, optimizing the sexual function of a patient requires more than one visit. With surgery and radiation, expertise is critical to you obtaining the best care. I see more than 1,000 patients per year who suffer erection problems because of prostate cancer treatments and there are many physicians throughout the United States who see very large numbers of patients in the same situation.

IV. Re-establishing a Good Sex Life

Most physicians know little about ED and its treatment, especially when it comes to relationship issues. Seeking the aid of a certified sex therapist is the quickest route to resolving bedroom relationship issues. The "sex conversation" is very difficult to conduct in 10 to 15 minutes. It is a very sensitive topic and, whether your partner is present or not, it is a difficult conversation. However, experienced sexual medicine physicians are used to discussing these issues and it is our task to do whatever we can to restore intimacy to the relationship.

In large centers, many sexual medicine physicians work alongside a sexual psychologist. At Memorial Sloan-Kettering, I have the luxury of working alongside Christian Nelson PhD. Every new patient or couple is seen by Dr. Nelson so that he can triage the key issues in the relationship. This discussion is far more productive if the partner is present. I believe this combined approach is the best way to assess the sexual problems in any given patient or couple.

Ralph and Barbara Alterowitz have written two excellent books. The first is entitled *Intimacy with Impotence* and the second, *The Lovin' Ain't Over: the Couple's Guide to Better Sex after Prostate Disease*. In this book, they talk about changing the relationship from a RUT to a CREST relationship. RUT stands for routine, unappreciated, and tired. This is the typical scenario for couples who have been together many years, who have many external pressures—children, finances, or work. On the other hand, trying to re-establish a CREST relationship, which stands for creativity, respect, excitement, sensitivity, and togetherness, is often a challenge. Ralph and Barbara discuss the ability to have a wonderfully physically intimate relationship in the absence of an erection. While this is attainable for some couples, for most men, the presence of an erection is psychologically critical to the satisfaction in their sexual relationships. It is difficult, although not possible, for a 65–year-old man who spent 50 years with good erections to suddenly transform his sexual relationship, in the absence of erection, into a fulfilling one. However, as I previously mentioned, 95% of patients who walk into my office are able to get erections hard enough for sexual intercourse, whether it be using a medication or device. Thus, I would contend that the re-establishment of intimacy is not only based on re-inventing how you make love, but also how to optimize integration of your medical aid, whether it be a pill, a suppository, an injection, or a device, into your sexual relationship.

Stan Althof PhD, who is an esteemed psychologist researcher from Florida, talks about factors that contribute to the high drop-out rate in medical therapy for erectile dysfunction. He attributes it to poorly managed or unresolved anger, power control issues, resentment on behalf of the partner, and sometimes the patient himself. These issues are impacted by the length of time the couple has not had sex before resuming sexual relations, the man's approach to resuming sex life with his partner, the partner's physical and emotional readiness to resume love making, the man's expectation of how the medications will change his life, the meaning for each partner of using a medication or device, whether there are any unconventional sexual arousal patterns in the man, and the quality of the couple's non-sexual relationship.

It is my experience that the longer a couple goes without having any form of physical intimacy, the more difficult it is for them to break the cycle and to re-establish it. This is one of the reasons why we like to see men early after surgery or radiation so that there is no interference in the flow of their sexual relationships. Having this conversation with the patient and using medication to help restore his erections, albeit artificially but temporarily, may go a long way toward reducing the resentment and disappointment that occurs in some partners.

I encourage men to go slowly in the pursuit of sexual intercourse during the period of time when physical relations resume. I encourage men to have initial penetration without the penis and to graduate to penile penetration once the woman is comfortable. Some couples will use vaginal dilators for this purpose. These are easily found on the internet. These objects come in graded sizes so a woman starts with a small one and moves up to larger versions as she becomes more comfortable. The partner's readiness to resume love making is a critical component of the re-establishment of intimacy. It is not uncommon for men to tell me, "Well, the injections work perfectly. I get a fully rigid erection, but my wife is turned off by the needle." It is always difficult for me to decipher whether this is actually the case or whether the wife is tacitly telling him that she has lost interest in having sexual relations.

When men are using aid to obtain erections, physicians should try to define the partner's take on this. For example, it is common for a couple to come in to see me where the partner is unhappy about the man using a pill because she is unclear as to whether it is the pill or her that is arousing him. This is easy to answer because men cannot get erections with Viagra, Levitra, or Cialis unless they are aroused. These pills work on chemicals that get released in the penis during sexual stimulation, so it is easy to tell the partner that it is she who is stimulating him and not the pill. This is far more difficult to answer when men are using penile injections as injections start an erection even in the absence of sexual stimulation. However, for most men, the level of rigidity and the duration of erection that they obtain with penis injections is directly linked to how turned on they are.

The quality of the couple's non-sexual relationship is a significant predictor of resumption of sexual activity. It is not uncommon for women to say to me that their interest in sex would be far greater if they felt that they were valued or treated better at home outside of the bedroom. Sometimes, women are looking for something as simple as a man helping out with the household chores and the kids, and demonstrating spontaneous thoughtfulness. Ralph and Barbara Alterowitz in their books talk about six steps to successful satisfying sexual relationships: ensuring the quality of the relationship, becoming fit for sex, creating a loving environment, relearning loving, warming up for loving, and then actual sex.

The critical step to getting back to close to where you were before in your sexual relationship is to open a dialogue with your partner. There are a number of steps involved in having this conversation. However, it is striking how many have not the first idea how to go about this. These are beyond the scope of this book but I refer you to the Alteropwitzes' books, which describe these steps in detail.

An understanding of where you as a couple came from is important. What was your sex life previously? Obviously, if you were having sex four times a year, then expecting to have sex weekly after surgery or radiation is not realistic. However, if you were very sexually active before treatment, then there is every reason in the world why you should be considering moving back to that level of activity.

Accepting that your sexual relationship may be different after surgery or radiation therapy is important. It is uncommon for men to return to the same level of erection hardness that they had before treatment without the use of medication. However, it is very common for men to get back to fully functional levels with or without the use of medication, whether it is a pill or an injection. The fact that you need to use a medication will alter the pattern of your sexual relationship. Accepting this and integrating these aids into your relationship, and relearning how to make love is an important component of getting back to satisfactory relations.

Moving your focus from erection is also a useful tool in the initial stages when sex is being resumed. I encourage all couples to spend the first few encounters focusing not on intercourse but on what is termed sexual outercourse. Kissing and cuddling and non-penetration-based activities, such as oral sex, massage, and direct finger clitoral stimulation are useful steps to take before launching back into penetrative relations.

Finally, what about sex and the single man? Not every man who is diagnosed with prostate cancer or who have been treated for prostate cancer has a partner. Indeed, it is not uncommon for me to hear from a man that they had a partner up until the time of their diagnosis or treatment, but then the relationship split up. Sometimes this relationship is broken up by the partner because of her fear or her inability to cope with his cancer diagnosis and the effects of treatment. Sometimes, however, the relationship is broken up by the patient as he fears for his future sexual activity and his inability to fulfill his partner physically. This is a very complicated issue and many large cancer centers have post-treatment resource programs which specialize in counseling men on dating and disclosure. There is no correct answer to the question, "When should I bring up my diagnosis of cancer and when should I discuss my problems with erections with a new partner?" This will depend on many factors, including what you and your partner are like. It is impressive to me, however, how often men will tell me that when they started dating and had disclosed that they have erection problems, how supportive their new partners were. One of the great concerns for a single man is that the absence of a partner may interfere with his interest or ability to comply with our penile rehabilitation program where we ask men to obtain erections on a regular basis in the early stages after surgery to protect erectile tissue. For men with and without partners, I spend the first year focusing not on sexual intercourse, but more on getting erections as a rehabilitation strategy.

SUGGESTED READING

I have attempted to list seminal medical papers on the various topics in each chapter to aid you in your decision-making regarding treatment of your prostate cancer and potential post-treatment problems. Most of these medical journal articles should be available online using most search engines, and if not, they will be available at the National Library of Medicine (www.pubmed.org).

Chapter 1: The Basics Of Sexual Function

Atlas of Male Sexual Dysfunction. Edited by Tom Lue MD. *Current Medicine*, 2004

Contemporary Diagnosis and Management of Male Erectile Dysfunction. Tom Lue MD. *Handbooks In Health Care Company*, 2005

Chapter 2: Prostate Enlargement and Sexual Dysfunction

Atlas of Clinical Urology (the Prostate). Edited by E. Darracott Vaughan MD. *Current Medicine*, 1999.

Baniel, J., Israilov, S., Shmueli, J., Segenreich, E., Livne, P.M.: Sexual Function in 131 Patients with Benign Prostatic Hyperplasia before Prostatectomy. *Eur Urol*, 38: 53, 2000

Barry, M. J., Fowler, F. J., Jr., O'Leary, M.P. et al.: The American Urological Association symptom index for benign prostatic hyperplasia. The Measurement Committee of the American Urological Association. *Journal of Urology*, 148: 1549, 1992

Beduschi, M. C., Oesterling.J.E.: Transurethral Needle Ablation of the Prostate: A Minimally Invasive Treatment for Symptomatic Benign Prostatic Hyperplasia. Mayo Clinic Proceedings, 73: 696, 1998

Birkhoff, J. D., Weiderhorn, A.R., Hamilton, M.L., et al.: Natural history of benign prostatic hypertrophy and acute urinary retention. *Urology*, 7: 48, 1976

Boyle, P., Gould, A.L., Roehrborn, C.G.: Prostate volume predicts outcome of treatment of benign prostatic hyperplasia with finesteride: Meta-analysis of randomized clinical trials. *Urology*, 48: 398, 1996

Braun, M., Wassmer, G., Klotz, T., Reifenrath, B., Mathers, M., Engelmann.U.: Epidemiology of erectile dysfunction: results of the "Cologne Male Survey". *International Journal of Impotence Research*, 12: 305, 2000

Braun, M. H., Sommer, F., Haupt, G. et al.: Lower urinary tract symptoms and erectile dysfunction: co-morbidity or typical "Aging Male" symptoms? Results of the "Cologne Male Survey." *European Urology*, 44: 588, 2003

Burger, B., Weidner.W., Altwein, J.E.: Prostate and Sexuality: An Overview. *European Urology*, 35: 177, 1999

Carraro, J. C., Raynaud, J.P., Koch, G.,et al.,: Comparison of phytotherapy (Permixon) with finesteride in the treatment of benign prostatic hyperplasia: a randomized international study of 1,098 patients. *Prostate*, 29: 231, 1996

Cohen, N. P., Mawas, A., Gibbons.B.: TURP can improve your sex life. *Journal of Urology*, 165 (suppl 5): 366, 2001

Dahlstrand, C., Walden, M., Geirsson, G., et al.,: Transurethral microwave thermotherapy versus transurethral resection for symptomatic benign prostatic obstruction: A prospective randomized study with a 2–year follow-up. *British Journal of Urology*, 76: 614, 1995

Ernst, E.: Harmless Herbs? *American Journal of Medicine*, 104: 170, 1998

Feldman, H. A., Goldstein, I., Hatzichristou, D.G., et al.,: Impotence and its medical and psychological correlates: results of the Massachusetts male aging study. *Journal of Urology*, 151: 54, 1994

SUGGESTED READING

Girman, C. J., Jacobsen, S. J., Rhodes, T. et al.: Association of health-related quality of life and benign prostatic enlargement. *European Urology*, 35: 277, 1999

Girman, C. J., Jacobsen, S. J., Tsukamoto, T. et al.: Health-related quality of life associated with lower urinary tract symptoms in four countries. *Urology*, 51: 428, 1998

Hansen, B. L.: Lower urinary tract symptoms (LUTS) and sexual function in both sexes. *European Urology*, 46: 229, 2004

Plosker, G. L., Brogden, R.N.: Serenoa repens (Permixon). A review of its pharmacology and therapeutic efficacy in benign prostatic hyperplasia. *Drugs Aging*, 9: 379, 1996

Sairam, K., Kulinskaya, E., McNicholas, T. A. et al.: Sildenafil influences lower urinary tract symptoms. *BJU Int*, 90: 836, 2002

Schiff, J. S., Mulhall, J.P.: The Link between LUTS and ED: Basic And Clinical Scientific Evidence. *Journal of Andrology*, 25: 470, 2004

Vallancien, G., Emberton, M., Harving, N. et al.: Sexual dysfunction in 1,274 European men suffering from lower urinary tract symptoms. *Journal of Urology*, 169: 2257, 2003

Wasson, J. H., Reda, D.J., Bruskewitz, R.C., et al.: A comparison of transurethral surgery with watchful waiting for moderate symptoms of benign prostatic hyperplasia. The Veterans Affairs Cooperative Study Group on Transurethral Resection of the Prostate. *New England Journal of Medicine*, 332: 75, 1995

Wilt, T. J., Ishani, A., Stark, G., et al.: Saw palmetto extracts for treatment of benign prostatic hyperplasia: a systematic review. *Journal of the American Medical Association*, 280: 1604, 1998

Zlotta, A. R., Schulman, C.C.: BPH and Sexuality. *European Urology*, 36(suppl 1): 107, 1999

Chapter 3: Deciding On a Treatment

Dr. Peter Scardino's *Prostate Book*. Chapter 12. Avery, 2005

Memorial Sloan Kettering Cancer Center Nomogram Website. www.mskcc.org/mskcc/html/10088.cfm

Begg, C. B., Riedel, E. R., Bach, P. B. et al.: Variations in morbidity after radical prostatectomy. *New England Journal of Medicine*, 346: 1138, 2002

Bianco, F. J., Jr., Kattan, M. W., Scardino, P. T. et al.: Radical prostatectomy nomograms in black American men: accuracy and applicability. *Journal of Urology*, 170: 73, 2003

Cagiannos, I., Karakiewicz, P., Eastham, J. A. et al.: A preoperative nomogram identifying decreased risk of positive pelvic lymph nodes in patients with prostate cancer. *Journal of Urology*, 170: 1798, 2003

Chun, F. K., Karakiewicz, P. I., Briganti, A. et al.: Prostate cancer nomograms: an update. *European Urology*, 50: 914, 2006

D'Amico, A. V., Whittington, R., Malkowicz, S. B. et al.: Biochemical outcome after radical prostatectomy, external beam radiation therapy, or interstitial radiation therapy for clinically localized prostate cancer. *Journal of the American Medical Association*, 280: 969, 1998

Di Blasio, C. J., Rhee, A. C., Cho, D. et al.: Predicting clinical end points: treatment nomograms in prostate cancer. *Seminars in Oncology*, 30: 567, 2003

Diblasio, C. J., Kattan, M. W.: Use of nomograms to predict the risk of disease recurrence after definitive local therapy for prostate cancer. *Urology*, 62 Suppl 1: 9, 2003

Fleming, C., Wasson, J. H., Albertsen, P. C. et al.: A decision analysis of alternative treatment strategies for clinically localized prostate cancer. Prostate Patient Outcomes Research Team. *Journal of the American Medical Association*, 269: 2650, 1993

Fryback, D. G., Albertsen, P. C., Storer, B. E.: Prostatectomy and survival among men with clinically localized prostate cancer. *Journal of the American Medical Association*, 276: 1723, 1996

Gomella, L. G., Albertsen, P. C., Benson, M. C. et al.: The use of video-based patient education for shared decision-making in the treatment of prostate cancer. *Seminars in Urologic Oncology*, 18: 182, 2000

Graefen, M., Karakiewicz, P. I., Cagiannos, I. et al.: A validation of two preoperative nomograms predicting recurrence following radical prostatectomy in a cohort of European men. *Urologic Oncology*, 7: 141, 2002

Graefen, M., Ohori, M., Karakiewicz, P. I. et al.: Assessment of the enhancement in predictive accuracy provided by systematic biopsy in predicting outcome for clinically localized prostate cancer. *Journal of Urology*, 171: 200, 2004

Hamilton, A. S., Stanford, J. L., Gilliland, F. D. et al.: Health outcomes after external-beam radiation therapy for clinically localized prostate cancer: results from the Prostate Cancer Outcomes Study. *Journal of Clinical Oncology*, 19: 2517, 2001

Holmberg, L., Bill-Axelson, A., Helgesen, F. et al.: A randomized trial comparing radical prostatectomy with watchful waiting in early prostate cancer. *New England Journal of Medicine*, 347: 781, 2002

Kattan, M. W.: Nomograms are superior to staging and risk grouping systems for identifying high-risk patients: preoperative application in prostate cancer. *Current Opinion in Urology*, 13: 111, 2003

Kattan, M. W.: Nomograms Are Difficult to Beat. *European Urology*, 2007

Kattan, M. W., Eastham, J. A., Wheeler, T. M. et al.: Counseling men with prostate cancer: a nomogram for predicting the presence of small, moderately differentiated, confined tumors. *Journal of Urology*, 170: 1792, 2003

Kattan, M. W., Scardino, P. T.: Prediction of progression: nomograms of clinical utility. *Clinical Prostate Cancer*, 1: 90, 2002

Kattan, M. W., Scardino, P. T.: Evidence for the usefulness of nomograms. *Nature Clinical Practice Urology*, 4: 638, 2007

Kattan, M. W., Zelefsky, M. J., Kupelian, P. A. et al.: Pretreatment nomogram that predicts 5–year probability of metastasis following three-dimensional conformal radiation therapy for localized prostate cancer. *Journal of Clinical Oncology*, 21: 4568, 2003

Koh, H., Kattan, M. W., Scardino, P. T. et al.: A nomogram to predict seminal vesicle invasion by the extent and location of cancer in systematic biopsy results. *Journal of Urology* 170: 1203, 2003

Nam, R. K., Toi, A., Klotz, L. H. et al.: Assessing individual risk for prostate cancer. *Journal of Clinical Oncology*, 25: 3582, 2007

Ohori, M., Kattan, M. W., Koh, H. et al.: Predicting the presence and side of extracapsular extension: a nomogram for staging prostate cancer. *Journal of Urology*, 171: 1844, 2004

Onel, E., Hamond, C., Wasson, J. H. et al.: Assessment of the feasibility and impact of shared decision-making in prostate cancer. *Urology*, 51: 63, 1998

Roach, M., 3rd, Weinberg, V., Nash, M. et al.: Defining high risk prostate cancer with risk groups and nomograms: implications for designing clinical trials. *Journal of Urology*, 176: S16, 2006

Ross, P. L., Gerigk, C., Gonen, M. et al.: Comparisons of nomograms and urologists' predictions in prostate cancer. *Seminars in Urologic Oncology*, 20: 82, 2002

Stephenson, A. J., Scardino, P. T., Eastham, J. A. et al.: Preoperative nomogram predicting the 10–year probability of prostate cancer recurrence after radical prostatectomy. *Journal of the National Cancer Institute*, 98: 715, 2006

Chapter 4: Radical Prostatectomy and Sexual Function

Aboseif, S., Shinohara, K., Breza, J. et al.: Role of penile vascular injury in erectile dysfunction after radical prostatectomy. *Br J Urol*, 73: 75, 1994

Ahlering, T. E., Eichel, L., Chou, D. et al.: Feasibility study for robotic radical prostatectomy cautery-free neurovascular bundle preservation. *Urology*, 65: 994, 2005

Ahlering, T. E., Eichel, L., Edwards, R. et al.: Impact of obesity on clinical outcomes in robotic prostatectomy. *Urology*, 65: 740, 2005

Anastasiadis, A. G., Salomon, L., Katz, R. et al.: Radical retropubic versus laparoscopic prostatectomy: a prospective comparison of functional outcome. *Urology*, 62: 292, 2003

Arredondo, S. A., Elkin, E. P., Marr, P. L. et al.: Impact of comorbidity on health-related quality of life in men undergoing radical prostatectomy: data from CaPSURE. *Urology*, 67: 559, 2006

Badani, K. K., Kaul, S., Menon, M.: Evolution of robotic radical prostatectomy: assessment after 2,766 procedures. *Cancer*, 110: 1951, 2007

Bates, T. S., Wright, M. P., Gillatt, D. A.: Prevalence and impact of incontinence and impotence following total prostatectomy assessed anonymously by the ICS-male questionnaire. *European Urology*, 33: 165, 1998

Begg, C. B., Riedel, E. R., Bach, P. B. et al.: Variations in morbidity after radical prostatectomy. *New England Journal of Medicine* 346: 1138, 2002

Bianco, F. J., Jr., Kattan, M. W., Scardino, P. T.: PSA velocity and prostate cancer. *New England Journal of Medicine*, 351: 1800, 2004

Bianco, F. J., Jr., Kattan, M. W., Scardino, P. T. et al.: Radical prostatectomy nomograms in black American men: accuracy and applicability. *Journal of Urology*, 170: 73, 2003

Bianco, F. J., Jr., Scardino, P. T., Eastham, J. A.: Radical prostatectomy: long-term cancer control and recovery of sexual and urinary function ("trifecta"). *Urology*, 66: 83, 2005

Borden, L. S., Jr., Kozlowski, P. M., Porter, C. R. et al.: Mechanical failure rate of da Vinci robotic system. Canadian *Journal of Urology*, 14: 3499, 2007

SUGGESTED READING

Breza, J., Aboseif, S. R., Orvis, B. R. et al.: Detailed anatomy of penile neurovascular structures: surgical significance. *Journal of Urology*, 141: 437, 1989

Burnett, A. L.: Rationale for cavernous nerve restorative therapy to preserve erectile function after radical prostatectomy. *Urology*, 61: 491, 2003

Burnett, A. L.: Neuroprotection and nerve grafts in the treatment of neurogenic erectile dysfunction. *Journal of Urology*, 170: S31, 2003

Chang SS, P. M., Smith JA Jr.: Intraoperative nerve stimulation predicts postoperative potency. *Urology*, 58: 594, 2001

Cooperberg, M. R., Broering, J. M., Litwin, M. S. et al.: The contemporary management of prostate cancer in the United States: lessons from the cancer of the prostate strategic urologic research endeavor (CapSURE), a national disease registry. *J Urol*, 171: 1393, 2004

Costello, A. J.: Beyond marketing: the real value of robotic radical prostatectomy. *BJU International*, 96: 1, 2005

Eggener, S. E., Scardino, P. T., Carroll, P. R. et al.: Focal therapy for localized prostate cancer: a critical appraisal of rationale and modalities. *Journal of Urology*, 178: 2260, 2007

Eggener, S. E., Yossepowitch, O., Serio, A. M. et al.: Radical prostatectomy shortly after prostate biopsy does not affect operative difficulty or efficacy. *Urology*, 69: 1128, 2007

Ficarra, V., Cavalleri, S., Novara, G. et al.: Evidence from robot-assisted laparoscopic radical prostatectomy: a systematic review. *European Urology*, 51: 45, 2007

Fowler, F. J., Barry, M.J., Lu-Yao, G., et. al.: Patient-reported complications and follow-up treatment after radical prostatectomy. The national medicare experience: 1988–1990 (updated June 1993). *Urology*, 42: 622, 1993

Goeman, L., Salomon, L., La De Taille, A. et al.: Long-term functional and oncological results after retroperitoneal laparoscopic prostatectomy according to a prospective evaluation of 550 patients. *World Journal of Urology*, 24: 281, 2006

Greenlee, R. T., Murray, T., Bolden, S., Wingo, P.A.: Cancer statistics 2006. *Ca: a Cancer Journal for Clinician*, 2006

Guillonneau, B.: To demonstrate the benefits of laparoscopic radical prostatectomy. *European Urology*, 50: 1160, 2006

Guillonneau, B. D.: Laparoscopic versus robotic radical prostatectomy. *Nature Clinical Practice Urology*, 2: 60, 2005

Martinez-Salamanca, J. I., Rao, S., Ramanathan, R. et al.: Nerve advancement with end-to-end reconstruction after partial neurovascular bundle resection: a feasibility study. *Journal of EndoUrology*, 21: 830, 2007

Masterson, T. A., Stephenson, A. J., Scardino, P. T. et al.: Recovery of erectile function after salvage radical prostatectomy for locally recurrent prostate cancer after radiotherapy. *Urology*, 66: 623, 2005

Mayer, E. K., Winkler, M. H., Aggarwal, R. et al.: Robotic prostatectomy: the first UK experience. *International Journal of Medical Robotics*, 2: 321, 2006

Menon, M., Shrivastava, A., Kaul, S. et al.: Vattikuti Institute prostatectomy: contemporary technique and analysis of results. *European Urology*, 51: 648, 2007

Mikhail, A. A., Song, D. H., Zorn, K. C. et al.: Sural nerve grafting in robotic laparoscopic radical prostatectomy: interim report. *Journal of EndoUrology*, 21: 1547, 2007

Mulhall, J. P.: Deciphering erectile dysfunction drug trials. *Journal of Urology* 170: 353, 2003

Mulhall, J. P.: Cavernous nerve stimulation and interposition grafting: a critical assessment and future perspectives. Reviews in *Urology*, 7 Suppl 2: S18, 2005

Mulhall, J. P., Graydon, R. J.: The hemodynamics of erectile dysfunction following nerve-sparing radical retropubic prostatectomy. *International Journal of Impotence Research*, 8: 91, 1996

Mulhall, J. P., Montorsi, F.: Evaluating preference trials of oral phosphodiesterase 5 inhibitors for erectile dysfunction. *European Urology*, 49: 30, 2006

Mulhall, J. P., Secin, F. P., Guillonneau, B.: Artery Sparing Radical Prostatectomy—Myth or Reality? *Journal of Urology*, 2008

Myers, R. P.: Radical prostatectomy: pertinent surgical anatomy. *Urologic Clinics of North America.*, 2: 1, 1994

Nosnik, I. P., Gan, T. J., Moul, J. W.: Open radical retropubic prostatectomy 2007: the true minimally invasive surgery for localized prostate cancer? *Expert Reviews in Anticancer Therapy*, 7: 1309, 2007

Polascik, T. J., Walsh, P. C.: Radical retropubic prostatectomy: the influence of accessory pudendal arteries on the recovery of sexual function. *Journal of Urology*, 154: 150, 1995

Quinlan, D. M., Nelson, R. J., Walsh, P. C.: Cavernous nerve grafts restore erectile function in denervated rats. *Journal of Urology*, 145: 380, 1991

SUGGESTED READING

Rabbani, F., Stapleton, A.M.F, Kattan, M.W., et. al.: Factors predicting recovery of erections after radical prostatectomy. *Journal of Urology* 164: 1929, 2000

Ramanathan, R., Mulhall, J., Rao, S. et al.: Predictive correlation between the International Index of Erectile Function (IIEF) and Sexual Health Inventory for Men (SHIM): implications for calculating a derived SHIM for clinical use. *Journal of Sexual Medicine*, 4: 1336, 2007

Rocco, B., Djavan, B.: Robotic prostatectomy: fact or fiction? *Lancet*, 369: 723, 2007

Rozet, F., Galiano, M., Cathelineau, X. et al.: Extraperitoneal laparoscopic radical prostatectomy: a prospective evaluation of 600 cases. *Journal of Urology*, 174: 908, 2005

Sala, E., Akin, O., Moskowitz, C. S. et al.: Endorectal MR imaging in the evaluation of seminal vesicle invasion: diagnostic accuracy and multivariate feature analysis. *Radiology*, 238: 929, 2006

Saranchuk, J. W., Kattan, M. W., Elkin, E. et al.: Achieving optimal outcomes after radical prostatectomy. *J Clin Oncol*, 23: 4146, 2005

Scardino, P.: Update: NCCN prostate cancer Clinical Practice Guidelines. *J National Comprehensive Cancer Network*, 3 Suppl 1: S29, 2005

Scardino, P. T., Kim, E.D.: Rationale for and results of nerve grafting during radical prostatectomy. *Urology*, 57: 1016, 2001

Scardino, P. T.: Intoxicated by technology: are we keeping our eyes on the prize? *Nature Clinical Practice Urology*, 4: 231, 2007

Secin, F. P., Koppie, T. M., Scardino, P. T. et al.: Bilateral cavernous nerve interposition grafting during radical retropubic prostatectomy: Memorial Sloan-Kettering Cancer Center experience. *Journal of Urology*, 177: 664, 2007

Secin, F. P., Touijer, K., Mulhall, J. et al.: Anatomy and preservation of accessory pudendal arteries in laparoscopic radical prostatectomy. *European Urology* 51: 1229, 2007

Siegel, R., Moul, J.W., Spevak, M., et. al.: The development of erectile dysfunction in men treated for prostate cancer. *Journal of Urology* 165: 430, 2001

Tal, R., Mulhall, J. P.: Sexual health issues in men with cancer. *Oncology* (Williston Park), 20: 294, 2006

Teloken, P., Valenzuela, R., Parker, M. et al.: The correlation between erectile function and patient satisfaction. *Journal of Sexual Medicine* 4: 472, 2007

Touijer, K., Guillonneau, B.: Laparoscopic radical prostatectomy: a critical analysis of surgical quality. *European Urology*, 49: 625, 2006

Van der Aa, F., Joniau, S., De Ridder, D. et al.: Potency after unilateral nerve sparing surgery: a report on functional and oncological results of unilateral nerve sparing surgery. *Prostate Cancer Prostatic Dis*, 6: 61, 2003

Vickers, A. J., Bianco, F. J., Jr., Boorjian, S. et al.: Does a delay between diagnosis and radical prostatectomy increase the risk of disease recurrence? *Cancer*, 106: 576, 2006

Vickers, A. J., Bianco, F. J., Serio, A. M. et al.: The surgical learning curve for prostate cancer control after radical prostatectomy. *J National Cancer Institute*, 99: 1171, 2007

Walsh, P. C., Marschke, P., Ricker, D., et. al.: Patient-reported urinary continence and sexual function after anatomic radical prostatectomy. *Urology*, 55: 58, 2000

Walsh, P. C.: Nerve grafts are rarely necessary and are unlikely to improve sexual function in men undergoing anatomic radical prostatectomy. *Urology*, 57: 1020, 2001

Walsh, P. C.: The discovery of the cavernous nerves and development of nerve sparing radical retropubic prostatectomy. *J Urol*, 177: 1632, 2007

Walsh P.C., M. P., Catalona WJ, Lepor H, Martin S, Myers RP, Steiner MS.: Efficacy of first-generation Cavermap to verify location and function of cavernous nerves during radical prostatectomy: a multi-institutional evaluation by experienced surgeons. *Urology*, 57: 491, 2001

Yossepowitch, O., Eggener, S. E., Bianco, F. J., Jr. et al.: Radical prostatectomy for clinically localized, high-risk prostate cancer: critical analysis of risk assessment methods. *Journal of Urology* 178: 493, 2007

Zorn, K. C., Gofrit, O. N., Orvieto, M. A. et al.: Da Vinci robot error and failure rates: single institution experience on a single three-arm robot unit of more than 700 consecutive robot-assisted laparoscopic radical prostatectomies. *Journal of EndoUrology*, 21: 1341, 2007

Chapter 5: Prostate Radiation Therapy and Sexual Function

al-Abany, M., Steineck, G., Agren Cronqvist, A. K. et al.: Improving the preservation of erectile function after external beam radiation therapy for prostate cancer. *Radiotherapy Oncology*, 57: 201, 2000

Albert, M., Tempany, C. M., Schultz, D. et al.: Late genitourinary and gastrointestinal toxicity after magnetic resonance image-guided prostate

SUGGESTED READING

brachytherapy with or without neoadjuvant external beam radiation therapy. *Cancer*, 98: 949, 2003

Krisch, E. B., Koprowski, C. D.: Deciding on radiation therapy for prostate cancer: the physician's perspective. *Seminars in Urologic Oncology*, 18: 214, 2000

D'Amico, A. V.: Radiation and hormonal therapy for locally advanced and clinically localized prostate cancer. *Urology*, 60: 32, 2002

D'Amico, A. V., Manola, J., Loffredo, M. et al.: 6–month androgen suppression plus radiation therapy vs. radiation therapy alone for patients with clinically localized prostate cancer: a randomized controlled trial. *Journal of the American Medical Association*, 292: 821, 2004

Eggener, S. E., Roehl, K. A., Yossepowitch, O. et al.: Pre-diagnosis prostate specific antigen velocity is associated with risk of prostate cancer progression following brachytherapy and external beam radiation therapy. *Journal of Urology* 176: 1399, 2006

Frank, S. J., Grimm, P. D., Sylvester, J. E. et al.: Interstitial implant alone or in combination with external beam radiation therapy for intermediate-risk prostate cancer: a survey of practice patterns in the United States. *Brachytherapy*, 6: 2, 2007

Frank, S. J., Pisters, L. L., Davis, J. et al.: An assessment of quality of life following radical prostatectomy, high-dose external beam radiation therapy and brachytherapy iodine implantation as monotherapies for localized prostate cancer. *Journal of Urology* 177: 2151, 2007

Haliloglu, A., Baltaci, S., Yaman, O.: Penile length changes in men treated with androgen suppression plus radiation therapy for local or locally advanced prostate cancer. *Journal of Urology*, 177: 128, 2007

Kao, J., Turian, J., Meyers, A. et al.: Sparing of the penile bulb and proximal penile structures with intensity-modulated radiation therapy for prostate cancer. British Journal of *Radiology*, 77: 129, 2004

Lai, S., Lai, H., Lamm, S. et al.: Radiation therapy in non-surgically-treated non-metastatic prostate cancer: geographic and demographic variation. *Urology*, 57: 510, 2001

Montie, J. E.: Follow-up after radical prostatectomy or radiation therapy for prostate cancer. *Urologic Clinics of North America*, 21: 673, 1994

Montie, J. E., Hussain, M.: Outcomes for radiation therapy after radical prostatectomy for prostate cancer: what really matters? *BJU International*, 100: 485, 2007

Mulhall, J. P., Yonover, P., Sethi, A. et al.: Radiation exposure to the corporeal bodies during 3–dimensional conformal radiation therapy for prostate cancer. *Journal of Urology* 167: 539, 2002

Ohebshalom, M., Parker, M., Guhring, P. et al.: The efficacy of sildenafil citrate following radiation therapy for prostate cancer: temporal considerations. *Journal of Urology*, 174: 258, 2005

Patel, A. R., Sandler, H. M., Pienta, K. J.: Radiation Therapy Oncology Group 0521: a phase III randomized trial of androgen suppression and radiation therapy versus androgen suppression and radiation therapy followed by chemotherapy with docetaxel/prednisone for localized, high-risk prostate cancer. *Clinical Genitourinary Cancer*, 4: 212, 2005

Perez, C. A., Michalski, J. M., Mansur, D. et al.: Three-dimensional conformal therapy versus standard radiation therapy in localized carcinoma of prostate: an update. *Clinical Prostate Cancer*, 1: 97, 2002

Pollack, J. M.: Radiation therapy options in the treatment of prostate cancer. *Cancer Investigation*, 18: 66, 2000

Potters, L.: Nomograms for clinically localized prostate cancer. Part II: radiation therapy. *Seminars in Urologic Oncology*, 20: 131, 2002

Potters, L., Freeman, K.: Prostatectomy, external beam radiation therapy, or brachytherapy for localized prostate cancer. *Journal of the American Medical Association*, 281: 1584; author reply 1585, 1999

Roach, M., DeSilvio, M., Valicenti, R. et al.: Whole-pelvis, "mini-pelvis," or prostate-only external beam radiotherapy after neoadjuvant and concurrent hormonal therapy in patients treated in the Radiation Therapy Oncology Group 9413 trial. *International Journal of Radiation Oncology Biology and Physics*, 66: 647, 2006

Roach, M., Lu, J., Pilepich, M. V. et al.: Race and survival of men treated for prostate cancer on radiation therapy oncology group phase III randomized trials. *Journal of Urology*, 169: 245, 2003

Sanchez-Ortiz, R. F., Broderick, G. A., Rovner, E. S. et al.: Erectile function and quality of life after interstitial radiation therapy for prostate cancer. *International Journal of Impotence Research*, 12 Suppl 3: S18, 2000

Stein, M. E., Boehmer, D., Kuten, A.: Radiation therapy in prostate cancer. *Cancer Research*, 175: 179, 2007

Stephenson, A. J., Scardino, P. T., Kattan, M. W. et al.: Predicting the outcome of salvage radiation therapy for recurrent prostate cancer after radical prostatectomy. *Journal of Clinical Oncology*, 25: 2035, 2007

Sylvester, J., Blasko, J. C., Grimm, P. D. et al.: Short-course androgen ablation combined with external-beam radiation therapy and low-dose-rate permanent brachytherapy in early-stage prostate cancer: a matched subset analysis. *Molecular Urology*, 4: 155, 2000

Sylvester, J., Blasko, J. C., Grimm, P. D. et al.: Neoadjuvant Androgen Ablation Combined with External-Beam Radiation Therapy and Permanent Interstitial Brachytherapy Boost in Localized Prostate Cancer. *Molecular Urology*, 3: 231, 1999

Valicenti, R. K., Bissonette, E. A., Chen, C. et al.: Longitudinal comparison of sexual function after 3–dimensional conformal radiation therapy or prostate brachytherapy. *Journal of Urology*, 168: 2499, 2002

Valicenti, R. K., Winter, K., Cox, J. D. et al.: RTOG 94–06: is the addition of neoadjuvant hormonal therapy to dose-escalated 3D conformal radiation therapy for prostate cancer associated with treatment toxicity? *International Journal of Radiation Oncology Biology Physics*, 57: 614, 2003

Yeoh, E. E., Holloway, R. H., Fraser, R. J. et al.: Hypofractionated versus conventionally fractionated radiation therapy for prostate carcinoma: updated results of a phase III randomized trial. *International Journal of Radiation Oncology Biology Physics*, 66: 1072, 2006

Yonemoto, L. T., Slater, J. D., Rossi, C. J., Jr. et al.: Combined proton and photon conformal radiation therapy for locally advanced carcinoma of the prostate: preliminary results of a phase I/II study. *International Journal of Radiation Oncology Biology Physics*, 37: 21, 1997

Yuen, J., Rodrigues, G., Trenka, K. et al.: Comparing two strategies of dynamic intensity modulated radiation therapy (dIMRT) with 3–dimensional conformal radiation therapy (3DCRT) in the hypofractionated treatment of high-risk prostate cancer. *Radiation Oncology*, 3: 1, 2008

Zelefsky, M. J., Fuks, Z., Hunt, M. et al.: High-dose intensity modulated radiation therapy for prostate cancer: early toxicity and biochemical outcome in 772 patients. *International Journal of Radiation Oncology Biology Physics*, 53: 1111, 2002

Zietman, A. L., Chung, C. S., Coen, J. J. et al.: 10–year outcome for men with localized prostate cancer treated with external radiation therapy: results of a cohort study. *Journal of Urology*, 171: 210, 2004

Chapter 6: Hormone Therapy and Sexual Function

Bahnson, R.: Androgen deprivation therapy for prostate cancer. *Journal of Urology*, 178: 1148, 2007

Berthelet, E., Pickles, T., Lee, K. W. et al.: Long-term androgen deprivation therapy improves survival in prostate cancer patients presenting with prostate-specific antigen levels > 20 ng/mL. *International Journal of Radiation Oncology Biology Physics*, 63: 781, 2005

Black, P. C., Basen-Engquist, K., Wang, X. et al.: A randomized prospective trial evaluating testosterone, haemoglobin kinetics and quality of life, during and after 12 months of androgen deprivation after prostatectomy: results from the Postoperative Adjuvant Androgen Deprivation trial. *BJU International*, 100: 63, 2007

Boccon-Gibod, L., Hammerer, P., Madersbacher, S. et al.: The role of intermittent androgen deprivation in prostate cancer. *BJU International*, 100: 738, 2007

Bylow, K., Mohile, S. G., Stadler, W. M. et al.: Does androgen-deprivation therapy accelerate the development of frailty in older men with prostate cancer?: a conceptual review. *Cancer*, 110: 2604, 2007

Chen, A. C., Petrylak, D. P.: Complications of androgen-deprivation therapy in men with prostate cancer. *Current Urology Reports*, 6: 210, 2005

de Leval, J., Boca, P., Yousef, E. et al.: Intermittent versus continuous total androgen blockade in the treatment of patients with advanced hormone-naive prostate cancer: results of a prospective randomized multicenter trial. *Clinical Prostate Cancer*, 1: 163, 2002

Famili, P., Cauley, J. A., Greenspan, S. L.: The effect of androgen deprivation therapy on periodontal disease in men with prostate cancer. *Journal of Urology*, 177: 921, 2007

Fridmans, A., Chertin, B., Koulikov, D. et al.: Reversibility of androgen deprivation therapy in patients with prostate cancer. *Journal of Urology*, 173: 784, 2005

Gomella, L. G.: Contemporary use of hormonal therapy in prostate cancer: managing complications and addressing quality-of-life issues. *BJU International*, 99 Suppl 1: 25, 2007

Gulley, J. L., Figg, W. D., Steinberg, S. M. et al.: A prospective analysis of the time to normalization of serum androgens following 6 months of androgen deprivation therapy in patients on a randomized phase III

SUGGESTED READING

clinical trial using limited hormonal therapy. *Journal of Urology* 173: 1567, 2005

Haidar, A., Yassin, A., Saad, F. et al.: Effects of androgen deprivation on glycemic control and on cardiovascular biochemical risk factors in men with advanced prostate cancer with diabetes. *Aging Male*, 10: 189, 2007

Hanks, G. E., Pajak, T. F., Porter, A. et al.: Phase III trial of long-term adjuvant androgen deprivation after neoadjuvant hormonal cytoreduction and radiotherapy in locally advanced carcinoma of the prostate: the Radiation Therapy Oncology Group Protocol 92–02. *Journal of Clinical Oncology*, 21: 3972, 2003

Hellerstedt, B. A., Pienta, K. J.: The truth is out there: an overall perspective on androgen deprivation. *Urologic Oncology*, 21: 272, 2003

Holmes, L., Jr., Chan, W., Jiang, Z. et al.: Effectiveness of androgen deprivation therapy in prolonging survival of older men treated for locoregional prostate cancer. *Prostate Cancer Prostatic Diseases*, 10: 388, 2007

Hussain, S. A., Weston, R., Stephenson, R. N. et al.: Immediate dual energy X-ray absorptiometry reveals a high incidence of osteoporosis in patients with advanced prostate cancer before hormonal manipulation. *BJU International*, 92: 690, 2003

Israeli, R. S., Ryan, C. W., Jung, L. L.: Managing bone loss in men with locally advanced prostate cancer receiving androgen deprivation therapy. *Journal of Urology*, 179: 414, 2008

Keating, N. L., O'Malley, A. J., McNaughton-Collins, M. et al.: Use of androgen deprivation therapy for metastatic prostate cancer in older men. *BJU International*, 2008

Kumar, S., Shelley, M., Harrison, C. et al.: Neo-adjuvant and adjuvant hormone therapy for localised and locally advanced prostate cancer. Cochrane Database Systematic Review: CD006019, 2006

Lamb, D. S., Denham, J. W., Mameghan, H. et al.: Acceptability of short-term neo-adjuvant androgen deprivation in patients with locally advanced prostate cancer. *Radiotherapy Oncology*, 68: 255, 2003

Lopez, A. M., Pena, M. A., Hernandez, R. et al.: Fracture risk in patients with prostate cancer on androgen deprivation therapy. *Osteoporosis International*, 16: 707, 2005

Makarov, D. V., Humphreys, E. B., Mangold, L. A. et al.: The natural history of men treated with deferred androgen deprivation therapy in whom metastatic prostate cancer developed following radical prostatectomy. *Journal of Urology*, 179: 156, 2008

Miyamoto, H., Messing, E. M., Chang, C.: Does androgen deprivation improve treatment outcomes in patients with low-risk and intermediate-risk prostate cancer? *Nature Clinical Practice Oncology*, 2: 236, 2005

Opfermann, K. J., Lai, Z., Essenmacher, L. et al.: Intermittent hormone therapy in non-metastatic prostate cancer. *Clinical Genitourinary Cancer*, 5: 138, 2006

Polascik, T. J.: Bone health in prostate cancer patients receiving androgen-deprivation therapy: the role of bisphosphonates. *Prostate Cancer Prostatic Dis*eases, 2007

Rashid, M. H., Chaudhary, U. B.: Intermittent androgen deprivation therapy for prostate cancer. *Oncologist*, 9: 295, 2004

Roach, M., 3rd, Bae, K., Speight, J. et al.: Short-term neoadjuvant androgen deprivation therapy and external-beam radiotherapy for locally advanced prostate cancer: long-term results of RTOG 8610. *Journal of Clinical Oncology*, 26: 585, 2008

Ryan, C. J., Small, E. J.: Early versus delayed androgen deprivation for prostate cancer: new fuel for an old debate. *Journal of Clinical Oncology*, 23: 8225, 2005

Saigal, C. S., Gore, J. L., Krupski, T. L. et al.: Androgen deprivation therapy increases cardiovascular morbidity in men with prostate cancer. *Cancer*, 110: 1493, 2007

Salminen, E., Portin, R., Korpela, J. et al.: Androgen deprivation and cognition in prostate cancer. British Journal of *Cancer*, 89: 971, 2003

Sharifi, N., Dahut, W. L., Figg, W. D.: Secondary hormonal therapy for prostate cancer: what lies on the horizon? *BJU International*, 101: 271, 2008

Singer, E. A., Golijanin, D. J., Miyamoto, H. et al.: Androgen deprivation therapy for prostate cancer. *Expert Opinion Pharmacotherapy*, 9: 211, 2008

Smith, M. R.: The role of bisphosphonates in men with prostate cancer receiving androgen deprivation therapy. *Oncology* (Williston Park), 18: 21, 2004

Smith, M. R.: Androgen deprivation therapy for prostate cancer: new concepts and concerns. *Current Opinion Endocrinology Diabetes Obesity*, 14: 247, 2007

Tiguert, R., Rigaud, J., Lacombe, L. et al.: Neoadjuvant hormone therapy before salvage radiotherapy for an increasing post-radical prostatectomy serum prostate specific antigen level. *Journal of Urology*, 170: 447, 2003

SUGGESTED READING

Tunn, U.: The current status of intermittent androgen deprivation (IAD) therapy for prostate cancer: putting IAD under the spotlight. *BJU International*, 99 Suppl 1: 19, 2007

van Andel, G., Kurth, K. H.: The impact of androgen deprivation therapy on health related quality of life in asymptomatic men with lymph node positive prostate cancer. *European Urology*, 44: 209, 2003

Youssef, E., Tekyi-Mensah, S., Hart, K. et al.: Intermittent androgen deprivation for patients with recurrent/metastatic prostate cancer. American *Journal of Clinical Oncology*, 26: e119, 2003

Zeliadt, S. B., Potosky, A. L., Penson, D. F. et al.: Survival benefit associated with adjuvant androgen deprivation therapy combined with radiotherapy for high- and low-risk patients with nonmetastatic prostate cancer. *International Journal of Radiation Oncology Biology Physics*, 66: 395, 2006

Chapter 7: Penile Rehabilitation and Preservation

Bannowsky, A., Schulze, H., van der Horst, C. et al.: Nocturnal tumescence: a parameter for postoperative erectile integrity after nerve sparing radical prostatectomy. *Journal of Urology*, 175: 2214, 2006

Briganti, A., Gallina, A., Salonia, A. et al.: Reliability of classification of erectile function domain of the international index of erectile function in patients affected by localized prostate cancer who are candidates for radical prostatectomy. *Urology*, 66: 1140; author reply 1140, 2005

Briganti, A., Salonia, A., Gallina, A. et al.: Management of erectile dysfunction after radical prostatectomy in 2007. *World Journal of Urology*, 25: 143, 2007

Ferrini, M. G., Davila, H. H., Kovanecz, I. et al.: Vardenafil prevents fibrosis and loss of corporal smooth muscle that occurs after bilateral cavernosal nerve resection in the rat. *Urology*, 68: 429, 2006

Foresta, C., Lana, A., Cabrelle, A. et al.: PDE-5 inhibitor, Vardenafil, increases circulating progenitor cells in humans. *International Journal of Impotence Research*, 17: 377, 2005

Ghofrani, H. A., Voswinckel, R., Reichenberger, F. et al.: Differences in hemodynamic and oxygenation responses to three different phosphodiesterase-5 inhibitors in patients with pulmonary arterial hypertension: a randomized prospective study. *Journal of the American College of Cardiology*, 44: 1488, 2004

Gontero, P., Fontana, F., Bagnasacco, A. et al.: Is there an optimal time for intracavernous prostaglandin E1 rehabilitation following nonnerve sparing radical prostatectomy? Results from a hemodynamic prospective study. *Journal of Urology*, 169: 2166, 2003

Gontero, P., Kirby, R.: Early rehabilitation of erectile function after nerve-sparing radical prostatectomy: what is the evidence? *BJU International*, 93: 916, 2004

Iacono, F., Giannella, R., Somma, P. et al.: Histological alterations in cavernous tissue after radical prostatectomy. *Journal of Urology*, 173: 1673, 2005

Kovanecz, I., Rambhatla, A., Ferrini, M. et al.: Long-term continuous sildenafil treatment ameliorates corporal veno-occlusive dysfunction (CVOD) induced by cavernosal nerve resection in rats. *International Journal of Impotence Research*, 2007

Kovanecz, I., Rambhatla, A., Ferrini, M. G. et al.: Chronic daily tadalafil prevents the corporal fibrosis and veno-occlusive dysfunction that occurs after cavernosal nerve resection. *BJU International*, 101: 203, 2008

Kukreja, R. C.: Cardiovascular protection with sildenafil following chronic inhibition of nitric oxide synthase. *British Journal of Pharmacology*, 2007

Leungwattanakij, S., Bivalacqua, T. J., Usta, M. F. et al.: Cavernous neurotomy causes hypoxia and fibrosis in rat corpus cavernosum. *Journal of Andrology*, 24: 239, 2003

Montorsi, F., Briganti, A., Salonia, A. et al.: Current and future strategies for preventing and managing erectile dysfunction following radical prostatectomy. *European Urology*, 45: 123, 2004

Montorsi, F., Guazzoni, G., Strambi, L. F. et al.: Recovery of spontaneous erectile function after nerve-sparing radical retropubic prostatectomy with and without early intracavernous injections of alprostadil: results of a prospective, randomized trial. *Journal of Urology*, 158: 1408, 1997

Montorsi, F., Salonia, A., Zanoni, M. et al.: Counselling the patient with prostate cancer about treatment-related erectile dysfunction. *Current Opinion in Urology*, 11: 611, 2001

Moreland, R. B.: Is there a role of hypoxemia in penile fibrosis: a viewpoint presented to the Society for the Study of Impotence. *International Journal of Impotence Research*, 10: 113, 1998

Mulhall, J.P, Mueller, A., Donohue, J. F. et al.: The functional and structural consequences of cavernous nerve injury in the rat model are ameliorated by sildenafil citrate. *Journal of Sexual Medicine*, 2008

Mulhall, J.P., Land, S., Parker, M. et al.: The use of an erectogenic pharmacotherapy regimen following radical prostatectomy improves recovery of spontaneous erectile function. *Journal of Sexual Medicine*, 2: 532, 2005

Mulhall, J. P., Graydon, R. J.: The hemodynamics of erectile dysfunction following nerve-sparing radical retropubic prostatectomy. *International Journal of Impotence Research*, 8: 91, 1996

Padma-Nathan, H., McCullough, A., Giuliano, F., et. al.: Nightly postoperative sildenafil dramatically improves the return of spontaneous erections following a bilateral nerve-sparing radical prostatectomy (abstract). *Journal of Urology*, 2003

Raja, S. G.: Cardioprotection with sildenafil: implications for clinical practice. *Current Medicine Chemistry*, 13: 3155, 2006

Rosano, G. M., Aversa, A., Vitale, C. et al.: Chronic treatment with tadalafil improves endothelial function in men with increased cardiovascular risk. *European Urology*, 47: 214, 2005

Salloum, F. N., Takenoshita, Y., Ockaili, R. A. et al.: Sildenafil and vardenafil but not nitroglycerin limit myocardial infarction through opening of mitochondrial K(ATP) channels when administered at reperfusion following ischemia in rabbits. *Journal of Molecular Cell Cardiology*, 42: 453, 2007

Salonia, A., Gallina, A., Briganti, A. et al.: Remembered International Index of Erectile Function Domain Scores Are Not Accurate in Assessing Preoperative Potency in Candidates for Bilateral Nerve-Sparing Radical Retropubic Prostatectomy. *Journal of Sexual Medicine*, 2008

Salonia, A., Zanni, G., Gallina, A. et al.: Baseline potency in candidates for bilateral nerve-sparing radical retropubic prostatectomy. *European Urology*, 50: 360, 2006

Schwartz, E. J., Wong, P., Graydon, R. J.: Sildenafil preserves intracorporeal smooth muscle after radical retropubic prostatectomy. *Journal of Urology*, 171: 771, 2004

Tal, R., Donohue, J.F., Akin-Olugbade, Y., et al.: The effect of hyperbaric oxygen therapy on erectile fucntion recovery in the rat cavernous nerve injury model. *Journal of Urology*, 175: 223, 2006

User, H. M., Hairston, J. H., Zelner, D. J. et al.: Penile weight and cell subtype specific changes in a post-radical prostatectomy model of erectile dysfunction. *Journal of Urology*, 169: 1175, 2003

Vignozzi, L., Filippi, S., Morelli.A., et al: Effect of chronic tadalafil administration on penile hypoxia induced by cavernous neurotomy in the rat. *Journal of Sexual Medicine*, 3: 419, 2006

Wayman, C., Burcden, A., Casey, J.: Sildenafil increases erection hardness by potentiating pudendal artery blood flow and intracavernosal pressure in the anesthetized dog. *Journal of Sexual Medicine*., 3: 222, 2005

Chapter 8: Miscellaneous Problems

Abouassaly, R., Lane, B.R., Lakin, M.M., Klein, A.N., and Gill, I.S.: Ejaculatory incontinence after radical prostatectomy: a review of 26 cases. *Urology*, 68:1248, 2006

Barnas, J., Parker, M., Guhring, P., Mulhall, J.P.: The utility of tamsulosin in the management of orgasm-associated pain: a pilot analysis. *European Urology*., 47: 361, 2005

Barnas, J. L., Pierpaoli, S., Ladd, P., Valenzuela, R., Aviv, N., Parker, M., et al.: The prevalence and nature of orgasmic dysfunction after radical prostatectomy. *BJU International*, 94: 603, 2004

Bongenhielm, U., Boissonade, F. M., Westermark, A. et al.: Sympathetic nerve sprouting fails to occur in the trigeminal ganglion after peripheral nerve injury in the rat. *Pain*, 82: 283, 1999

Choi, J. M., Nelson, C. J., Stasi, J. et al.: Orgasm-associated incontinence (climacturia) following radical pelvic surgery: rates of occurrence and predictors. *Journal of Urology*, 177: 2223, 2007

Ciancio, S. J., Kim, E. D.: Penile fibrotic changes after radical retropubic prostatectomy. *BJU International*, 85: 101, 2000

Demyttenaere, K., and Huygens, R.: Painful ejaculation and urinary hesitancy in association with antidepressant therapy: relief with tamsulosin. *European Neuropsychopharmacology*, 12: 337, 2002

Dunsmuir, W. D., Emberton, M.: Surgery, drugs, and the male orgasm. *British Medical Journal*, 314: 319, 1997

Fraiman, M. C., Lepor, H., McCullough, A. R.: Changes in Penile Morphometrics in Men with Erectile Dysfunction after Nerve-Sparing Radical Retropubic Prostatectomy. *Molecular Urology*, 3: 109, 1999

Helgason, A. R., Adolfsson, J., Dickman, P. et al.: Sexual desire, erection, orgasm and ejaculatory functions and their importance to elderly Swedish men: a population-based study. *Age Ageing*, 25: 285, 1996

Hendry, W. F., Althof, S.E., Benson, G.S., et al.: Male orgasmic and ejaculatory disorders. In: Erectile Dysfunction. Edited by A. Jardin, Wagner, G., Khoury, S., Guiliano, F., Padma-Nathan, H., and Rosen, R. Plymouth, UK: Plymbridge Distributors, pp. 477–506, 2000

Koeman, M., Van Driel, M.F., Weijmar Schultz, W.C.M., and Mensink, H.J.A. : Orgasm after radical prostatectomy. *British Journal of Urology*, 77: 861, 1996

Lee, J., Fleshner, N,. Lee, C., and Hersey, K. : Climacturia following radical prostatectomy: incidence and risk factors. *Journal of Urology*, 176:2562, 2006

Mah, K., and Binik, Y.M.: The nature of human orgasm: a critical review of major trends. *Clinical Psychology Review*, 21: 823, 2001

McMahon, C. G., Abdo, C., Incrocci, L., Perelman, M., Rowland, D., Waldinger, M., and Xin, Z.C.: Disorders of orgasm and ejaculation in men. *Journal of Sexual Medicine*, 1: 58, 2004

Mulhall, J. P.: Penile length changes after radical prostatectomy. *BJU Int*, 96: 472, 2005

Munding, M. D., Wessells, H. B., Dalkin, B. L.: Pilot study of changes in stretched penile length 3 months after radical retropubic prostatectomy. *Urology*, 58: 567, 2001

Savoie, M., Kim, S. S., Soloway, M. S.: A prospective study measuring penile length in men treated with radical prostatectomy for prostate cancer. *Journal of Urology*, 169: 1462, 2003

Zhou, S., Chen, L. S., Miyauchi, Y. et al.: Mechanisms of cardiac nerve sprouting after myocardial infarction in dogs. *Circulation Research*, 95: 76, 2004

Chapter 9: Pills

Ahn, G. J., Yu, J. Y., Choi, S. M. et al.: Chronic administration of phosphodiesterase 5 inhibitor improves erectile and endothelial function in a rat model of diabetes. *Int J Androl*, 28: 260, 2005

Bella, A. J., Brant, W. O., Lue, T. F. et al.: Non-arteritic anterior ischemic optic neuropathy (NAION) and phosphodiesterase type-5 inhibitors. *Can J Urol*, 13: 3233, 2006

Bella, A. J., Deyoung, L. X., Al-Numi, M. et al.: Daily administration of phosphodiesterase type 5 inhibitors for urological and nonurological indications. *Eur Urol*, 52: 990, 2007

Blander, D. S., Sanchez-Ortiz, R. F., Wein, A. J. et al.: Efficacy of sildenafil in erectile dysfunction after radical prostatectomy. *Int J Impot Res*, 12: 165, 2000

Boorjian, S., Hopps, C. V., Ghaly, S. W. et al.: The utility of sildenafil citrate for infertile men with sexual dysfunction: a pilot study. *BJU Int*, 100: 603, 2007

Boyce, E. G., Umland, E. M.: Sildenafil citrate: a therapeutic update. *Clin Ther*, 23: 2, 2001

Briganti, A., Salonia, A., Gallina, A. et al.: Drug Insight: oral phosphodiesterase type 5 inhibitors for erectile dysfunction. *Nat Clin Pract Urol*, 2: 239, 2005

Brock, G., Nehra, A., Lipshultz, L. I. et al.: Safety and efficacy of vardenafil for the treatment of men with erectile dysfunction after radical retropubic prostatectomy. *J Urol*, 170: 1278, 2003

Carson, C. C., 3rd: Sildenafil: a 4-year update in the treatment of 20 million erectile dysfunction patients. *Curr Urol Rep*, 4: 488, 2003

Carson, C. C., Lue, T. F.: Phosphodiesterase type 5 inhibitors for erectile dysfunction. *BJU Int*, 96: 257, 2005

Crowe, S. M., Streetman, D. S.: Vardenafil treatment for erectile dysfunction. *Ann Pharmacother*, 38: 77, 2004

Feng, M. I., Huang, S., Kaptein, J. et al.: Effect of sildenafil citrate on postradical prostatectomy erectile dysfunction. *J Urol*, 164: 1935, 2000

Gresser, U., Gleiter, C. H.: Erectile dysfunction: comparison of efficacy and side effects of the PDE-5 inhibitors sildenafil, vardenafil and tadalafil—review of the literature. *Eur J Med Res*, 7: 435, 2002

Hatzimouratidis, K.: Sildenafil in the treatment of erectile dysfunction: an overview of the clinical evidence. *Clin Interv Aging*, 1: 403, 2006

Hauri, D.: Erectile dysfunction after radical prostatectomy and its treatment. *Urol Int*, 71: 235, 2003

Hong, E. K., Lepor, H., McCullough, A. R.: Time-dependent patient satisfaction with sildenafil for erectile dysfunction (ED) after nerve-sparing radical retropubic prostatectomy (RRP). *Int J Impot Res*, 11 Suppl 1: S15, 1999

SUGGESTED READING

Kendirci, M., Hellstrom, W. J.: Current concepts in the management of erectile dysfunction in men with prostate cancer. *Clin Prostate Cancer*, 3: 87, 2004

Kostis, J. B., Jackson, G., Rosen, R. et al.: Sexual dysfunction and cardiac risk (the Second Princeton Consensus Conference). *Am J Cardiol*, 96: 313, 2005

Kovanecz, I., Rambhatla, A., Ferrini, M. et al.: Long-term continuous sildenafil treatment ameliorates corporal veno-occlusive dysfunction (CVOD) induced by cavernosal nerve resection in rats. *Int J Impot Res*, 2007

Lee, Y. H., Huang, J. K., Lu, C. M.: The impact on sexual function after nerve sparing and non-nerve sparing radical retropubic prostatectomy. *J Chin Med Assoc*, 66: 13, 2003

Lin, J. S.: Erectile dysfunction after radical prostatectomy treatment and challenge. *J Chin Med Assoc*, 66: 2, 2003

Lowentritt, B. H., Scardino, P. T., Miles, B. J. et al.: Sildenafil citrate after radical retropubic prostatectomy. *J Urol*, 162: 1614, 1999

Lue, T. F.: Erectile dysfunction. *N Engl J Med*, 342: 1802, 2000

Matthew, A. G., Goldman, A., Trachtenberg, J. et al.: Sexual dysfunction after radical prostatectomy: prevalence, treatments, restricted use of treatments and distress. *J Urol*, 174: 2105, 2005

McCullough, A., Woo, K., Telegrafi, S. et al.: Is sildenafil failure in men after radical retropubic prostatectomy (RRP) due to arterial disease? Penile duplex Doppler findings in 174 men after RRP. *Int J Impot Res*, 14: 462, 2002

McCullough, A. R.: Prevention and management of erectile dysfunction following radical prostatectomy. *Urol Clin North Am*, 28: 613, 2001

McCullough, A. R., Levine, L. A., Padma-Nathan, H.: Return of Nocturnal Erections and Erectile Function after Bilateral Nerve-Sparing Radical Prostatectomy in Men Treated Nightly with Sildenafil Citrate: Subanalysis of a Longitudinal Randomized Double-Blind Placebo-Controlled Trial. *J Sex Med*, 5: 476, 2008

McMahon, C. G.: High-dose sildenafil citrate as a salvage therapy for severe erectile dysfunction. *Int J Impot Res*, 14: 533, 2002

McMahon, C. G., Samali, R., Johnson, H.: Efficacy, safety and patient acceptance of sildenafil citrate as treatment for erectile dysfunction. *J Urol*, 164: 1192, 2000

Merrick, G. S., Butler, W. M., Lief, J. H. et al.: Efficacy of sildenafil citrate in prostate brachytherapy patients with erectile dysfunction. *Urology*, 53: 1112, 1999

Montorsi, F., Burnett, A. L.: Erectile dysfunction after radical prostatectomy. *BJU Int*, 93: 1, 2004

Montorsi, F., Corbin, J., Phillips, S.: Review of phosphodiesterases in the urogenital system: new directions for therapeutic intervention. *J Sex Med*, 1: 322, 2004

Montorsi, F., McCullough, A.: Efficacy of sildenafil citrate in men with erectile dysfunction following radical prostatectomy: a systematic review of clinical data. *J Sex Med*, 2: 658, 2005

Montorsi, F., Nathan, H. P., McCullough, A. et al.: Tadalafil in the treatment of erectile dysfunction following bilateral nerve sparing radical retropubic prostatectomy: a randomized, double-blind, placebo controlled trial. *J Urol*, 172: 1036, 2004

Montorsi, F., Salonia, A., Zanoni, M. et al.: Counselling the patient with prostate cancer about treatment-related erectile dysfunction. *Curr Opin Urol*, 11: 611, 2001

Montorsi, F., Verheyden, B., Meuleman, E. et al.: Long-term safety and tolerability of tadalafil in the treatment of erectile dysfunction. *Eur Urol*, 45: 339, 2004

Mulcahy, J. J.: Erectile function after radical prostatectomy. *Semin Urol Oncol*, 18: 71, 2000

Mulhall, J., Althof, S. E., Brock, G. B. et al.: Erectile dysfunction: monitoring response to treatment in clinical practice—recommendations of an international study panel. *J Sex Med*, 4: 448, 2007

Mulhall, J., Barnas, J., Aviv, N. et al.: Sildenafil citrate response correlates with the nature and the severity of penile vascular insufficiency. *J Sex Med*, 2: 104, 2005

Mulhall, J., Land, S., Parker, M. et al.: The use of an erectogenic pharmacotherapy regimen following radical prostatectomy improves recovery of spontaneous erectile function. *J Sex Med*, 2: 532, 2005

Mulhall, J. P.: Understanding erectile dysfunction medication preference studies. *Curr Opin Urol*, 14: 367, 2004

Mulhall, J. P., Goldstein, I., Bushmakin, A. G. et al.: Validation of the erection hardness score. *J Sex Med*, 4: 1626, 2007

SUGGESTED READING

Mulhall, J. P., King, R., Kirby, M. et al.: Evaluating the Sexual Experience in Men: Validation of the Sexual Experience Questionnaire. *J Sex Med*, 2007

Mulhall, J. P., Levine, L. A., Junemann, K. P.: Erection hardness: a unifying factor for defining response in the treatment of erectile dysfunction. *Urology*, 68: 17, 2006

Mulhall, J. P., McLaughlin, T. P., Harnett, J. P. et al.: Medication utilization behavior in patients receiving phosphodiesterase type 5 inhibitors for erectile dysfunction. *J Sex Med*, 2: 848, 2005

Mulhall, J. P., Morgentaler, A.: Penile rehabilitation should become the norm for radical prostatectomy patients. *J Sex Med*, 4: 538, 2007

Mulhall, J. P., Simmons, J.: Assessment of comparative treatment satisfaction with sildenafil citrate and penile injection therapy in patients responding to both. *BJU Int*, 100: 1313, 2007

Muller, A., Shelton, J., Parker, M. et al.: Nitrate cessation profiles in men wishing to use sildenafil citrate. *Urology*, 69: 946, 2007

Muller, A., Smith, L., Parker, M. et al.: Analysis of the efficacy and safety of sildenafil citrate in the geriatric population. *BJU Int*, 100: 117, 2007

Musicki, B., Champion, H. C., Becker, R. E. et al.: Erection capability is potentiated by long-term sildenafil treatment: role of blood flow–induced endothelial nitric-oxide synthase phosphorylation. *Mol Pharmacol*, 68: 226, 2005

Nehra, A., Grantmyre, J., Nadel, A. et al.: Vardenafil improved patient satisfaction with erectile hardness, orgasmic function and sexual experience in men with erectile dysfunction following nerve sparing radical prostatectomy. *J Urol*, 173: 2067, 2005

Ogura, K., Ichioka, K., Terada, N. et al.: Role of sildenafil citrate in treatment of erectile dysfunction after radical retropubic prostatectomy. *Int J Urol*, 11: 159, 2004

Ohebshalom, M., Parker, M., Guhring, P. et al.: The efficacy of sildenafil citrate following radiation therapy for prostate cancer: temporal considerations. *J Urol*, 174: 258, 2005

Padma-Nathan, H.: PDE-5 Inhibitor Therapy for Erectile Dysfunction Secondary to Nerve-Sparing Radical Retropubic Prostatectomy. *Rev Urol*, 7 Suppl 2: S33, 2005

Raina, R., Lakin, M. M., Agarwal, A. et al.: Long-term effect of sildenafil citrate on erectile dysfunction after radical prostatectomy: 3-year follow-up. *Urology*, 62: 110, 2003

Schwartz, E. J., Wong, P., Graydon, R. J.: Sildenafil preserves intracorporeal smooth muscle after radical retropubic prostatectomy. *J Urol*, 171: 771, 2004

Seftel, A. D.: Circulating endothelial progenitor cells in subjects with erectile dysfunction. *J Urol*, 174: 656; discussion 656, 2005

Setter, S. M., Iltz, J. L., Fincham, J. E. et al.: Phosphodiesterase 5 inhibitors for erectile dysfunction. *Ann Pharmacother*, 39: 1286, 2005

Sharabi, F. M., Daabees, T. T., El-Metwally, M. A. et al.: Effect of sildenafil on the isolated rat aortic rings. *Fundam Clin Pharmacol*, 19: 449, 2005

Smith, L. J., Mulhall, J. P., Deveci, S. et al.: Sex after seventy: a pilot study of sexual function in older persons. *J Sex Med*, 4: 1247, 2007

Sussman, D. O.: Pharmacokinetics, pharmacodynamics, and efficacy of phosphodiesterase type 5 inhibitors. *J Am Osteopath Assoc*, 104: S11, 2004

Tal, R., Mulhall, J. P.: Sexual health issues in men with cancer. *Oncology* (Williston Park), 20: 294, 2006

Teloken, P., Valenzuela, R., Parker, M. et al.: The correlation between erectile function and patient satisfaction. *J Sex Med*, 4: 472, 2007

Teloken, P. E., Ohebshalom, M., Mohideen, N. et al.: Analysis of the Impact of Androgen Deprivation Therapy on Sildenafil Citrate Response Following Radiation Therapy for Prostate Cancer. *J Urol*, 178: 2521, 2007

Yavuzgil, O., Altay, B., Zoghi, M. et al.: Endothelial function in patients with vasculogenic erectile dysfunction. *Int J Cardiol*, 103: 19, 2005

Zagaja, G. P., Mhoon, D. A., Aikens, J. E. et al.: Sildenafil in the treatment of erectile dysfunction after radical prostatectomy. *Urology*, 56: 631, 2000

Zippe, C. D., Raina, R., Thukral, M. et al.: Management of erectile dysfunction following radical prostatectomy. *Curr Urol Rep*, 2: 495, 2001

Chapter 10: Urethral Suppositories

Briganti, A., Salonia, A., Gallina, A. et al.: Management of erectile dysfunction after radical prostatectomy in 2007. *World Journal of Urology*, 25: 143, 2007

Burnett, A. L.: Vasoactive pharmacotherapy to cure erectile dysfunction: fact or fiction? *Urology*, 65: 224, 2005

SUGGESTED READING

Costabile, R. A., Spevak, M., Fishman, I. J. et al.: Efficacy and safety of transurethral alprostadil in patients with erectile dysfunction following radical prostatectomy. *Journal of Urology*, 160: 1325, 1998

Hellstrom, W. J., Bennett, A. H., Gesundheit, N. et al.: A double-blind, placebo-controlled evaluation of the erectile response to transurethral alprostadil. *Urology*, 48: 851, 1996

Jaffe, J. S., Antell, M. R., Greenstein, M. et al.: Use of intraurethral alprostadil in patients not responding to sildenafil citrate. *Urology*, 63: 951, 2004

McMahon, C. G.: Current concepts in the management of post-radical prostatectomy impotence. *Current Opinion in Urology*, 8: 535, 1998

Mulhall, J. P., Jahoda, A. E., Ahmed, A. et al.: Analysis of the consistency of intraurethral prostaglandin E(1) (MUSE) during at-home use. *Urology*, 58: 262, 2001

Mydlo, J. H., Viterbo, R., Crispen, P.: Use of combined intracorporal injection and a phosphodiesterase-5 inhibitor therapy for men with a suboptimal response to sildenafil and/or vardenafil monotherapy after radical retropubic prostatectomy. *BJU International*, 95: 843, 2005

Mydlo, J. H., Volpe, M. A., Macchia, R. J.: Initial results utilizing combination therapy for patients with a suboptimal response to either alprostadil or sildenafil monotherapy. *European Urology*, 38: 30, 2000

Nehra, A., Blute, M. L., Barrett, D. M. et al.: Rationale for combination therapy of intraurethral prostaglandin E(1) and sildenafil in the salvage of erectile dysfunction patients desiring noninvasive therapy. *International Journal of Impotence Research*, 14 Suppl 1: S38, 2002

Padma-Nathan, H., Hellstrom, W. J., Kaiser, F. E. et al.: Treatment of men with erectile dysfunction with transurethral alprostadil. Medicated Urethral System for Erection (MUSE) Study Group. *New England Journal of Medicine*, 336: 1, 1997

Peterson, C. A., Bennett, A. H., Hellstrom, W. J. et al.: Erectile response to transurethral alprostadil, prazosin and alprostadil-prazosin combinations. *Journal of Urology*, 159: 1523, 1998

Raina, R., Agarwal, A., Ausmundson, S. et al.: Long-term efficacy and compliance of MUSE for erectile dysfunction following radical prostatectomy: SHIM (IIEF-5) analysis. *International Journal of Impotence Research*, 17: 86, 2005

Raina, R., Nandipati, K. C., Agarwal, A. et al.: Combination therapy: medicated urethral system for erection enhances sexual satisfaction in sildenafil citrate failure following nerve-sparing radical prostatectomy. *Journal of Andrology*, 26: 757, 2005

Raina, R., Pahlajani, G., Agarwal, A. et al.: The early use of transurethral alprostadil after radical prostatectomy potentially facilitates an earlier return of erectile function and successful sexual activity. *BJU International*, 100: 1317, 2007

Tam, P. Y., Keller, T., Poppiti, R. et al.: Hemodynamic effects of transurethral alprostadil measured by color duplex ultrasonography in men with erectile dysfunction. *Journal of Urology*, 160: 1321, 1998

Chapter 11: Penile Injections

Awad, H., El-Karaksy, A., Mostafa, T. et al.: Repeated intracorporeal self-injection: effect on peak systolic velocity and cavernosal artery diameter. *International Journal of Impotence Research* 19: 505, 2007

Brindley, G. S.: Maintenance treatment of erectile impotence by cavernosal unstriated muscle relaxant injection. *British Journal of Psychiatry*, 149: 210, 1986

Brock, G., Tu, L. M., Linet, O. I.: Return of spontaneous erection during long-term intracavernosal alprostadil (Caverject) treatment. *Urology*, 57: 536, 2001

de Meyer, J. M., Thibo, P.: The effect of re-dosing of vasodilators on the intracavernosal pressure and on the penile rigidity. *European Urology*, 33: 293, 1998

El-Sakka, A. I.: Intracavernosal prostaglandin E1 self vs. office injection therapy in patients with erectile dysfunction. *International Journal of Impotence Research*, 18: 180, 2006

Escrig, A., Marin, R., Mas, M.: Repeated PGE1 treatment enhances nitric oxide and erection responses to nerve stimulation in the rat penis by upregulating constitutive NOS isoforms. *Journal of Urology*, 162: 2205, 1999

Fugl-Meyer, A. R., et al.: On life satisfaction in male erectile dysfunction. *International Journal of Impotence Research*, 9: 141, 1997

Gheorghiu, S., Goldschalk, M.F., Gentili, A. Mulligan, T.: Quality of life in patients using self-admnistered intracavernosal injections of prostaglandin E1 for erectile dysfunction. *Journal of Urology*, 156: 80, 1996

Giuliano, F., Amar, E., Chevallier, D. et al.: How Urologists Manage Erectile Dysfunction after Radical Prostatectomy: A National Survey

SUGGESTED READING

(REPAIR) by the French Urological Association. *Journal of Sexual Medicine*, 5: 448, 2008

Gontero, P., Fontana, F., Zitella, A. et al.: A prospective evaluation of efficacy and compliance with a multistep treatment approach for erectile dysfunction in patients after non-nerve sparing radical prostatectomy. *BJU International*, 95: 359, 2005

Hatzichristou, D. G., et al.: Sildenafil versus intracavernous injection therapy: efficacy and preference in patients on intracavernous injection for more than 1 year. *Journal of Urology*, 164: 1197, 2000

Kaplan, H. S.: The combined use of sex therapy and intrapenile injections in the treatment of impotence. *Journal of Sex and Marital Therapy*, 16: 195, 1990

Khan, M. A., Raistrick, M., Mikhailidis, D. P. et al.: MUSE: clinical experience. *Current Medical Research Opinion*, 18: 64, 2002

Kromann-Andersen, B.: Intracavernosal pharmacotherapy with injection pen. *Lancet*, 1: 54, 1988

Kunelius, P., Lukkarinen, O.: Intracavernous self-injection of prostaglandin E1 in the treatment of erectile dysfunction. *International Journal of Impotence Research*, 11: 21, 1999

Linet, O. I., Neff, L. L.: Intracavernous prostaglandin E1 in erectile dysfunction. *Clinical Investigation*, 72: 139, 1994

Linet, O. I., Ogrinc, F. G.: Efficacy and safety of intracavernosal alprostadil in men with erectile dysfunction. The Alprostadil Study Group. *New England Journal of Medicine*, 334: 873, 1996

Montorsi, F., Salonia, A., Deho, F. et al.: Pharmacological management of erectile dysfunction. *BJU International*, 91: 446, 2003

Mulhall, J. P., Simmons, J.: Assessment of comparative treatment satisfaction with sildenafil citrate and penile injection therapy in patients responding to both. *BJU Int*, 100: 1313, 2007

Mulhall, J. P.: Intracavernosal injection therapy: a practical guide. *Techniques in Urology*, 3: 129, 1997

Mulhall, J. P., Abdel-Moneim, A., Abobakr, R. et al.: Improving the accuracy of vascular testing in impotent men: correcting hemodynamic alterations using a vasoactive medication re-dosing schedule. *Journal of Urology*, 166: 923, 2001

Mulhall, J. P., Jahoda, A. E., Cairney, M. et al.: The causes of patient dropout from penile self-injection therapy for impotence. *Journal of Urology*, 162: 1291, 1999

Perimenis, P., Gyftopoulos, K., Athanasopoulos, A. et al.: Diabetic impotence treated by intracavernosal injections: high treatment compliance and increasing dosage of vaso-active drugs. *European Urology*, 40: 398, 2001

Perimenis, P., Konstantinopoulos, A., Perimeni, P. P. et al.: Long-term treatment with intracavernosal injections in diabetic men with erectile dysfunction. *Asian Journal of Andrology*, 8: 219, 2006

Pierpaoli, S. M., Mulhall, J. P.: A positive urine opiate screen following intracavernosal papaverine injection. *Journal of Urology*, 159: 1299, 1998

Purvis, K., Egdetveit, I., Christiansen, E.: Intracavernosal therapy for erectile failure—impact of treatment and reasons for drop-out and dissatisfaction. *International Journal of Impotence Research*, 11: 287, 1999

Rowland, D. L., Boedhoe, H. S., Dohle, G. et al.: Intracavernosal self-injection therapy in men with erectile dysfunction: satisfaction and attrition in 119 patients. *International Journal of Impotence Research*, 11: 145, 1999

Shokeir, A. A., Alserafi, M. A., Mutabagani, H.: Intracavernosal versus intraurethral alprostadil: a prospective randomized study. *BJU International*, 83: 812, 1999

Szasz, G., Stevenson, R. W., Lee, L. et al.: Induction of penile erection by intracavernosal injection: a double-blind comparison of phenoxybenzamine versus papaverine-phentolamine versus saline. *Archives of Sexual Behavior*, 16: 371, 1987

van der Windt, F., Dohle, G. R., van der Tak, J. et al.: Intracavernosal injection therapy with and without sexological counselling in men with erectile dysfunction. *BJU International*, 89: 901, 2002

Virag, R.: Intracavernous injection of papaverine for erectile failure. *Lancet*, 2: 938, 1982

Virag, R.: Comments from Ronald Virag on intracavernous injection: 25 years later. *Journal of Sexual Medicine*, 2: 289, 2005

Willke, R. J., Glick, H. A., McCarron, T. J. et al.: Quality of life effects of alprostadil therapy for erectile dysfunction. *Journal of Urology*, 157: 2124, 1997

Chapter 12: Vacuum Devices

Aloui, R., Iwaz, J., Kokkidis, M. J. et al.: A new vacuum device as alternative treatment for impotence. *British Journal of Urology*, 70: 652, 1992

SUGGESTED READING

Bosshardt, R. J., Farwerk, R., Sikora, R. et al.: Objective measurement of the effectiveness, therapeutic success and dynamic mechanisms of the vacuum device. *British Journal of Urology*, 75: 786, 1995

Bratton, R. L., Cassidy, H. D.: Vacuum erection device use in elderly men: a possible severe complication. *Journal of the American Board of Family Practice*, 15: 501, 2002

Broderick, G. A., Allen, G., McClure, R. D.: Vacuum tumescence devices: the role of papaverine in the selection of patients. *Journal of Urology*, 145: 284, 1991

Broderick, G. A., McGahan, J. P., Stone, A. R. et al.: The hemodynamics of vacuum constriction erections: assessment by color Doppler ultrasound. *Journal of Urology*, 147: 57, 1992

Chen, J., Godschalk, M. F., Katz, P. G. et al.: Combining intracavernous injection and external vacuum as treatment for erectile dysfunction. *Journal of Urology*, 153: 1476, 1995

Chen, J., Mabjeesh, N. J., Greenstein, A.: Sildenafil versus the vacuum erection device: patient preference. *Journal of Urology*, 166: 1779, 2001

Dall'era, J. E., Mills, J. N., Koul, H. K. et al.: Penile rehabilitation after radical prostatectomy: important therapy or wishful thinking? *Reviews in Urology*, 8: 209, 2006

Derouet, H., Caspari, D., Rohde, V. et al.: Treatment of erectile dysfunction with external vacuum devices. *Andrologia*, 31 Suppl 1: 89, 1999

Dutta, T. C., Eid, J. F.: Vacuum constriction devices for erectile dysfunction: a long-term, prospective study of patients with mild, moderate, and severe dysfunction. *Urology*, 54: 891, 1999

Ganem, J. P., Lucey, D. T., Janosko, E. O. et al.: Unusual complications of the vacuum erection device. *Urology*, 51: 627, 1998

Gilbert, H. W., Gingell, J. C.: Vacuum constriction devices: second-line conservative treatment for impotence. *British Journal of Urology*, 70: 81, 1992

Glugla, M., Draznin, B.: Treatment of impotence with vacuum-operated erection assistance device. *Diabetes Care*, 11: 445, 1988

Gontero, P., Fontana, F., Zitella, A. et al.: A prospective evaluation of efficacy and compliance with a multistep treatment approach for erectile dysfunction in patients after non-nerve sparing radical prostatectomy. *BJU International*, 95: 359, 2005

Hakim, L. S., Munarriz, R. M., Kulaksizoglu, H. et al.: Vacuum erection associated impotence and Peyronie's disease. *Journal of Urology*, 155: 534, 1996

Katz, P. G., Haden, H. T., Mulligan, T. et al.: The effect of vacuum devices on penile hemodynamics. *Journal of Urology*, 143: 55, 1990

Kava, B. R.: Advances in the Management of Post-Radical Prostatectomy Erectile Dysfunction: Treatment Strategies When PDE-5 Inhibitors Don't Work. *Reviews in Urology*, 7 Suppl 2: S39, 2005

Kendirci, M., Bejma, J., Hellstrom, W. J.: Update on erectile dysfunction in prostate cancer patients. *Current Opinion in Urology*, 16: 186, 2006

Kim, J. H., Carson, C. C., 3rd: Development of Peyronie's disease with the use of a vacuum constriction device. *Journal of Urology*, 149: 1314, 1993

Kohler, T. S., Pedro, R., Hendlin, K. et al.: A pilot study on the early use of the vacuum erection device after radical retropubic prostatectomy. *BJU International* 100: 858, 2007

Korenman, S. G., Viosca, S. P.: Use of a vacuum tumescence device in the management of impotence in men with a history of penile implant or severe pelvic disease. *Journal of the American Geriatric Society*, 40: 61, 1992

Levine, L. A.: External devices for treatment of erectile dysfunction. *Endocrine*, 23: 157, 2004

Levine, L. A., Dimitriou, R. J.: Vacuum constriction and external erection devices in erectile dysfunction. *Urologic Clinics of North America*, 28: 335, 2001

Lewis, R. W., Witherington, R.: External vacuum therapy for erectile dysfunction: use and results. *World Journal of Urology*, 15: 78, 1997

Marmar, J. L., DeBenedictis, T. J., Praiss, D. E.: The use of a vacuum constrictor device to augment a partial erection following an intracavernous injection. *Journal of Urology*, 140: 975, 1988

McMahon, C. G.: Nonsurgical treatment of cavernosal venous leakage. *Urology*, 49: 97, 1997

Miles, C. L., Candy, B., Jones, L. et al.: Interventions for sexual dysfunction following treatments for cancer. Cochrane Database Syst Rev: CD005540, 2007

Oakley, N., Moore, K. T.: Vacuum devices in erectile dysfunction: indications and efficacy. *British Journal of Urology*, 82: 673, 1998

Raina, R., Agarwal, A., Ausmundson, S. et al.: Early use of vacuum constriction device following radical prostatectomy facilitates early sexual activity and potentially earlier return of erectile function. *International Journal of Importence Research*, 18: 77, 2006

Salvatore, F. T., Sharman, G. M., Hellstrom, W. J.: Vacuum constriction devices and the clinical urologist: an informed selection. *Urology*, 38: 323, 1991

Turner, L. A., Althof, S. E., Levine, S. B. et al.: External vacuum devices in the treatment of erectile dysfunction: a one-year study of sexual and psychosocial impact. *Journal of Sex and Marital Therapy*, 17: 81, 1991

Chapter 13: Penile Implants

Akin-Olugbade, O., Parker, M., Guhring, P. et al.: Determinants of patient satisfaction following penile prosthesis surgery. *Journal of Sexual Medicine*, 3: 743, 2006

Anastasiadis, A. G., Wilson, S. K., Burchardt, M. et al.: Long-term outcomes of inflatable penile implants: reliability, patient satisfaction and complication management. Current Opinion *Urology*, 11: 619, 2001

Brinkman, M. J., Henry, G. D., Wilson, S. K. et al.: A survey of patients with inflatable penile prostheses for satisfaction. *Journal of Urology*, 174: 253, 2005

Carson, C. C.: Penile prosthesis implantation: surgical implants in the era of oral medication. *Urologic Clinics of North America*, 32: 503, 2005

Cutando-Soriano, A., Galindo-Moreno, P.: Antibiotic prophylaxis in dental patients with body prostheses. *Medicine Oral*, 7: 348, 2002

Deveci, S., Martin, D., Parker, M. et al.: Penile length alterations following penile prosthesis surgery. *European Urology*, 51: 1128, 2007

Henry, G. D., Wilson, S. K., Delk, J. R., 2nd et al.: Penile prosthesis cultures during revision surgery: a multicenter study. *Journal of Urology*, 172: 153, 2004

Henry, G. D., Wilson, S. K., Delk, J. R., 2nd et al.: Revision washout decreases penile prosthesis infection in revision surgery: a multicenter study. *Journal of Urology*, 173: 89, 2005

Ilbeigi, P., Sadeghi-Nejad, H., Kim, M.: Retained rear-tip extenders in redo penile prosthesis surgery: a case for heightened suspicion and thorough physical examination. *Journal of Sexual Medicine*, 2: 149, 2005

Kumar, R., Nehra, A.: Dual implantation of penile and sphincter implants in the post-prostatectomy patient. *Current Urology Reports*, 8: 477, 2007

Milbank, A. J., Montague, D. K., Angermeier, K. W. et al.: Mechanical failure of the American Medical Systems Ultrex inflatable penile prosthesis: before and after 1993 structural modification. *Journal of Urology*, 167: 2502, 2002

Mireku-Boateng, A. O., Dennery, M., Littlejohn, J.: Use of sildenafil in penile implant patients. *Urology International*, 66: 149, 2001

Mireku-Boateng, A. O., Oben, F.: Surgical outcome of radical retropubic prostatectomy is not adversely affected by preexisting three-piece inflatable penile implant. *Urology International*, 74: 221, 2005

Montague, D. K., Angermeier, K. W.: Contemporary aspects of penile prosthesis implantation. Urology International 70: 141, 2003

Montorsi, F., Deho, F., Salonia, A. et al.: Penile implants in the era of oral drug treatment for erectile dysfunction. *BJU International*, 94: 745, 2004

Mulcahy, J. J., Wilson, S. K.: Current use of penile implants in erectile dysfunction. *Current Urology Reports*, 7: 485, 2006

Mulhall, J., Ahmed, A., Anderson, M.: Penile prosthetic surgery for Peyronie's disease: defining the need for intraoperative adjuvant maneuvers. *Journal of Sexual Medicine*, 1: 318, 2004

Mulhall, J. P., Ahmed, A., Branch, J. et al.: Serial assessment of efficacy and satisfaction profiles following penile prosthesis surgery. *Journal of Urology*, 169: 1429, 2003

Mulhall, J. P., Bloom, K.: Comparison of in-patient and out-patient penile prosthesis surgery. *International Journal of Impotence Research*, 13: 251, 2001

Pescatori, E. S., Goldstein, I.: Intraluminal device pressures in 3–piece inflatable penile prostheses: the "pathophysiology" of mechanical malfunction. *Journal of Urology*, 149: 295, 1993

Rajpurkar, A., Bianco, F. F., Jr., Al-Omar, O. et al.: Fate of the retained reservoir after replacement of 3–piece penile prosthesis. *Journal of Urology*, 172: 664, 2004

Rhee, E. Y.: Technique for concomitant implantation of the penile prosthesis with the male sling *Journal of Urology*, 173: 925, 2005

Wilson, S. K., Cleves, M. A., Delk, J. R., 2nd: Ultrex cylinders: problems with uncontrolled lengthening (the S-shaped deformity). *Journal of Urology*, 155: 135, 1996

Wilson, S. K., Cleves, M. A., Delk, J. R., 2nd: Comparison of mechanical reliability of original and enhanced Mentor Alpha I penile prosthesis. *Journal of Urology*, 162: 715, 1999

Wilson, S. K., Delk, J. R., 2nd, Mulcahy, J. J. et al.: Upsizing of inflatable penile implant cylinders in patients with corporal fibrosis. *Journal of Sexual Medicine*, 3: 736, 2006

Wilson, S. K., Delk, J. R., Salem, E. A. et al.: Long-term survival of inflatable penile prostheses: single surgical group experience with 2,384 first-time implants spanning two decades. *Journal of Sexual Medicine*, 4: 1074, 2007

Wilson, S. K., Henry, G. D., Delk, J. R., Jr. et al.: The mentor Alpha 1 penile prosthesis with reservoir lock-out valve: effective prevention of auto-inflation with improved capability for ectopic reservoir placement. *Journal of Urology*, 168: 1475, 2002

Wilson, S. K., Zumbe, J., Henry, G. D. et al.: Infection reduction using antibiotic-coated inflatable penile prosthesis. *Urology*, 70: 337, 2007

Chapter 14: Future Therapies for Sexual Problems

Baumhakel, M., Werner, N., Bohm, M. et al.: Circulating endothelial progenitor cells correlate with erectile function in patients with coronary heart disease. *European Heart Journal*, 27: 2184, 2006

Bella, A. J., Lin, G., Cagiannos, I. et al.: Emerging neuromodulatory molecules for the treatment of neurogenic erectile dysfunction caused by cavernous nerve injury. Asian *Journal of Andrology*, 10: 54, 2008

Bennett, N. E., Kim, J. H., Wolfe, D. P. et al.: Improvement in erectile dysfunction after neurotrophic factor gene therapy in diabetic rats. *Journal of Urology*, 173: 1820, 2005

Bivalacqua, T. J., Deng, W., Kendirci, M. et al.: Mesenchymal stem cells alone or ex vivo gene modified with endothelial nitric oxide synthase reverse age-associated erectile dysfunction. *American Journal of Physiology of the Heart and Circulatory Physiol*, 292: H1278, 2007

Bivalacqua, T. J., Strong, T. D.: The use of gene transfer technology to study the pathophysiology of erectile dysfunction. *Journal Sexual Medicine*, 5: 268, 2008

Bivalacqua, T. J., Usta, M. F., Champion, H. C. et al.: Gene transfer of endothelial nitric oxide synthase partially restores nitric oxide synthesis and erectile function in streptozotocin diabetic rats. *Journal of Urology*, 169: 1911, 2003

Briganti, A., Chun, F. K., Salonia, A. et al.: A comparative review of apomorphine formulations for erectile dysfunction: recommendations for use in the elderly. *Drugs Aging*, 23: 309, 2006

Brock, G.: The evolution of ED therapy in the 21st century. *European Urology*, 50: 1157, 2006

Burnett, A. L.: Neuroprotection and nerve grafts in the treatment of neurogenic erectile dysfunction. *Journal of Urology*, 170: S31, 2003

Burnett, A. L., Kramer, M. F., Dalrymple, S. et al.: Nonimmunosuppressant immunophilin ligand GPI-1046 does not promote in vitro growth of prostate cancer cells. *Urology*, 65: 1003, 2005

Burnett, A. L., Lue, T. F.: Neuromodulatory therapy to improve erectile function recovery outcomes after pelvic surgery. *Journal of Urology*, 176: 882, 2006

Carson, C. C., 3rd: Central nervous system-acting agents and the treatment of erectile and sexual dysfunction. *Current Urology Reports*, 8: 472, 2007

Chancellor, M. B., Tirney, S., Mattes, C. E. et al.: Nitric oxide synthase gene transfer for erectile dysfunction in a rat model. *BJU International*, 91: 691, 2003

Chen, Y., Li, S. X., Yao, L. S. et al.: Valsartan treatment reverses erectile dysfunction in diabetic rats. *Int J Impot Res*, 19: 366, 2007

Christ, G. J.: Gene therapy: future strategies and therapies. *Drugs Today* (Barc), 36: 175, 2000

Christ, G. J.: Frontiers in gene therapy for erectile dysfunction. *International Journal of Impotence Research*, 15 Suppl 5: S33, 2003

Christ, G. J.: Gene therapy treatments for erectile and bladder dysfunction. *Current Urology Reports*, 5: 52, 2004

Christ, G. J.: siRNA for erectile dysfunction. *Journal of Urology*, 174: 819, 2005

Dean, R. C., Lue, T. F.: Neuroregenerative strategies after radical prostatectomy. Reviews in *Urology*, 7 Suppl 2: S26, 2005

Deng, W., Bivalacqua, T. J., Hellstrom, W. J. et al.: Gene and stem cell therapy for erectile dysfunction. *International Journal of Impotence Research*, 17 Suppl 1: S57, 2005

Diamond, L. E., Earle, D. C., Garcia, W. D. et al.: Co-administration of low doses of intranasal PT-141, a melanocortin receptor agonist, and sildenafil to men with erectile dysfunction results in an enhanced erectile response. *Urology*, 65: 755, 2005

SUGGESTED READING

Diamond, L. E., Earle, D. C., Rosen, R. C. et al.: Double-blind, placebo-controlled evaluation of the safety, pharmacokinetic properties and pharmacodynamic effects of intranasal PT-141, a melanocortin receptor agonist, in healthy males and patients with mild-to-moderate erectile dysfunction. *International Journal of Impotence Research*, 16: 51, 2004

Donatucci, C. F., Greenfield, J. M.: Recovery of sexual function after prostate cancer treatment. *Current Opinion in Urology*, 16: 444, 2006

Fadini, G. P., Agostini, C., Avogaro, A.: Endothelial progenitor cells and erectile dysfunction. *European Heart Journal*, 28: 639, 2007

Foresta, C., Caretta, N., Lana, A. et al.: Circulating endothelial progenitor cells in subjects with erectile dysfunction. *International Journal of Impotence Research*, 17: 288, 2005

Foresta, C., Ferlin, A., De Toni, L. et al.: Circulating endothelial progenitor cells and endothelial function after chronic tadalafil treatment in subjects with erectile dysfunction. *International Journal of Impotence Research*, 18: 484, 2006

Gholami, S. S., Rogers, R., Chang, J. et al.: The effect of vascular endothelial growth factor and adeno-associated virus-mediated brain-derived neurotrophic factor on neurogenic and vasculogenic erectile dysfunction induced by hyperlipidemia. *Journal of Urology*, 169: 1577, 2003

Giuliano, F.: Control of penile erection by the melanocortinergic system: experimental evidences and therapeutic perspectives. *Journal of Andrology*, 25: 683, 2004

Gontero, P., D'Antonio, R., Pretti, G. et al.: Clinical efficacy of Apomorphine SL in erectile dysfunction of diabetic men. *International Journal of Impotence Research*, 17: 80, 2005

Gonzalez-Cadavid, N. F., Rajfer, J.: Therapy of erectile dysfunction: potential future treatments. *Endocrine*, 23: 167, 2004

Hadley, M. E., Dorr, R. T.: Melanocortin peptide therapeutics: historical milestones, clinical studies and commercialization. *Peptides*, 27: 921, 2006

Hagemann, J. H., Berding, G., Bergh, S. et al.: Effects of visual sexual stimuli and apomorphine SL on cerebral activity in men with erectile dysfunction. *European Urology*, 43: 412, 2003

Hatzimouratidis, K., Hatzichristou, D. G.: Looking to the future for erectile dysfunction therapies. *Drugs*, 68: 231, 2008

Hedlund, P.: PT-141 Palatin. Current Opinion in Investigational Drugs, 5: 456, 2004

Jiang, R., Chen, J. H., Jin, J. et al.: Ultrastructural comparison of penile cavernous tissue between hypertensive and normotensive rats. *International Journal of Impotence Research*, 17: 417, 2005

Kendirci, M., Teloken, P. E., Champion, H. C. et al.: Gene therapy for erectile dysfunction: fact or fiction? *European Urology*, 50: 1208, 2006

King, S. H., Mayorov, A. V., Balse-Srinivasan, P. et al.: Melanocortin receptors, melanotropic peptides and penile erection. *Current Topics in Medical Chemistry*, 7: 1098, 2007

Melman, A.: Gene transfer for the therapy of erectile dysfunction: progress in the 21st century. *International Journal of Impotence Research*, 18: 19, 2006

Melman, A., Bar-Chama, N., McCullough, A. et al.: hMaxi-K gene transfer in males with erectile dysfunction: results of the first human trial. *Human Gene Therapy*, 17: 1165, 2006

Mills, J. N., Barqawi, A., Koul, S. et al.: The molecular basis of erectile dysfunction: from bench to bedside. Reviews in *Urology*, 7: 128, 2005

Mills, J. N., Dall'Era, J. E., Carlsen, S. N. et al.: Gene therapy for erectile dysfunction. *Pharmacogenomics*, 8: 979, 2007

Molinoff, P. B., Shadiack, A. M., Earle, D. et al.: PT-141: a melanocortin agonist for the treatment of sexual dysfunction. *Ann New York Academy of Sciences*, 994: 96, 2003

Mulhall, J.: Neuroimmunophilin ligands protect cavernous nerves after crush injury in the rat: new experimental paradigms. *European Urology*, 51: 1488, 2007

Nossaman, B. D., Gur, S., Kadowitz, P. J.: Gene and stem cell therapy in the treatment of erectile dysfunction and pulmonary hypertension; potential treatments for the common problem of endothelial dysfunction. *Current Gene Therapy*, 7: 131, 2007

Perimenis, P., Markou, S., Gyftopoulos, K. et al.: Efficacy of apomorphine and sildenafil in men with nonarteriogenic erectile dysfunction. A comparative crossover study. *Andrologia*, 36: 106, 2004

Pfaus, J., Giuliano, F., Gelez, H.: Bremelanotide: an overview of preclinical CNS effects on female sexual function. *Journal of Sexual Medicine*, 4 Suppl 4: 269, 2007

Rajfer, J.: Growth factors and gene therapy for erectile dysfunction. Reviews in *Urology*, 2: 34, 2000

Rogers, R. S., Graziottin, T. M., Lin, C. S. et al.: Intracavernosal vascular endothelial growth factor (VEGF) injection and adeno-associated

SUGGESTED READING

virus-mediated VEGF gene therapy prevent and reverse venogenic erectile dysfunction in rats. *International Journal of Impotence Research*, 15: 26, 2003

Rosen, R. C., Diamond, L. E., Earle, D. C. et al.: Evaluation of the safety, pharmacokinetics and pharmacodynamic effects of subcutaneously administered PT-141, a melanocortin receptor agonist, in healthy male subjects and in patients with an inadequate response to Viagra. *International Journal of Impotence Research*, 16: 135, 2004

Schiff, J. D., Mulhall, J. P.: Neuroprotective strategies in radical prostatectomy. *BJU International*, 95: 11, 2005

Schultheiss, D.: Regenerative medicine in andrology: Tissue engineering and gene therapy as potential treatment options for penile deformations and erectile dysfunction. *European Urology*, 46: 162, 2004

Sezen, S. F., Hoke, A., Burnett, A. L. et al.: Immunophilin ligand FK506 is neuroprotective for penile innervation. *Nature Medicine*, 7: 1073, 2001

Sievert, K. D., Amend, B., Stenzl, A.: Tissue engineering for the lower urinary tract: a review of a state-of-the-art approach. *European Urology*, 52: 1580, 2007

Sommer, F., Engelmann, U.: Future options for combination therapy in the management of erectile dysfunction in older men. *Drugs Aging*, 21: 555, 2004

Strong, T. D., Gebska, M. A., Burnett, A. L. et al.: Endothelium-specific gene and stem cell-based therapy for erectile dysfunction. *Asian Journal of Andrology*, 10: 14, 2008

Uthayathas, S., Karuppagounder, S. S., Tamer, S. I. et al.: Evaluation of neuroprotective and anti-fatigue effects of sildenafil. *Life Sciences*, 81: 988, 2007

Valentine, H., Chen, Y., Guo, H. et al.: Neuroimmunophilin ligands protect cavernous nerves after crush injury in the rat: new experimental paradigms. *European Urology*, 51: 1724, 2007

Xie, D., Annex, B. H., Donatucci, C. F.: Growth factors for therapeutic angiogenesis in hypercholesterolemic erectile dysfunction. *Asian Journal of Andrology*, 10: 23, 2008

Yetik-Anacak, G., Catravas, J. D.: Nitric oxide and the endothelium: history and impact on cardiovascular disease. *Vascular Pharmacology*, 45: 268, 2006

Chapter 15: Testosterone and the Prostate

Agarwal, P. K., Oefelein, M. G.: Testosterone replacement therapy after primary treatment for prostate cancer. *Journal of Urology*, 173: 533, 2005

Baum, N. H., Torti, D. C.: Managing hot flashes in men being treated for prostate cancer. *Geriatrics*, 62: 18, 2007

Bohle, A.: Preoperative serum testosterone level as an independent predictor of treatment failure following radical prostatectomy. International Brazilian *Journal of Urology*, 33: 731, 2007

Crawford, E. D., Barqawi, A. B., O'Donnell, C. et al.: The association of time of day and serum testosterone concentration in a large screening population. *BJU International*, 100: 509, 2007

Ebling, D. W., Ruffer, J., Whittington, R. et al.: Development of prostate cancer after pituitary dysfunction: a report of 8 patients. *Urology*, 49: 564, 1997

Eskelinen, S. I., Vahlberg, T. J., Isoaho, R. E. et al.: Associations of sex hormone concentrations with health and life satisfaction in elderly men. *Endocrine Practice*, 13: 743, 2007

Gleave, M., Qian, J., Andreou, C. et al.: The effects of the dual 5 alpha-reductase inhibitor dutasteride on localized prostate cancer—results from a 4–month pre-radical prostatectomy study. *Prostate*, 66: 1674, 2006

Heracek, J., Richard, H., Martin, H. et al.: Tissue and serum levels of principal androgens in benign prostatic hyperplasia and prostate cancer. *Steroids*, 72: 375, 2007

Hoffman, M. A., DeWolf, W. C., Morgentaler, A.: Is low serum free testosterone a marker for high-grade prostate cancer? *Journal of Urology*, 163: 824, 2000

Isom-Batz, G., Bianco, F. J., Jr., Kattan, M. W. et al.: Testosterone as a predictor of pathological stage in clinically localized prostate cancer. *Journal of Urology*, 173: 1935, 2005

Katz, A., Katz, A., Burchill, C.: Androgen therapy: testing before prescribing and monitoring during therapy. *Canadian Family Physician*, 53: 1936, 2007

Kaufman, J. M., Graydon, R. J.: Androgen replacement after curative radical prostatectomy for prostate cancer in hypogonadal men. *Journal of Urology*, 172: 920, 2004

SUGGESTED READING

Lazarou, S., Reyes-Vallejo, L., Morgentaler, A.: Wide variability in laboratory reference values for serum testosterone. *Journal of Sexual Medicine*, 3: 1085, 2006

Loughlin, K. R.: Testosterone replacement therapy. A rush to judgment? *Journal of Urology*, 172: 827, 2004

Madersbacher, S., Schatzl, G., Bieglmayer, C. et al.: Impact of radical prostatectomy and TURP on the hypothalamic-pituitary-gonadal hormone axis. *Urology*, 60: 869, 2002

Massengill, J. C., Sun, L., Moul, J. W. et al.: Pretreatment total testosterone level predicts pathological stage in patients with localized prostate cancer treated with radical prostatectomy. *Journal of Urology*, 169: 1670, 2003

Miller, L. R., Partin, A. W., Chan, D. W. et al.: Influence of radical prostatectomy on serum hormone levels. *Journal of Urology*, 160: 449, 1998

Morgentaler, A.: Testosterone and prostate cancer: an historical perspective on a modern myth. *European Urology*, 50: 935, 2006

Morgentaler, A.: Testosterone replacement therapy and prostate risks: where's the beef? Canadian *Journal of Urology*, 13 Suppl 1: 40, 2006

Morgentaler, A.: Testosterone deficiency and prostate cancer: emerging recognition of an important and troubling relationship. *European Urology*, 52: 623, 2007

Morgentaler, A.: Cultural biases and scientific squabbles: the challenges to acceptance of testosterone therapy as a mainstream medical treatment. *Aging Male*, 10: 1, 2007

Morgentaler, A., Rhoden, E. L.: Prevalence of prostate cancer among hypogonadal men with prostate-specific antigen levels of 4.0 ng/mL or less. *Urology*, 68: 1263, 2006

Reyes-Vallejo, L., Lazarou, S., Morgentaler, A.: Subjective sexual response to testosterone replacement therapy based on initial serum levels of total testosterone. *Journal of Sexual Medicine*, 4: 1757, 2007

Rhoden, E. L., Morgentaler, A.: Testosterone replacement therapy in hypogonadal men at high risk for prostate cancer: results of 1 year of treatment in men with prostatic intraepithelial neoplasia. *Journal of Urology*, 170: 2348, 2003

Rhoden, E. L., Morgentaler, A.: Treatment of testosterone-induced gynecomastia with the aromatase inhibitor, anastrozole. *International Journal of Impotence Research*, 16: 95, 2004

Rhoden, E. L., Morgentaler, A.: Risks of testosterone-replacement therapy and recommendations for monitoring. *New England Journal of Medicine*, 350: 482, 2004

Saad, F., Gooren, L., Haider, A. et al.: Effects of testosterone gel followed by parenteral testosterone undecanoate on sexual dysfunction and on features of the metabolic syndrome. *Andrologia*, 40: 44, 2008

San Francisco, I. F., Regan, M. M., Dewolf, W. C. et al.: Low age adjusted free testosterone levels correlate with poorly differentiated prostate cancer. *Journal of Urology*, 175: 1341, 2006

Shariat, S. F., Lamb, D. J., Roehrborn, C. G. et al.: Potentially harmful effect of a testosterone dietary supplement on prostate cancer growth and metastasis. *Archives of Internal Medicine*, 168: 235, 2008

Spark, R. F.: Testosterone, diabetes mellitus, and the metabolic syndrome. *Current Urology Reports*, 8: 467, 2007

Syme, D. B., Corcoran, N. M., Bouchier-Hayes, D. M. et al.: The effect of androgen status on the structural and functional success of cavernous nerve grafting in an experimental rat model. *Journal of Urology*, 177: 390, 2007

Teloken, C., Da Ros, C. T., Caraver, F. et al.: Low serum testosterone levels are associated with positive surgical margins in radical retropubic prostatectomy: hypogonadism represents bad prognosis in prostate cancer. *Journal of Urology*, 174: 2178, 2005

Weiss, J. M., Huang, W. Y., Rinaldi, S. et al.: Endogenous sex hormones and the risk of prostate cancer: A prospective study. *International Journal of Cancer*, 2008

Yamamoto, S., Yonese, J., Kawakami, S. et al.: Preoperative serum testosterone level as an independent predictor of treatment failure following radical prostatectomy. *European Urology*, 52: 696, 2007

Yang, X. J., Lecksell, K., Short, K. et al.: Does long-term finasteride therapy affect the histologic features of benign prostatic tissue and prostate cancer on needle biopsy? PLESS Study Group. Proscar Long-Term Efficacy and Safety Study. *Urology*, 53: 696, 1999

Zhang, P. L., Rosen, S., Veeramachaneni, R. et al.: Association between prostate cancer and serum testosterone levels. *Prostate*, 53: 179, 2002

Chapter 16: Getting Back a Sex Life

Althof, S. E., Leiblum, S. R., Chevret-Measson, M. et al.: Psychological and interpersonal dimensions of sexual function and dysfunction. *Journal of Sexual Medicine*, 2: 793, 2005

Alterowitz, R., Alterowitz, B. Intimacy with impotence. First DaCapo Life Long Books, Cambridge, Massachussets, 2004

Alterowitz, R., Alterowitz, B. The lovin' ain't over: a couple's guide to better sex after prostate disease. Health Education Literary Publisher, Westbury, New York

Anand, M. The Art of Sexual Magic. Putnam Sons, New York, 1995

Azar, M., Noohi, S., Shafiee Kandjani, A. R.: Relationship between female sexual difficulties and mental health in patients referred to two public and private settings in Tehran, Iran. *Journal of Sex Medicine*, 4: 1262, 2007

Bancroft, J., Janssen, E., Strong, D. et al.: The relation between mood and sexuality in heterosexual men. *Archives of Sexual Behavior*, 32: 217, 2003

Ben-Zion, I., Rothschild, S., Chudakov, B. et al.: Surrogate versus couple therapy in vaginismus. *Journal of Sexual Medicine*, 4: 728, 2007

Bergamnn, M.S. The anatomy of loving. Fawcett Columbine, New York, 1987.

Bokhour, B. G., Clark, J. A., Inui, T. S. et al.: Sexuality after treatment for early prostate cancer: exploring the meanings of "erectile dysfunction". *Journal of General Internal Medicine*, 16: 649, 2001

Bradford, A., Meston, C.: Correlates of placebo response in the treatment of sexual dysfunction in women: a preliminary report. *Journal of Sexual Medicine*, 4: 1345, 2007

Camacho, M. E., Reyes-Ortiz, C. A.: Sexual dysfunction in the elderly: age or disease? *International Journal of Impotence Research*, 17 Suppl 1: S52, 2005

Canada, A. L., Neese, L. E., Sui, D. et al.: Pilot intervention to enhance sexual rehabilitation for couples after treatment for localized prostate carcinoma. *Cancer*, 104: 2689, 2005

Clark, J. A., Inui, T. S., Silliman, R. A. et al.: Patients' perceptions of quality of life after treatment for early prostate cancer. *Journal of Clinical Oncology*, 21: 3777, 2003

Clayton, A. H.: Epidemiology and neurobiology of female sexual dysfunction. *Journal Sexual Medicine*, 4 Suppl 4: 260, 2007

Derby, C. A., Mohr, B. A., Goldstein, I. et al.: Modifiable risk factors and erectile dysfunction: can lifestyle changes modify risk? *Urology*, 56: 302, 2000

Dunn, M. E.: Restoration of couple's intimacy and relationship vital to reestablishing erectile function. *Journal of the American Osteopathic Association*, 104: S6, 2004

Esposito, K., Ciotola, M., Marfella, R. et al.: The metabolic syndrome: a cause of sexual dysfunction in women. *International Journal of Impotence Research*, 17: 224, 2005

Esposito, K., Giugliano, D.: Obesity, the metabolic syndrome, and sexual dysfunction. *International Journal of Impotence Research*, 17: 391, 2005

Feldman, H. A., Goldstein, I., Hatzichristou, D. G. et al.: Impotence and its medical and psychosocial correlates: results of the Massachusetts Male Aging Study. *J Urol*, 151: 54, 1994

Feldmann, J., Middleman, A. B.: Adolescent sexuality and sexual behavior. *Current Opinion Obstetrics Gynecology*, 14: 489, 2002

Garos, S., Kluck, A., Aronoff, D.: Prostate cancer patients and their partners: differences in satisfaction indices and psychological variables. *Journal of Sexual Medicine*, 4: 1394, 2007

Goldstein, I.: Female sexual dysfunction and the central nervous system. *Journal of Sexual Medicine*, 4 Suppl 4: 255, 2007

Goldstein, I.: Current management strategies of the postmenopausal patient with sexual health problems. *Journal of Sexual Medicine*, 4 Suppl 3: 235, 2007

Graziottin, A.: Prevalence and evaluation of sexual health problems—HSDD in Europe. *Journal of Sexual Medicine*, 4 Suppl 3: 211, 2007

Howe, D.L. Prostate and me: a couple deals with prostate cancer.

Jenkins, R., Schover, L. R., Fouladi, R. T. et al.: Sexuality and health-related quality of life after prostate cancer in African-American and white men treated for localized disease. *Journal of Sex and Marital Therapy*, 30: 79, 2004

Johannes, C. B., Araujo, A. B., Feldman, H. A. et al.: Incidence of erectile dysfunction in men 40 to 69 years old: longitudinal results from the Massachusetts male aging study. *J Urol*, 163: 460, 2000

Jongpipan, J., Charoenkwan, K.: Sexual function after radical hysterectomy for early-stage cervical cancer. *Journal of Sexual Medicine*, 4: 1659, 2007

Kingsberg, S.: Testosterone treatment for hypoactive sexual desire disorder in postmenopausal women. *Journal of Sexual Medicine*, 4 Suppl 3: 227, 2007

Kingsberg, S. A.: The testosterone patch for women. *International Journal of Impotence Research*, 17: 465, 2005

Larsson, I., Svedin, C. G.: Sexual experiences in childhood: young adults' recollections. *Archives of Sexual Behavior*, 31: 263, 2002

Laumann, E. O., Michael, R. T., Gagnon, J. H.: A political history of the national sex survey of adults. *Family Planning Perspectives*, 26: 34, 1994

Laumann, E. O., Nicolosi, A., Glasser, D. B. et al.: Sexual problems among women and men aged 40–80 y: prevalence and correlates identified in the Global Study of Sexual Attitudes and Behaviors. *International Journal of Impotence Research*, 17: 39, 2005

Laumann, E. O., Paik, A., Glasser, D. B. et al.: A cross-national study of subjective sexual well-being among older women and men: findings from the Global Study of Sexual Attitudes and Behaviors. *Archives of Sexual Behavior*, 35: 145, 2006

Laumann, E. O., Paik, A., Glasser, D. B. et al.: A Cross-National Study of Subjective Sexual Well-Being among Older Women and Men: Findings from the Global Study of Sexual Attitudes and Behaviors. *Archives of Sexual Behavior*, 2006

Laumann, E. O., Paik, A., Rosen, R. C.: Sexual dysfunction in the United States: prevalence and predictors. *Journal of the American Medical Association*, 281: 537, 1999

Leiblum, S. R.: After sildenafil: bridging the gap between pharmacologic treatment and satisfying sexual relationships. *Journal of Clinical Psychiatry*, 63 Suppl 5: 17, 2002

Leiblum, S., Sachs, J. Getting the sex you want. ASJA Press, Lincoln, Nebraska, 2001

Lindau, S. T., Schumm, L. P., Laumann, E. O. et al.: A study of sexuality and health among older adults in the United States. *New England Journal of Medicine*, 357: 762, 2007

Mah, K., Binik, Y. M.: Do all orgasms feel alike? Evaluating a two-dimensional model of the orgasm experience across gender and sexual context. *Journal of Sex Research*, 39: 104, 2002

Malatesta, V. J.: Sexual problems, women and aging: an overview. *Journal of Women and Aging*, 19: 139, 2007

McCabe, M. P.: Intimacy and quality of life among sexually dysfunctional men and women. *Journal of Sex and Marital Therapy*, 23: 276, 1997

McKee, A. L., Jr., Schover, L. R.: Sexuality rehabilitation. *Cancer*, 92: 1008, 2001

Mehta, A., Bachmann, G.: Premenopausal women with sexual dysfunction: the need for a bladder function history. *Journal of Sexual Medicine*, 5: 407, 2008

Meyer, T. L., Cheng, T. L.: Unveiling the secrecy behind masturbation. *Pediatrics Review*, 23:148, 2002

Monturo, C. A., Rogers, P. D., Coleman, M. et al.: Beyond sexual assessment: lessons learned from couples post-radical prostatectomy. *Journal of the American Academy of Nurse Practitioners*, 13: 511, 2001

Moreira, E. D., Jr., Brock, G., Glasser, D. B. et al.: Help-seeking behaviour for sexual problems: the global study of sexual attitudes and behaviors. *International Journal of Clinical Practice*, 59: 6, 2005

Neese, L. E., Schover, L. R., Klein, E. A. et al.: Finding help for sexual problems after prostate cancer treatment: a phone survey of men's and women's perspectives. *Psychooncology*, 12: 463, 2003

Nicolosi, A., Laumann, E. O., Glasser, D. B. et al.: Sexual behavior and sexual dysfunctions after age 40: the global study of sexual attitudes and behaviors. *Urology*, 64: 991, 2004

Nusbaum, M. R.: Therapeutic options for patients returning to sexual activity. *Journal of the American Osteopathic Association*, 104: S2, 2004

Olarinoye, J., Olarinoye, A.: Determinants of Sexual Function among Women with Type 2 Diabetes in a Nigerian Population. *Journal of Sexual Medicine*, 2007

Panzer, C., Wise, S., Fantini, G. et al.: Impact of oral contraceptives on sex hormone-binding globulin and androgen levels: a retrospective study in women with sexual dysfunction. *Journal of Sexual Medicine*, 3: 104, 2006

Papaharitou, S., Nakopoulou, E., Kirana, P. et al.: Women's sexual concerns: data analysis from a help-line. *Journal of Sexual Medicine*, 2: 652, 2005

Penney, A. How to make love to a man. Gramercy Books, New York 1981

Perez, M. A., Skinner, E. C., Meyerowitz, B. E.: Sexuality and intimacy following radical prostatectomy: patient and partner perspectives. *Health Psychology*, 21: 288, 2002

Piccinino, L. J., Mosher, W. D.: Trends in contraceptive use in the United States: 1982–1995. *Family Planning Perspectives*, 30: 4, 1998

SUGGESTED READING

Ponholzer, A., Temml, C., Rauchenwald, M. et al.: Is the metabolic syndrome a risk factor for female sexual dysfunction in sexually active women? *International Journal of Impotence Research*, 20: 100, 2008

Pope, K. S., Levenson, H., Schover, L. R.: Sexual intimacy in psychology training: results and implications of a national survey. *American Psychologist*, 34: 682, 1979

Rice, D.: Say yes to intimacy. Treatment options for erectile dysfunction. *Diabetes Self Management*, 21: 81, 2004

Robinson, B. B., Bockting, W. O., Rosser, B. R. et al.: The Sexual Health Model: application of a sexological approach to HIV prevention. *Health Education Research*, 17: 43, 2002

Ryan, G. Reclaiming male sexuality. Evans, New York, 1997

Sadovsky, R., Nusbaum, M.: Sexual health inquiry and support is a primary care priority. *Journal of Sexual Medicine*, 3: 3, 2006

Sand, M., Fisher, W. A.: Women's endorsement of models of female sexual response: the nurses' sexuality study. *Journal of Sexual Medicine*, 4: 708, 2007

Schover, L. R.: Sexuality and fertility in urologic cancer patients. *Cancer*, 60: 553, 1987

Schover, L. R.: Sexual rehabilitation after treatment for prostate cancer. *Cancer*, 71: 1024, 1993

Schover, L. R., Fouladi, R. T., Warneke, C. L. et al.: The use of treatments for erectile dysfunction among survivors of prostate carcinoma. *Cancer*, 95: 2397, 2002

Schover, L. R., Fouladi, R. T., Warneke, C. L. et al.: Defining sexual outcomes after treatment for localized prostate carcinoma. *Cancer*, 95: 1773, 2002

Schover, L. R., Fouladi, R. T., Warneke, C. L. et al.: Seeking help for erectile dysfunction after treatment for prostate cancer. *Archives of Sexual Behavior*, 33: 443, 2004

Schover, L. R., LoPiccolo, J.: Treatment effectiveness for dysfunctions of sexual desire. *Journal of Sex and Marital Therapy*, 8: 179, 1982

Schwarz, E. R., Kapur, V., Bionat, S. et al.: The prevalence and clinical relevance of sexual dysfunction in women and men with chronic heart failure. *International Journal of Impotence Research*, 20: 85, 2008

Schwenkhagen, A.: Hormonal changes in menopause and implications on sexual health. *Journal of Sexual Medicine*, 4 Suppl 3: 220, 2007

Seal, B. N., Meston, C. M.: The impact of body awareness on sexual arousal in women with sexual dysfunction. *Journal of Sexual Medicine*, 4: 990, 2007

Smith, L. J., Mulhall, J. P., Deveci, S. et al.: Sex after seventy: a pilot study of sexual function in older persons. *Journal of Sexual Medicine*, 4: 1247, 2007

Spark, R. F.: Intrinsa fails to impress FDA advisory panel. *International Journal of Impotence Research*, 17: 283, 2005

Verit, F. F., Verit, A.: Validation of the female sexual function index in women with chronic pelvic pain. *Journal of Sexual Medicine*, 4: 1635, 2007

Weijmar Schultz, W., Basson, R., Binik, Y. et al.: Women's sexual pain and its management. *Journal of Sexual Medicine*, 2: 301, 2005

Wierman, M., Basson, R., Davis, S. et al.: Are the endocrine society's clinical practice guidelines on androgen therapy in women misguided? A commentary-response. *Journal of Sexual Medicine*, 4: 1782, 2007

Youngkin, E. Q.: The myths and truths of mature intimacy: mature guidance for nurse practitioners. *Advanced Nurse Practice*, 12: 45, 2004

RESOURCES

Dr. Peter Scardino's Prostate Book. **Avery Books, New York, 2005**

Dr. Patrick Walsh's Guide To Surviving Prostate Cancer. **Warner Books, New York, 2001**

These two books are the seminal works on the treatments for prostate cancer and deciding which to pursue. While they address sexual function briefly, the focus of the books is not this topic.

www.drcatalona.com

This site, written by one of the world's leaders in prostate cancer diagnosis and radiation prostectomy, is full of very useful and practical advice about prostate cancer and its treatment.

Man to Man. **Michael Korda. Vintage Books, New York, 1997**

One man's personal account of his journey through prostate cancer diagnosis and treatment.

The Lovin' Ain't Over. **Ralph and Barbara Alterowitz.**

This book is an excellent guide to overcoming the psychological aspects of post-prostatectomy sexual dysfunction, written by a couple who has been down this road. www.renewintimacy.org

www.peyroniesassociation.org

The premier site on the internet for unbiased educational material for the man with Peyronie's disease. This is a non-profit organization known as the Association of Peyronie's Disease Advocates (APDA). There is a forum for chatting with other men who have Peyronie's disease and an option to submit questions and have them answered by experts in the field of Peyronie's disease.

www.sexhealthmatters.org

The patient website of the Sexual Medicine Society of North America, the group of urologists devoted to research in and the care of sexual disorders. This is the premier group in the world for the dissemination of credible information on sexual health issues. There is a very useful "locate a doctor" feature and information from news and medical journals posted regularly on the site.

www.issm.info

This site run by the International Society of Sexual Medicine is useful for international readers.

www.mskcc.org

The official website of Memorial Sloan-Kettering Cancer Center. There is much information for patients on many forms of cancer. This site houses the home of the prediction model (nomogram) site at www.nomograms.org.

www.urologyhealth.org

This site is the patient education site for the American Urological Association (AUA), whose main website can be found at www.auanet.org.

www.nci.nih.gov

The website of the National Cancer Institute of the National Institutes for Health. Much information on cancer and its treatment.

www.nccn.org

The National Comprehensive Cancer Network is a group of leading cancer centers, and this site provides guidelines for treatment of a variety of cancers.

www.cancer.org

The American Cancer Society is the leading private cancer organization in the USA.

www.clinicaltrials.gov

This site houses information on trials being conducted nationally for all diseases, including prostate cancer.

www.prostatecancerfoundation.org

This site belongs to the Prostate Cancer Foundation, which donates money for prostate cancer research and also promotes public awareness of prostate cancer.

www.webMD.com

This is a very useful commercial site for obtaining basic information on many health topics. While relatively superficial, it is an excellent brief resource.

www.USToo.com

The premier support group network for men with prostate Cancer, untreated and treated. There are many chapters throughout the country.

www.phoenix5.org

Another excellent support site for men with prostate cancer.

www.malecare.org

A site for patients with prostate cancer run by men with prostate cancer. Much useful information on treatments. This group also runs local support groups.

GLOSSARY

Accessory Pudendal Arteries • arteries that travel close to the prostate, which can be injured at the time of radical prostatectomy and may be exposed to radiation during radiation therapy for prostate cancer.

ACTIS Band • a rubber band placed over the base of the penis to either augment erection or prevent orgasm associated incontinence (climacturia).

ADT • aka androgen deprivation therapy. Medications used to cut off the production of testosterone in a variety of circumstances (high grade prostate cancer before prostate radiation, metastatic prostate cancer).

Adrenal Glands • organs positioned just above the kidneys which produce a variety of hormones including cortisol and testosterone.

Adrenaline • known as the "flight or fight" hormone. Chemical produced under stress, anxiety, fatigue. This is the most anti-erection chemical the body produces.

Alpha Blockers • a class of drugs which are used primarily for benign prostate enlargement (BPH). This class includes medications such as Hytrin, Cardura, Flomax, and Uroxatral.

Alpha-Adrenergic Agonists • a class of drugs used to reverse erection. This class includes neosynephrine which is injected into the penis for prolonged erection. The nasal decongestant pseudo-ephedrine (Sudafed) also belongs in this class.

Androgens • a class of hormones which derive its name fro the effects of these hormones on male sexual organs. The group includes testosterone, DHT, androstenedione.

Anorgasmia • absence of orgasm.

Anti-Androgens • a class of drugs which are used to block the action of testosterone on the prostate and other organs in men with metastatic prostate cancer.

BPH • aka benign prostatic hyperplasia. This refers to the benign enlargement of the prostate that occurs in all men eventually.

Brachytherapy • the technical term for radiation seed placement.

Cavernosal Artery • the tiny artery that travels through the center of the erection chamber (corpus cavernosum) that carries blood into the penis during erection.

Cavernous Nerves • the nerves that course alongside the prostate which are vital for erection, that are traumatized during prostatectomy and exposed to radiation during prostate cancer treatment.

cGMP • aka cyclic GMP. The chemical which when accumulated in the corpus cavernousm causes erectile tissue to relax, blood to flow into the penis and erection to occur.

Climacturia • refers to the leakage of urine at the time of orgasm (also known as orgasm associated incontinence)

Corpus Cavernosum • the erection chamber of which there are two (corpora cavernosa), which house the erectile tissue and spaces that fill with blood during erection.

Corpus Spongiosum • the third chamber in the penis which houses the urethra and is not a major part of erection

Cryotherapy • a treatment using very low temperatures to freeze the prostate and kill cancer.

DHT • aka dihydrotestosterone. This is a breakdown product of testosterone and is the major androgen in the prostate. This is the hormone that is involved in male pattern baldness and BPH. 5–alpha reductase inhibitor medications (Proscar, Avodart) block the production of this chemical.

GLOSSARY

Doppler Ultrasound • an ultrasound using Doppler effect to measure velocity of blood flow in the erection arteries to diagnose the cause of erectile dysfunction.

Emissary Veins • a series of veins on the penis which transport blood away from the erection chamber.

Endothelium • the cell layer which lines blood vessels in the body as well as the lacunar spaces inside the erection chamber. The health of this tissue is critical to erectile function.

Estrogen • a hormone which is the predominant sex hormone in women but present in small amounts in men. Elevated levels of estrogen result in the development of breast tissue (gynecomastia).

5–Alpha Reductase • the enzyme which degrades testosterone to DHT, which can be blocked to prevent DHT production.

Foley Catheter • a tube that is placed into the bladder to drain urine. This tube is left in place for 1–2 weeks after radical prostatectomy surgery.

Gleason Grade • the pathology system used to grade the aggressiveness of prostate cancer.

Gynecomastia • term referring to the development of breast tissue in men.

Hypogonadism • term referring to low testosterone levels associated with symptoms such as low sex drive, decreased energy, decreased strength and endurance and loss of muscle mass.

IIEF • aka the International Index of Erectile Function. This is the gold standard questionnaire to assess erectile function.

IMRT • aka intensity modulated radiation therapy. A modern, highly focused form of radiation, designed to deliver higher doses and minimize side effects.

Intralesional Injections • a treatment of Peyronie's disease, whereby medication is injected into the scar (plaque) in an effort to either stall the progress of the condition or reverse the penile deformity.

In-Vitro Fertilization • aka IVF. A form of assisted reproduction that uses eggs extracted from a woman and sperm procured from a man. Sperm is joined with the eggs in a Petri dish (conventional IVF) or a sperm is injected into an egg (intracytoplasmic sperm injection, aka ICSI).

IPSS • aka the International Prostate Symptom Score. The gold standard questionnaire used to assess urinary function in a man.

Lacunar Spaces • aka sinusoids. The spaces within the erection chamber (corpus cavernosum) which contract in the flaccid state and relax in the erect state to fill up with blood.

Leydig Cells • cells within the testicle, positioned between the sperm producing tubules, whose function is to produce testosterone.

LH • aka Luteinizing Hormone. Produced by the pituitary gland in the brain. Its function is to stimulate Leydig cells to produce testosterone.

LHRH • aka Luteinizing Hormone Releasing Hormone. Produced by the hypothalamus in the brain. Its function is to stimulate the pituitary gland to produce LH.

Libido • aka sex drive.

Lymphocele • a collection of lymph fluid. May be seen after lymph gland removal associated with radical prostatectomy surgery.

LUTS • aka Lower Urinary Tract Symptoms. This term refers to a constellation of symptoms such as poor urinary stream, frequency and urgency of urination, getting up at night to urinate, difficulty starting urinary stream.

Metastatic Cancer • cancer that has spread beyond its primary site.

MRI • aka magnetic resonance imaging. A for of imaging that does not use X-rays, which is excellent at looking at the body's tissues, in particular the prostate.

MUSE • aka medicated urethral system for erection. A small suppository about the size of a grain of rice that is placed into the urethra (urine channel) in an effort to produce an erection.

Multifocality • the idea that cancer may be in multiple places within an organ.

Multimodal Strategy • a treatment strategy combining different modalities of treatment (for example, chemotherapy plus radiation therapy).

GLOSSARY

Nerve Grafting • the technique of grafting live nerve tissue in between the ends of the cavernous (erection) nerves in an effort to minimize erectile problems after radical prostatectomy.

Nerve Sparing • the concept of minimizing trauma to the cavernous (erection) nerves. Described for the first time in 1982 by Dr. Patrick Walsh at Johns Hopkins, this technique revolutionized the ability of surgeons to have men experience recovery of erections after radical prostatectomy.

Neuromodulators • a group of medications used to either prevent in jury to nerves or increase the regenerative capability of nerves after trauma.

Neurovascular Bundle • the term given to the nerve bundle in association with its blood vessels. The neurovascular bundle runs alongside the prostate and they are therefore exposed to some degree of trauma at the time of radical prostatectomy.

Nitric Oxide • aka NO. THE chemical responsible for erection.

Nocturia • term give to act of having to break sleep to urinate.

Nomogram • term given to a mathematical model that predicts a specific outcome, for example, erectile function recovery after radical prostatectomy.

OAI • aka orgasm associated incontinence. See *Climacturia*.

Oncologist • a physician specializing in the treatment of patients with cancer.

Osteoporosis • term given to significant decrease in bone density, which increases the risk for fractures of the hip, forearm as well as loss of height due to compression of the vertebral bodies. A less severe form of this is known as *osteopenia*.

PDE5 Inhibitors • a class of medications that block the enzyme PDE5, which is the enzyme that breaks down cGMP, the erection-producing chemical. By blocking PDE5, PDE5 inhibitors allow accumulation of cGMP thus promoting the development and maintenance of erection.

Penile Injections • aka intracavernosal injections. A well recognized treatment for erectile problems, whereby a tiny needle is placed into the side of the penile shaft that produces an erection in 5 minutes for the majority of men using them.

Penile Prostheses • plastic devices placed into the penis to allow men with severe erectile problems to have sexual intercourse.

Penile Rehabilitation • the idea that we can use medications or devices to prevent erectile tissue damage after radical prostatectomy or radiation to maximize the chances of erectile function recovery.

Peyronie's Disease • a scarring condition of the penis which results in penile deformity (usually curvature).

Phenylephrine • a medication given by penile injection to reverse a prolonged erection.

PIN • aka prostate intra-epithelial neoplasia. A pre-cancerous condition in the prostate which warrants close monitoring of the patient.

Pituitary Gland • a pea-sized organ on the undersurface of the brain which produces several critical hormones for survival including LH (for testosterone production) and FSH (for fertility).

Placebo • a sugar pill used in controlled trials to help define the true effectiveness of a drug.

Positive Margin • a state where cancer cells have been left behind at the time of radical prostatectomy.

Premature Ejaculation • defined by the International Society for Sexual medicine as "a male sexual dysfunction characterized by ejaculation which always or nearly always occurs prior to or within about one minute of vaginal penetration; and inability to delay ejaculation on all or nearly all vaginal penetrations; and negative personal consequences, such as distress, bother, frustration and/or the avoidance of sexual intimacy"

Priapism • defined as an erection of penetration hardness lasting longer than 4 hours.

Proctitis • inflammation of the rectum (as occurs in some men after radiation therapy for prostate cancer).

Prostaglandin E • a chemical that promotes erection and may be protective of erectile tissue.

PSA • aka prostate specific antigen. A blood test for this is the standard screen for the presence of prostate cancer.

GLOSSARY

Pulmonary Embolus • a blood clot that migrates to the lungs, which can be fatal if large.

Randomized, Controlled • a study where patients are assigned to different groups,

Trial • often including a placebo-treated group, in an effort to accurately define the effect of a treatment without bias. •

Retrograde Ejaculation • the term given to the process whereby semen passes backwards into the bladder.

Seed Implantation • • see *Brachtherapy*

Semen • aka seminal fluid. The fluid containing sperm that is ejaculated at orgasm

Sex Therapist • a mental health professional that specializes in the treatment of patients with sexual problems.

Sperm Banking • the process of procuring sperm and having it frozen (cryo-preserved) for future in vitro fertilization.

Sperm Extraction • the process of extracting sperm (usually from the testicle) for use with in vitro fertilization, usually from men who cannot produce sperm through ejaculation.

Spermatic Cord • the structure upon which the testicle hangs in the scrotum. It contains arteries, veins, nerves as well as the vas deferens.

SSRIs • aka Selective Serotonin Re-Uptake Inhibitors. A class of medications used primarily for the treatment of depression. This class includes Prozac, Zoloft, Paxil, Luvox, Celexa, Lexapro, among others.

Statins • a class of medications used to treat high cholesterol and triglycerides. This class includes Lipitor, Crestor, Zocor, pravachol, simvastatin among others.

Testosterone • the primary male sex hormone critical to several bodily functions

Testosterone Supplementation • the administration of testosterone (or similar products) to raise the level of testosterone in the blood.

Titration • term given to the dose-by-dose adjustment of a medication.

Trandermal Therapy • the application of medicated gels to the skin for the treatment of a number of medical conditions.

Transurethral Surgery • surgical procedures conducted through the urethra using fiberoptic instruments to treat conditions of the urethra, prostate or bladder.

Urethra • medical term given to the urine channel, which passes from the bladder to the tip of the penis.

Urinary Incontinence • leak of urine most often due to defective urinary sphincter or an overactive bladder.

Urinary Retention • term given to the complete inability to pass urine. This condition is painful and requires emergent passage of a catheter into the bladder to drain it.

Urinoma • a collection of urine anywhere in the body other than the kidney or bladder.

Vacuum Erection Device • device that uses a vacuum to draw blood into the penis to help with erection.

Vas Deferens • tube-like structure which carries sperm from the testicle to the prostate. Surgical closure of this is known as a vasectomy.

Venous Leak • the condition resulting from a defective valve in the erection chamber resulting in leakage of blood from the erection chamber back into the general circulation, resulting in poor erection hardness and poor sustaining capability of erection.

Watchful Waiting • term given to active surveillance of a man with prostate cancer usually reserved or men with tiny amounts of cancer of low aggressiveness.

INDEX

5–alpha reductase inhibitors, 22–24
   how they work, 23
   side effects, 24
   using to reduce PSA levels, 23
aging and sexual function, 229–232
alcohol, limiting intake of, 21
alpha blockers (medications), 11, 21–24, 79, 80, 113
   difference between older and newer, 22
   how they work, 22
   side effects, 22
androgen deprivation therapy (ADT), 85–89
   See also hormone therapy
   advantages of, 86–88
   anti-androgens, 87
   semen production and, 91
anesthesia
   potential risks of, 36
   radical prostatectomy and, 55
anorgasmia, 112
anti-androgens, 87–88

benign prostate enlargement. *See* BPH/LUTS
benign prostatic hyperplasia. *See* BPH/LUTS
bibliography (suggested reading), 241–288
bladder
   bladder stones, 21
   changes in the bladder muscle, 20–21
BPH/LUTS
   circulatory process and, 11
   contributors to, 20
   impact on erectile function, 27–29
   lower urinary tract symptoms, 18–19, 28–29
   medications for, 21–24
   patient's bother index, 21
   questionnaire to take, 19–20
   studies on, 27–28
   suggested reading, 241–243
   surgical treatments, 24–27
   symptoms of, 18–19
   urinary retention and, 20
brachytherapy (radiation therapy), 74, 77–79

caffeine, limiting intake of, 21
Cardura (doxazosin). *See* alpha blockers
catherization, urinary retention and, 20

Caverject (medication), 146, 147–152
   effectiveness of, 148
   side effects, 149–152
   standard dose, 148
chemical castration. *See* androgen deprivation therapy
Cialis. *See* Viagra like medications
climacturia. *See* orgasm associated incontinence
cryosurgery (cryotherapy), 62

deep venous thrombosis (DVT), 36–37, 64
diabetes, and erectile dysfunction, 14
dysorgasmia (orgasmic pain), 113

ED. *See* erectile dysfunction
ejaculation, 10–12, 121–122. *See also* semen
   after radical prostatectomy, 11, 121–122
   premature ejaculation, 130–133
enlarged prostate. *See* BPH/LUTS
erectile dysfunction (ED), 13–15
   adrenaline, part it plays, 33–34
   causes of, 14
   defined, 13
   diabetes and, 14
   discussing with your doctor, 233–235
   future drug therapies to treat, 197–199
   International Index of Erectile Function, 47–48
   lower urinary tract symptoms and, 28–29
   predicting rates for recovery, 48–50, 65–67
   questionnaire, 49–50
   radiation therapy and, 83–84
   role surgeon plays, 57, 69
   statistics, 13, 235
   surgeries that can cause, 14

erections
   consistency of erections, 70
   erectile function after surgery, 67–71
   following hormone therapy, 91–93
   gels to help with, 197
   how they work, 7–8, 32–33
   older men vs. younger men, 65–66
   quality of, 69–70

female sexual dysfunction, 231–232
fertility options, 121–122
   in-vitro fertilization (IVF), 10
Flomax (tamsulosin). *See* alpha blockers
future therapies, 193–203
   drugs for erectile dysfunction, 197–199
   drugs for nerve protection, 193–196
   growth factor therapy, 199–200
   multimodal therapy, 201–203
   stem cell therapy, 200–201
   suggested readings, 275–279

gene therapy, 199–200
   growth factor therapy and, 199–200
Gleason grading system, 23, 32, 40, 85, 86
glossary of terms, 291–298

high intensity focus ultrasound (HIFU), 62
hip fractures and low testosterone, 210
hormone therapy, 85–93
   advantages of, 86–88
   androgen deprivation therapy (ADT), 85–89
   before having radiation therapy, 79
   effect on sexual function, 91–93
   history of, 86, 167
   how it works, 86

INDEX

penile implants and, 173
side effects, 89–91
suggested reading, 254–257
Viagra like medications and, 93
why used, 85–86
hypogonadism, 208–209. *See also* testosterone
Hytrin (terazosin). *See* alpha blockers

IMRT (intensity modulated radiation therapy), 75–76, 79–80
in-vitro fertilization (IVF), 10
incontinence. *See* urine leakage during sex
International Prostate Symptoms Score, 30
intimacy, re-establishing. *See* sex life
intraurethral suppositories. *See* suppositories

Levitra. *See* Viagra like medications
libido. *See also* sexual function
age playing a factor, 229–231
factors impacting, 12–13
low sex drive, 12–13
and sex life, 230
testosterone levels and, 12–13, 91–93
LUTS (lower urinary tract symptoms). *See* BPH/LUTS

male pattern baldness, 23
male reproductive organs, 8–10
medications, 123–134. *See also* Viagra like medications
advantages of, 127–128
containing nitrates, 134
history of, 123
how they work, 124–125
premature ejaculation, 130–132
side effects, 128–129
suggested readings, 261–266
multimodal therapy, 201–203

MUSE (suppository). *See* suppositories

NAION (type of blindness), 130
nasal spray (future drug therapy), 198
nerve grafting, 61–62
nerve protection, drugs for, 193–196
nerve sparing, 58–62, 69
concept of, 54
grading system, 60
nerve grating, 61–62
nitrates, medications containing, 134
nocturia (urinary frequency), 19–20
nomograms (prediction models), 47–48
erectile function recovery and, 51–52, 71

orchiectomy, 86, 91. *See also* hormone therapy
orgasm associated incontinence (climacturia), 107–109
treatment for, 109–110
orgasms, 11–12
after prostatectomy, 111–113
aging process and, 231
diabetic men and, 111–112
erectile dysfunction and, 34
importance to men, 228–229
medication related, 111
orgasm associated incontinence, 107–109
penile sensation nerve injury, 111–112
problems having, 110–113
suggested reading, 260–261
osteopenia (osteoporosis), 90
testosterone and, 214

PDE5 inhibitors. *See* Viagra like medications
penile anatomy, 1–8
blood supply, 5–6
erection chambers, 2–4

erections, 7–8
external, 2
nerve supply, 6–7
tissue types, 2–5
penile curvature (Peyronie's disease), 116–121, 234
   case study, 117
   difficulty in having sexual intercourse, 116
   information about, 116
   pain from having, 116, 118
   surgical reconstruction, 120–121
   treatment for, 114, 118–120
   vacuum devices and, 161–162
penile implants, 167–192
   advances in, 168–171
   advantages/disadvantages, 168, 177, 190
   antibiotics and, 178
   auto-inflation, 186, 190
   candidates for, 171–173
   case study, 182
   caution regarding having other surgeries, 185
   choosing the right implant, 175–177
   complications, 168, 180, 181, 183–191
   device migration, 187
   device types, 174–175
   effect on sexual function, 168, 172–173
   erosion of implant, 186–187, 191
   history of, 167–168
   how it works, 171–172
   implant infection, 184–185, 190
   mechanical breakdown, 185–186, 190
   penile length changes, 188
   post-operative care, 181–183, 191–192
   preparing for surgery, 177–178
   radical prostatectomy and, 171, 172–173
   re-operation, 190
   reservoir herniation, 187
   salvage implant surgery, 185
   scrotal hematoma, 191
   suggested reading, 273–275
   surgery, 179–181
   what to expect, 191
penile injections, 141–158
   adrenaline and, 146, 153
   advantages/disadvantages, 142, 144
   anxiety about needle injections, 144, 147
   case studies, 150
   erectile function after, 153
   history of, 95–96, 141–142
   how they work, 143
   how to get the best from, 144–147
   instructions for ER staff, 157–158
   medications, 146–148, 152
      side effects, 143
      traveling with, 152–153
   needle injection training, 143–147, 155–156
   penile implants and, 172
   priapism and, 150–151
   suggested reading, 268–270
   uncircumcised men and, 147
penile length changes, 112–115
   radical prostatectomy and, 112
   shrinkage factor, 114–115
   studies on, 115
penile rehabilitation and preservation, 95–104
   case studies, 95–97, 102–103
   causes of erection tissue damage, 96–97
   concept of, 97–100
   current treatment program, 102
   erectile function after, 97–98
   evidence supporting, 96
   history of, 95–96
   non-pharmacological approaches, 104

INDEX

pharmacological approaches, 99–101
side effects, 149–152
strategy for, 162–163
structure of the program, 100–103
suggested reading, 257–260
penis. *See*
  penile anatomy
  penile curvature
  penile implants
  penile injections
  penile length changes
  penile rehabilitation and preservation
Peyronie's Disease. *See* penile curvature
photodynamic (light) therapy, 62
pills. *See* Viagra like medications
premature ejaculation, 33–34, 130–133
  aging process and, 231
  medications to treat, 130–133
  most common cause of, 132
  SSRIs and, 132
priapism (erection lasting over 4 hours), 143–144, 150–151, 153, 156
  instructions for ER staff, 151
  preventing, 152
  Sudafed to treat, 151–152
prostate, 8–10
  anatomy of the, 8–9, 17–18
  biopsy, 40
  examination of, 234
  function of the, 18
  questionnaire on prostate symptoms, 19–20, 29, 30
  testosterone and the, 215–218
prostate cancer
  being diagnosed with, xix, 32–34
  clinical trials, 23
  grading system, 32
  prediction models for survival, 47–48, 51–52
  questionnaire, 49–50
  statistics on, xv, xix
  and testosterone, 215–218
prostate enlargement. *See also* BPH/LUTS
prostate radiation. *See* radiation therapy
prostatectomy, 24–25. *See also* radical prostatectomy
  laparoscopic, 64, 70
  laser, 24–25
  radical retropubic, 54, 57
  robotic, 42, 56–58, 64, 70
  suprapubic (simple), 24–25
PSA (prostate specific antigen, 18, 58
  reducing with medications, 23
  testosterone, 218–219

radiation oncologist, 78
radiation therapy, 73–84
  brachytherapy, 74, 77–79
  different types of, 75–78
  effect on sperm, 10
  ejaculatory fluid and, 80
  erectile function after, 38, 80–84, 99, 126
  history of, 73–74
  hormone therapy prior to receiving, 79
  how it works, 74–78
  IMRT, 38, 46, 75–76, 79–80
  penile implants and, 173
  side effects, 37–38, 78–80
  suggested reading, 250–253
  Viagra like medications after, 133
radical prostatectomy (surgical procedure), 24–25, 53–71
  case study, 218–219
  complications of surgery, 37, 64–65
  effect on reproductive organs, 9–10
  ejaculatory process and, 11, 121–122

erectile function after, 14–15, 25, 67–71, 97–98
experience of surgeon, 56
history of, 54
local therapies, 62
nerve sparing and, 60. 66. 125
orgasms after, 111–113
pain management, 63, 64
penile implants and, 171–173, 176
penile injections and, 154
penile length changes after, 112
predictors of erectile function, 48–52, 65–67
purpose of, 60–61
seeing doctor before, 100
suggested reading, 246–250
testosterone supplementation and, 217–218
vacuum devices and, 162–163
Viagra like medications after, 131
watchful waiting, 34
what is involved, 53–58
what to expect before and after, 62–64
which approach is best, 58
resources (web sites), 289–290

semen, 18. *See also* sperm
androgen deprivation and, 91
impact of prostate surgery on, 11
semen production and aging, 230–231
seminal vesicles, 9
sex drive. *See* libido
sex life. *See also* sexual function
frequency of sex, 227–228
importance of partner, 236–239
libido, how it works, 12–13
lifestyle factors, 230
normal sex life, 227–239
orgasms, importance for men, 228–229
re-establishing a good one, 236–239

sex and the single man, 239
sex without erections, 236
suggested reading, 236, 283–288
using sex aids, 236, 238
sexual function. *See also* sex life
androgen deprivation and, 91–93
case study (cancer diagnosis), 35
diagnosis of cancer, impact on, 32–35
effects of aging and, 229–232
ejaculation, 10–12, 121–122
erectile dysfunction, 13–15, 229
erections, 7–8
female sexual dysfunction, 231–232
full sexual health work-up, 232–235
hormone therapy and, 91–93
libido, how it works, 12–13
orgasm, 11–12
partner should be present on doctor visit, 235
penile anatomy, 1–8
physical exam with doctor, 234
premature ejaculation, 33–34, 130–133
psychological dimension, 237
radiation therapy and, 38, 80–84
radical prostatectomy and, 67–71
reproductive organs, 8–10
seeing a doctor for sexual problems, 232–235
sexual difficulties are common, 13–15
suggested reading, 241–243
urine leakage during sex, 105–110
sildenafil (Viagra). *See* Viagra like medications
sperm, 9–10
fertility options, 121–122
sperm extraction, 122
stem cell therapy, 200–201
suppositories (MUSE), 104, 135–139

INDEX

advantages/disadvantages, 137–138
dosage levels, 136–137
effectiveness of, 136
erectile function after, 137–138
history of, 135
how they work, 135–137
side effects/complications, 138–139
suggested reading, 266–268
Viagra users and, 137

testicles
and aging, 93, 230
chemotherapy and, 209
removal of, 86
small testicles, 93, 211, 217
testosterone and, 206–208, 230
testosterone supplementation, 218–223
testosterone, 205–225
after radical prostatectomy, 217–218
DHT causing prostate growth, 20, 23
estrogen and, 206–207
evaluation of low, 211–212, 224–225
hormone therapy and, 91–93
hypogonadism, 208–209
libido problems and, 12–13, 91–92
medical conditions associated with low, 208–209
patches and gels, 221–222
prostate cancer and, 215–218
questionnaire on testosterone deficiency, 224–225
symptoms of low, 209–211
testosterone supplementation
how it works, 218–222
monitoring, 223
risks and benefits of, 212–215
where it comes from, 206

treatments
complications of treatment, 36–38
deciding on a treatment, 31–33, 38
factors to consider, 38–42
future therapies, 193–203
hormone therapy, 85–93
impact of sexual function following diagnosis, 32–35
information to give doctor, 42–45
medications, 123–129
penile implants, 167–192
penile injections, 141–158
penile rehabilitation and preservation, 96–104
questions to ask doctor, 45–48
radiation therapy, 38
radical prostatectomy, 53–71
suggested readings, 243–246
suppositories, 104, 135–139
vacuum devices, 104, 159–165
TUIP (transurethral incision of the prostate), 26
TUMT (transurethral microwave therapy), 26–27
TUNA (transurethral needle aspiration), 26–27
TURP (transurethral resection of the prostate), 25–26
TUVAP (laser vaporization), 26

urethral suppositories. *See* suppositories
urinary problems
bladder stones, 21
frequency of urination, 21
medications to help treat, 29
radiation therapy and, 38
urinary incontinence, 37
urinary retention, 20
urine leakage during sex, 105–110
case study, 107–110
foreplay incontinence, 108, 109

how continence is achieved, 105–106
incontinence following prostatectomy, 106, 108
incontinence following radiation, 106, 108
orgasm associated incontinence, 107–109
treatments for, 110
urologists, specializing in sexual medicine, 232
Uroxatral (alfuzosin). *See* alpha blockers

vacuum devices, 104, 159–165
   advantages/disadvantages, 162–164
   complications, 163–164
   erectile function after, 163
   getting the best out of, 160–162
   history of, 159
   how they work, 159–162, 165
   how to use, 165
   penile curvature and, 161–162
   radical prostatectomy and, 162–163
   suggested reading, 270–273
   Viagra and, 163
Vancomycin (antibiotic), 178
venous leak, 93, 98, 171–172
Viagra like medications (PDE5 inhibitors), 60, 66, 69, 93, 96–97, 99, 101, 123–129
   arousal playing a factor in how effective, 237–239
   case studies, 131, 133
   differences and similarities in, 126–129
   future drug therapies, 193–203
   history of, 123
   how they work, 124–125
   incidence of heart attacks, 129–130
   neuromodulation and, 196
   patients least likely to respond to, 125–126
   penile implants for when pills fail, 171
   penile rehabilitation and preservation, 99–104
   proper use of, 233
   safety of, 129–130
   side effects, 128–130, 171
   studies on use of, 101–103
   suggested reading, 261–266
   taking after radiation therapy, 103, 133
   taking after radical prostatectomy, 131
   vacuum devices and, 163

web sites, 289–290

ABOUT THE AUTHOR

Dr. Mulhall is a native of Dublin, Ireland. He received his medical degree at University College Medical School in Dublin. He did his urology and sexual/reproductive medicine training in Connecticut and Boston. He is the Director of the Sexual and Reproductive Medicine Program in the Division of Urology at Memorial Sloan-Kettering Cancer Center in New York City. Dr Mulhall is the recipient of honors from several organizations, including awards from the Veterans Administration, the Sexual Medicine Society of North America, the International Society for Sexual Medicine, and the American Urological Association.

He sits on several committees of national and international organizations, including the board of directors of the Sexual Medicine Society of North America (SMSNA). He is an editor for several medical journals including the *Journal of Sexual Medicine*. Dr. Mulhall has published more than 150 papers in medical journals, has authored numerous book chapters and is author of the medical textbook *Sexual Function in the Prostate Cancer Patient*.

He is recognized as one of the world's authorities on sexual rehabilitation following treatment for prostate cancer. He is an internationally acclaimed speaker and educator and is frequently consulted by the media, including major network and cable news channels. He enjoys scuba diving and golf, although by his own admission, he is not expecting to be on the professional golf tour anytime soon. He lives with his wife Sarah and 6–year-old son Cameron in Purchase, New York.